To John:
With many thanks from
a friend for a truly stimulating
cooperation and a thorough support.

January 92

Chris [illegible]

G. Adler C. Beglinger (Eds.)

Cholecystokinin Antagonists in Gastroenterology

Basic and Clinical Status

Foreword by
Niklaus E. Gyr

With 47 Figures

Springer-Verlag
Berlin Heidelberg New York
London Paris Tokyo
Hong Kong Barcelona
Budapest

Professor Dr. med., GUIDO ADLER
Abteilung Innere Medizin I
Medizinische Klinik und Poliklinik
Oberer Eselsberg, Robert-Koch-Straße 8
W-7900 Ulm, FRG

Privatdozent Dr. med., CHRISTOPH BEGLINGER
Abteilung für Gastroenterologie
Universitätsklinik, Petersgraben 6
4031 Basel, Switzerland

ISBN 3-540-53582-9 Springer-Verlag Berlin Heidelberg New York
ISBN 0-387-53582-9 Springer-Verlag New York Berlin Heidelberg

Library of Congress Cataloging-in-Publication Data. Cholecystokinin antagonists in gastroenterology: basic and clinical status/G. Adler, C. Beglinger (eds.); foreword by Niklaus E. Gyr. p. cm. Includes index. ISBN 3-540-53582-9 (alk. paper). – ISBN 0-387-53582-9 (alk. paper) 1. Cholecystokinin – Antagonists – Therapeutic use – Testing. 2. Cholecystokinin – Physiological effect. 3. Gastrointestinal system – Diseases – Chemotherapy. I. Adler, G. II. Beglinger, C. (Christoph), 1950– . [DNLM: 1. Cholecystokinin – antagonists & inhibitors. 2. Cholecystokinin – physiology. WK 170 C5469] RC802.C46 1991 616.3 – dc20 DNLM/DLC for Library of Congress 91-4841 CIP

Typesetting: Best-set Typesetter Ltd., Hong Kong
19/3130-543210 – Printed on acid-free paper

Foreword

Cholecystokinin (CCK) was the third peptide to be described among the large variety of gastrointestinal hormones known today. It was originally extracted from the intestinal mucosa and shown to exert distinct stimulatory effects on gallbladder contraction and on pancreatic enzyme secretion. At the time of its detection, the situation appeared simple and straightforward – CCK and secretin were the hormonal regulators of pancreatic secretion and gallbladder contraction. A new hormonal concept replaced Pavlow's neuroregulatory scheme of exocrine pancreatic secretion. But things turned out to be much more complex. In fact, CCK has fooled biochemists, physiologists, and clinicians up to the present day. Not only have at least five physiologically important molecular forms been described, but CCK peptides have also been localized outside the gastrointestinal mucosa in the nerves of the gastrointestinal tract as well as in the peripheral and central nervous system. Thus, CCK, besides being a hormone, acts as neurotransmitter and might have a role as a neuroendocrine and paracrine substance as well. Moreover, measurement of CCK in plasma has posed serious technical problems and still remains cumbersome due to the heterogeneity of molecular forms and the close similarity of its carboxy-terminal end with that of gastrin. Difficulties with the synthesis of the larger forms of CCK33 have further complicated research. In this complex situation, the development and availability of specific and highly potent CCK receptor antagonists represents a real breakthrough. Using these antagonists, it has become possible to study the physiology and pathophysiology of CCK in the reverse way. Astonishingly enough, unexpected observations have been reported, such as the acceleration of colonic transit time and gastric emptying by CCK antagonists, while other functions of CCK, such as the stimulatory action on the gallbladder and pancreatic secretion, have been shown to be of physiological relevance. Interesting pharmacodynamic actions have been observed, such as the improvement of constipation in an elderly nursing home population and alleviation of biliary pain, which render the CCK receptor blockers clinically attractive.

The editors of this book, both experts in the field of gastrointestinal physiology, have accepted the challenge to collect the most up-to-date information on CCK research, especially focusing on the use of receptor blockers. A great number of leading scientists have accepted the invitation to contribute to this impressive compilation of data on CCK. The information presented will interest biochemists, physiologists, pharmacologists, and clinicians in equal measure. Again, with accumulation of knowledge it becomes obvious that there is an increasing demand for further research.

Niklaus E. Gyr
Medical Department
Kantonsspital Liestal
University of Basel
Switzerland

Preface

Appreciating the fact that many peptides from the gastrointestinal tract function as hormones and/or neurotransmitters has important implications. A good example is cholecystokinin (CCK), a peptide from the small intestinal mucosa and the nervous system with multiple functions on gastrointestinal secretions and motility. CCK causes the gallbladder to contract and the pancreas to secrete enzymes which, in turn, facilitate digestion. Because of the importance of regulatory peptides for body function, drugs that mimick or block their effects on receptors are important scientific tools, but may also be putative therapeutic agents. Developing compounds which can affect peptide systems has, however, been difficult. Recently, CCK has been used as a model for the development of different classes of CCK receptor antagonists. Several compounds have been synthesized and characterized in various animal models. Two emerged from these studies and have become available for testing in humans: loxiglumide (previously designated CR1505) and devazepide (also known as MK329 or L-364 718). The development of these compounds is a landmark for several reasons. Most importantly the work demonstrates that peptide receptors can be influenced by orally active, nonpeptidal drugs. In principal, this strategy should be possible with other peptides and it could be speculated that peptide antagonists will have the same impact in gastroenterological research and therapy as did the introduction of H_2 antagonists.

This book is devoted to the development and characterization of the CCK antagonists loxiglumide and devazepide. We have attempted to cover the advances in a number of areas. The first two parts of the book cover the biological characterization of CCK and chemistry of the new CCK antagonists. The following part is devoted to the physiological application of these new compounds, whereas in the last section we have tried to cover most of the areas of clinical importance. Whether the currently available CCK antagonists represent a new class of therapeutic drugs is speculation as they may not be sufficiently selective to be useful in clinical practice. There is, however, no doubt that further development is aimed at finding a dose or a compound that can selectively block a specific action.

We would like to thank all of the authors for the time they spent in preparing these articles. We hope that this volume will provide essential information on the role of CCK in health and disease and help to stimulate further research.

Ulm and Basel

GUIDO ADLER
CHRISTOPH BEGLINGER

Contents

Part III: Physiological Application of CCK Antagonists

Part IV: Clinical Potentials of CCK Antagonists

List of Contributors

You will find the addresses at the beginning of the respective contribution

Part I: Biology of CCK

Biochemistry of CCK

G.J. Dockray and A. Varro[1]

Introduction

The isolation of cholecystokinin (CCK) from porcine duodenum by Mutt and Jorpes [22] in the late 1960s provided the foundation for the very considerable advances in our understanding of the biochemistry of this substance that have taken place over the last 20 years. It also marked the culmination of what can now been seen as the pioneering phase in the development of our ideas of the hormonal regulation of digestion in the small intestine. Mutt and Jorpes demonstrated that the purified peptide stimulated both gall bladder contraction and pancreatic enzyme secretion and so left no doubt that these must be two properties of the same molecule, and not due to independent actions of separate hormones (CCK and pancreozymin) as had hitherto been supposed. They also made the important observation that the C-terminal tryptic peptide of CCK (CCK8) possessed both biological activities [22]. Four major biochemical developments have followed from the work of this period. First, it soon became clear that CCK was part of the same chemical family as the gastric hormone gastrin, and the amphibian peptide caerulein. Second, it became possible to develop antibodies to CCK, or synthetic fragments of it, that could be used for radioimmunoassay and immunohistochemistry. Third, CCK assays have in turn revealed new molecular forms, and have facilitated the discovery of CCK in previously unexpected places, notably the central nervous system. Fourth, with the later development of recombinant DNA techniques, the way became open for the elucidation of cDNA and gene sequences, and for studies of the control of CCK expression. Each of these topics will be considered here.

The CCK Family

The sequence of the C-terminal tryptic fragment of CCK described by Mutt and Jorpes was immediately seen to resemble that of gastrin, which had

[1] MRC Secretory Control Research Group, Department of Physiology, University of Liverpool, Liverpool, UK.

G. Adler and C. Beglinger (Eds.)
CCK Antagonists in Gastroenterology

CCK	- Arg - Asp - Tyr* - Met - Gly - **Trp - Met - Asp - Phe - NH$_2$**
G17	- Glu - Glu - Ala - Tyr* - Gly - **Trp - Met - Asp - Phe - NH$_2$**
Caerulein	- Gln - Asn - Tyr* - Thr - Gly - **Trp - Met - Asp - Phe - NH$_2$**
Chicken Gastrin	- His - Phe - Tyr* - Pro - Asp - **Trp - Met - Asp - Phe - NH$_2$**

Fig. 1. Amino acid sequence of C-terminal nonapeptide of CCK and related peptides. The common C-terminal tetrapeptide is identified in *bold type*. Note the position of the tyrosine residue which determines specificity at different receptor types (see text). The tyrosine (*indicated by**) is normally sulphated (although in gastrin about 50% of naturally occurring peptide is in the unsulphated form)

been reported somewhat earlier. Soon after, the amphibian skin peptide caerulein was characterized as a member of the same group [see 7]. The important common structural feature of these peptides is the C-terminal tetrapeptide Trp-Met-Asp-Phe-NH_2 (Fig. 1); this is preceded by a tyrosine-containing sequence in the configuration Tyr-X-Trp-(gastrin) or Tyr-X-X-Trp-(CCK/caerulein). The tyrosine is interesting because it occurs in the sulphated state. Virtually all naturally occurring CCK in brain and gut, and caerulein in amphibian skin, is in the sulphated form, but usually only about 50% of gastrin from normal antral mucosa is sulphated. The high affinity of CCK for gall bladder and pancreatic acinar cell receptors is conferred by a sulphated tyrosine at position 7 from the C-terminal. Desulphation, or shifting the tyrosine from this position, markedly reduces activity at these targets and produces a gastrin-like spectrum of actions (i.e. high potency for stimulation of acid secretion, low potency on gall bladder and pancreas). Recent studies on chicken gastrin provide an interesting exception to these generalizations [4]. Chicken gastrin, as its name suggests, stimulates gastric acid secretion (in birds and mammals) with high potency, but has low potency for stimulation of the pancreas and gall bladder. Its sequence, however, is CCK-like. It seems that, in this case, there is a Pro residue in the sequence Tyr-Pro-X-Trp-that serves the purpose of shifting the orientation of the side chain of the sulphated tyrosine residue relative to the C-terminal thereby changing selectivity for different receptor subtypes.

Molecular Forms of CCK

Mutt and Jorpes characterized CCK as a peptide of 33 residues (CCK33), and later a variant of 39 residues (CCK39) extended at the N-terminus was described [21]. Although CCK8 was quite widely used as a convenient synthetic analogue from about 1970 onwards, it was not immediately realized that this fragment might exist naturally in its own right. Chromatographic and radioimmunoassay studies first suggested that CCK might occur in brain as CCK8 [5,6,20,24], and this was verified by isolation and sequencing [8]. Subsequently, many different forms of CCK have been chemically characterized by isolation from either brain or gut. In man and pig the major forms are the peptides of 8, 33, 39 and 58 residues [9,14,28]. In rat intestine, CCK22 appears to be a relatively important form [12]. The smallest form to be chemically characterized is the C-terminal pentapeptide (gastrin or CCK5) [26], but as this has relatively low affinity for CCK receptors, its significance is not known. In addition to the major peptides a number of other forms have been chemically identified, e.g. CCK25, 18 and 7, but the significance of these forms is also unknown at present [23]. The different forms are produced by alternative processing of the CCK precursor, and their relative abundance varies between tissues, probably as a consequence of different patterns of post-translational processing (see below). The smaller forms are relatively acidic and are well extracted in boiling water, but the larger forms carry a net positive charge and are best extracted in acid.

The CCK Gene

Deschenes et al. [2] cloned DNA complimentary to the CCK mRNA from rat medullary thyroid carcinoma cell lines. The cDNA sequence indicated a single copy of CCK, a characteristic signal sequence and an overall precursor size of 115 residues (Fig. 2). Subsequently, homologous cDNA sequences for human, mouse and pig preproCCK have been elucidated [15,16,18]. The homology between these sequences is particularly striking in the CCK8 region, and in the immediate C- and N-terminal regions to it. The first genomic sequence was reported by Deschenes et al. [3] for material cloned from a rat liver genomic library using probes derived from the rat cDNA previously obtained by them. They identified three exons separated by two relatively large (approximately 1 and 5 kbp) introns. The first exon corresponds to the 5′ untranslated region, the second, to the signal sequence and the third, to most of the CCK33 region and the remaining C-terminal part of proCCK. The second and third exons of the human gene are similarly organized [27]. The transcription start site was identified 29 bp 3′ to a TATA-like sequence. A promoter region has been found within −144 bp of the transcription start site, although it has still to be characterized in detail. The available evidence suggests that there is a single gene which is expressed from the same start site in both CNS neurons and gut endocrine cells [15,16]. Recent studies suggest that transcription in gut endocrine cells is controlled by the luminal environment of the small intestine [19]. In

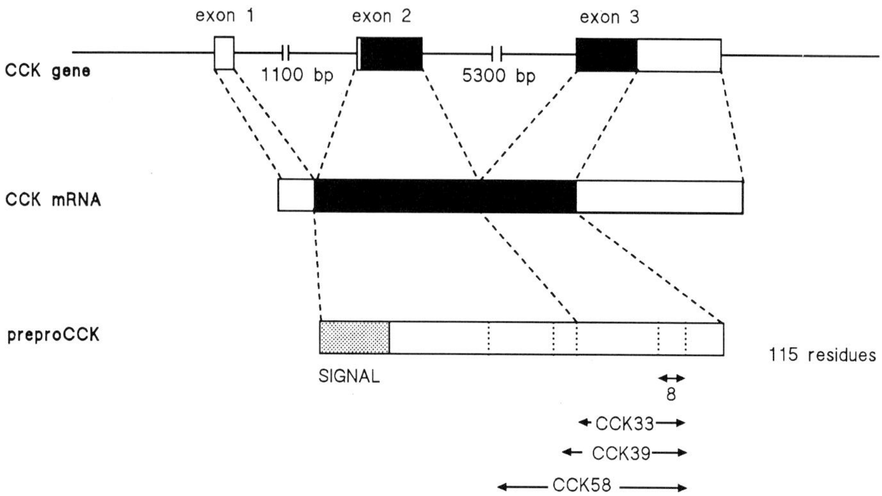

Fig. 2. Schematic representation of the CCK gene, CCK mRNA, and preproCCK showing their interrelationships and the relevant major biologically active products (CCK 8,33,39 and 58). *Shaded boxes* indicate nucleotide sequences that corresponded to the translated regions in preproCCK; *open boxes* indicate untranslated sequences, and the *stippled region* is the signal peptide

particular, trypsin inhibitors, which are known to act as CCK releasers, also increased rat small intestinal CCK mRNA, probably by increasing gene expression, although the cellular mechanisms mediating this effect are still not understood. Humoral factors are also important, and for example the levels of CCK mRNA in rat intestine have been reported to be depressed by somatostatin [17].

Post-Translational Processing

The conversion of preproCCK to its active products involves at least five different steps. Not all have been worked out in detail, but it is possible to deduce some of them by analogy with other well-studied peptides and from examination of naturally occurring fragments and forms. The first step involves removal of the signal sequence (probably residues 1–20 of preproCCK), and occurs in the endoplasmic reticulum. Thereafter proCCK enters the Golgi where tyrosine sulphation occurs. In addition to the tyrosine in the C-terminus of CCK, there are three other tyrosines in proCCK. One in the N-terminus of CCK39, and two in the extreme C-terminal region of the precursor. In three cases the tyrosine residue is preceded by one or more acidic residues, which is a consensus sequence for sulphation; all these tyrosines are virtually fully sulphated [13,29]. In the fourth case (the N-terminus of CCK39) the tyrosine is not preceded by acidic residues and is unsulphated.

The three remaining steps in CCK processing involve cleavage by endopeptidase and carboxypeptidase B-like enzymes and finally C-terminal amidation. The endopeptidase cleavage of proCCK is interesting in that in many instances, e.g. the N-terminal side of CCK8, 33, 39 and 58, the chain is cleaved at single Arg residues. In contrast, the cleavage at the C-terminus of the active forms occurs at a pair of arginines. Whether or not there are two different endopeptides involved remains uncertain. In any event, it is clear that after endopeptidase cleavage the remaining C-terminal arginine residues are removed by a carboxypeptidase B-like enzyme. The N-terminal fragments generated by cleavage to yield CCK8 have been characterized [1, 11]. The intermediates generated immediately prior to C-terminal amidation of the active forms, i.e. Gly-extended CCK, have also been characterized [25].

There seems to be general agreement that differences in the patterns of forms of CCK are found in brain and gut [6,10,24]. These are attributable to variation in post-translational processing pathways. In neurons CCK8 is a major product, and in endocrine cells the larger forms predominate. The affinity of different peptides for known CCK receptors is probably very similar. However, smaller peptides like CCK8 may be more readily cleared than larger forms on passage through the liver. For this reason CCK8 released from gut endocrine cells may make only a minor contribution to the total CCK activity in the systemic circulation.

Acknowledgements. The help of Christine Carter in the preparation of the manuscript is gratefully acknowledged.

References

1. Beinfeld MC (1985) Cholecystokinin (CCK) gene-related peptides: distribution and characterization of immunoreactive pro-CCK and an amino-terminal pro-CCK fragment in rat brain. Brain Res 344:351–355
2. Deschenes RJ, Lorenz LJ, Huan RS, Roos BA, Collier KJ, Dixon JE (1984) Cloning and sequence analysis of a cDNA encoding rat preprocholecystokinin. Proc Natl Acad Sci USA 81:726–730
3. Deschenes RJ, Huan RS, Funckes CL, Dixon JE (1985) A gene encoding rat cholecystokinin: isolation, nucleotide sequence and promotor activity. J Biol Chem 260:1280–1286
4. Dimaline R, Young J, Gregory H (1986) Isolation form chicken antrum and primary amino acid sequence of a novel 36-residue peptide of the gastrin/CCK family. FEBS Lett 205:318–322
5. Dockray GJ (1976) Immunochemical evidence of cholecystokinin-like peptides in brain. Nature 264:568–570
6. Dockray GJ (1977) Immunoreactive component resembling cholecystokinin octapeptide in intestine. Nature 270:359–361

7. Dockray GJ (1989) Comparative neuroendocrinology of gut peptides. In: Makhlouf GM (ed) The gastrointestinal system, vol 2. American Physiological Society, New York, pp. 133–170 (Handbook of physiology)
8. Dockray GJ, Gregory RA, Hutchison JB, Harris JI, Runswick MJ (1978) Isolation, structure and biological activity of two cholecystokinin octapeptides from sheep brain. Nature 274:711–713
9. Eberlein GA, Eysselein VE, Goebell H (1988) Cholecystokinin-58 is the major molecular form in man, dog and cat but not in pig, beef and rat intestine. Peptides 9:993–998
10. Eng J, Shina Y, Straus E, Yalow RS (1982) Post-translational processing of cholecystokinin in pig brain and gut. Proc Natl Acad Sci USA 79:6060–6064
11. Eng J, Shiina Y, Pan Y-CE, Blacher R, Chang M, Stein S, Yalow RS (1983) Pig brain contains cholecystokinin octapeptide and several cholecystokinin desoctapeptides. Proc Natl Acad Sci USA 80:6381–6385
12. Eng J, Du B-H, Pan Y-CE, Chang M, Hulmes JD, Yalow RS (1984) Purification and sequencing of a rat intestinal 22 amino acid C-terminal CCK fragment. Peptides 5:1203–1206
13. Eng J, Gubler U, Raufman J-P, Chang M, Hulmes JD, Pan Y-CE, Yalow RS (1986) Cholecystokinin-associated COOH-terminal peptides are fully sulfated in pig brain. Proc Natl Acad Sci USA 83:2832–2835
14. Eysselein VE, Reeve JR Jr, Shively JE, Miller C, Walsh JH (1984) Isolation of a large cholecystokinin precursor from canine brain. Proc Natl Acad Sci USA 81:6565–6568
15. Friedman J, Schneider BS, Powell D (1985) Differential expression of the mouse cholecystokinin gene during brain and gut development. Proc Natl Acad Sci USA 82:5593–5597
16. Gubler U, Chua AO, Hoffman BJ, Collier KJ, Eng J (1984) Cloned cDNA to cholecystokinin mRNA predicts an identical preprocholecystokinin in pig brain and gut. Proc Natl Acad Sci USA 81:4307–4310
17. Kanayama S, Liddle RA (1990) Somatostatin regulates duodenal cholecystokinin and somatostatin messenger RNA. Am J Physiol 258:G358–G364
18. Kuwano R, Araki K, Usui H, Fukui T, Ohtsuka E, Ikehara M, Takahashi Y (1984) Molecular cloning and nucleotide sequence of cDNA coding for rat brain cholecystokinin precursor. J Biochem 96:923–926
19. Liddle RA, Carter JD, McDonald AR (1988) Dietary regulation of rat intestinal cholecystokinin gene expression. J Clin Invest 81:2015–2019
20. Muller JE, Straus E, Yalow RS (1977) Cholecystokinin and its COOH-terminal octapeptide in the pig brain. Proc Natl Acad Sci USA 74:3035–3037
21. Mutt V (1976) Further investigations on intestinal hormonal polypeptides. Clin Endocrinol [Suppl] (Oxf) 6:175s–183s
22. Mutt V, Jorpes JE (1968) Structure of porcine cholecystokinin-pancreozymin. I. Cleavage with thrombin and with trypsin. Eur J Biochem 6:156–162
23. Reeve JR Jr, Eysselein V, Walsh JH (1986) New molecular forms of cholecystokinin: microsequence analysis of forms previously characterized by chromatographic methods. J Biol Chem 261:16392–16397
24. Rehfeld JF (1978) Immunochemical studies on cholecystokinin. II. Distribution and molecular heterogeneity in the central nervous system and small intestine of man and hog. J Biol Chem 253:4022–4030
25. Rehfeld JF, Hansen HF (1986) Characterization of preprocholecystokinin products in the porcine cerebral cortex: evidence of different processing pathways. J Biol Chem 261:5832–5840
26. Shively JE, Reeve JR Jr, Eysselein VE, Ben-Avram C, Vigna SR, Walsh JH (1987) CCK-5: sequence analysis of a small cholecystokinin from canine brain and intestine. Am J Physiol 252:G272–G275
27. Takahashi Y, Kato K, Hayashizaki Y, Wakabayashi T, Ohtsuka E, Matsuki S, Ikehara M, Matsubara K (1985) Molecular cloning of the human cholecystokinin

gene by use of a synthetic probe containing deoxyinosine. Proc Natl Acad Sci USA 82:1931–1935
28. Tatemoto K, Jörnvall H, Siimensmaa S, Hallden G, Mutt V (1984) Isolation and characterization of cholecystokinin-58 (CCK-58) from porcine brain. FEBS Letts 174:289–293
29. Varro A, Young J, Gregory H, Cseh J, Dockray GJ (1986) Isolation, structure and properties of the C-terminal flanking peptide of preprocholecystokinin from rat brain. FEBS Letts 204:386–390

The Morphological Localization of Cholecystokinin and Its Binding Sites in the Diffuse Neuroendocrine System

A.E. Bishop, Y.D. Zhao, D.R. Springall, and J.M. Polak[1]

Introduction

Cholecystokinin (CCK) clearly belongs to the group of substances known as brain-gut peptides; it functions both as a neuropeptide and a gut hormone. A major hindrance to the investigation of CCK localization has been the fact that its C-terminal pentapeptide is identical to that of another major gut peptide, gastrin. These amino acids are responsible for the biological activity of the peptides, with differential specificity of action being conferred by the adjacent residues. This common sequence led to much controversy concerning the activities and localizations of CCK and gastrin but the development of antibodies specific for defined regions of each peptide has helped to resolve many of the complications.

This chapter describes the localization of the various molecular forms of CCK and its mRNA in the cells of the diffuse neuroendocrine system and the morphological analysis of its target sites.

Technology

The cytological techniques employed for the morphological study of CCK and other peptides include:

1. Immunocytochemistry, used at both light and electron microscopical levels to establish the distribution of the peptide and its receptors.
2. In situ hybridization, for demonstration of peptide gene expression.
3. In vitro autoradiography, for examination of peptide receptors with respect to histology.

Localization of Peptides: Immunocytochemistry

Light Microscopy

Immunocytochemistry has been the major means of identifying the cells of origin of peptides. There was a considerable time interval between the

[1] Dept. of Histochemistry, Royal Postgraduate Medical School, Du Cane Road, London W12 ONN, UK.

G. Adler and C. Beglinger (Eds.)
CCK Antagonists in Gastrogenterology

discovery of gut hormones and the advent of reliable immunohistochemical methods. The slow progress was due to several factors. Primarily, extraction of peptides was difficult, both because of their rapid degradation and the diffuse nature of gut endocrine cells, and so there was a lack of appropriate antibodies. However, these problems were overcome, and today a wide range of antisera is available to whole sequences or fragments of natural and synthetic bioactive peptides and their precursors or variants. Several techniques are available for the immunocytochemistry of peptides [see 39]. These include methods which result in permanent stains, for example the unlabelled antibody enzyme [56] and avidin biotin complex [20] methods, and fluorescent labelling techniques [6]. The choice of method is usually open to individual preference but, in general, permanent stains are used in diagnostic histopathology whilst fluorescent techniques are preferred for immunocytochemistry of nerves as they render the morphology of fibres easier to discern.

Electron Microscopy

As with light microscopy, several methods have been developed for the immunocytochemistry of peptides at the ultrastructural level. Initially, electron microscopic profiles of peptide-producing cells were determined using the semithin-thin technique, which compares light microscopical immunostains with electron microscopy of the same cells in serial sections [40]. The major advance in this field was the use of the peroxidase-antiperoxidase method, as osmication renders diaminobenzidine electron-dense. Thus, it became possible to localize peptides to individual secretory granules in cells. However, the peroxidase-antiperoxidase method is limited; for example, the final reaction product can spread and obscure the cell ultrastructure. Also, a single cell can contain a heterogeneous population of granules, or co-storage of peptides can occur in a single granule. To study such occurrences, multiple simultaneous immunostains are needed, and they cannot be achieved with the peroxidase-antiperoxidase technique. The use of gold-labelled antisera removes these limitations. Colloidal gold is electron-dense, and a number of methods take advantage of this fact. These include the immunogold staining (IGS) technique, a simple, two-step method [9], and both the protein A gold [50] and the gold-labelled antigen detection (GLAD) [26] techniques. Multiple immunostains can be made using colloidal gold particles of different sizes.

Localization of Peptide Gene Expression: In Situ Hybridization

Immunocytochemistry localizes the final peptide product of enocrine cells, while in situ hybridization allows analysis of mRNA species directing peptide synthesis. Thus, using this method, information can be derived on the site, rate and control of peptide gene expression. In situ hybridization uses the capacity of complementary nucleic acid sequences to hybridize within a cell. Single or double stranded DNA or RNA probes can be used and are mostly radiolabelled and/or biotinylated to allow visualization of hybridization sites in tissue preparations [see 38].

Localization and Characterization of Peptide Binding Sites

The extensive literature on peptide binding sites mainly describes work on isolated cell or membrane preparations. Such an approach gives only limited information on the exact distribution of target cells and their anatomical relationships with other tissue structures; moreover, it is possible that receptor characteristics can be altered by the process of cell or membrane isolation. Morphological methods can be used to provide more detailed information on receptor distributions. Specific receptors can be immunostained using anti-idiotypic antibodies [13], but this method does not allow full analysis of receptor kinetics. The use of divalent ligand which binds to receptors and then is visualized using electron immunocytochemistry [25] is also limited in that no quantitative data can be derived; but it remains useful for tissues where only low numbers of active receptors are present and a very sensitive means of detection is needed.

In vitro autoradiography [62] has been used with great success for the localization and full kinetic characterization of peptide receptors, combined with histological analysis. Basically, the method involves incubation of a histological preparation with a radiolabelled peptide. Autoradiography is used to identify ligand binding sites. Autoradiographs can be generated on film or on emulsion-coated coverslips. The latter has the advantage of allowing comparison of the distribution of target cells with the general histology of the tissue preparation. The kinetics of the receptors can be studied using computerized image analysis of optical density in autoradiographs [see 43].

Cellular Localization of CCK

Brain-Gut Axis

The several forms of CCK which have been desribed in mammals show some evidence of differential distributions. In the gut, the major forms of CCK are CCK-33 (the original form identified by the arduous work of Mutt and Jorpes [33]) and the N-terminally extended molecules CCK-39 and CCK-58. In nervous tissue, the biologically active C-terminal octapeptide of CCK is the main form [11,46]. Molecular cloning has shown that both brain and gut contain a 114 amino acid precursor form of CCK [17] but the mechanisms underlying the differences in post-translational processing of this molecule in neuronal and endocrine cells have yet to be defined. Tetrin,

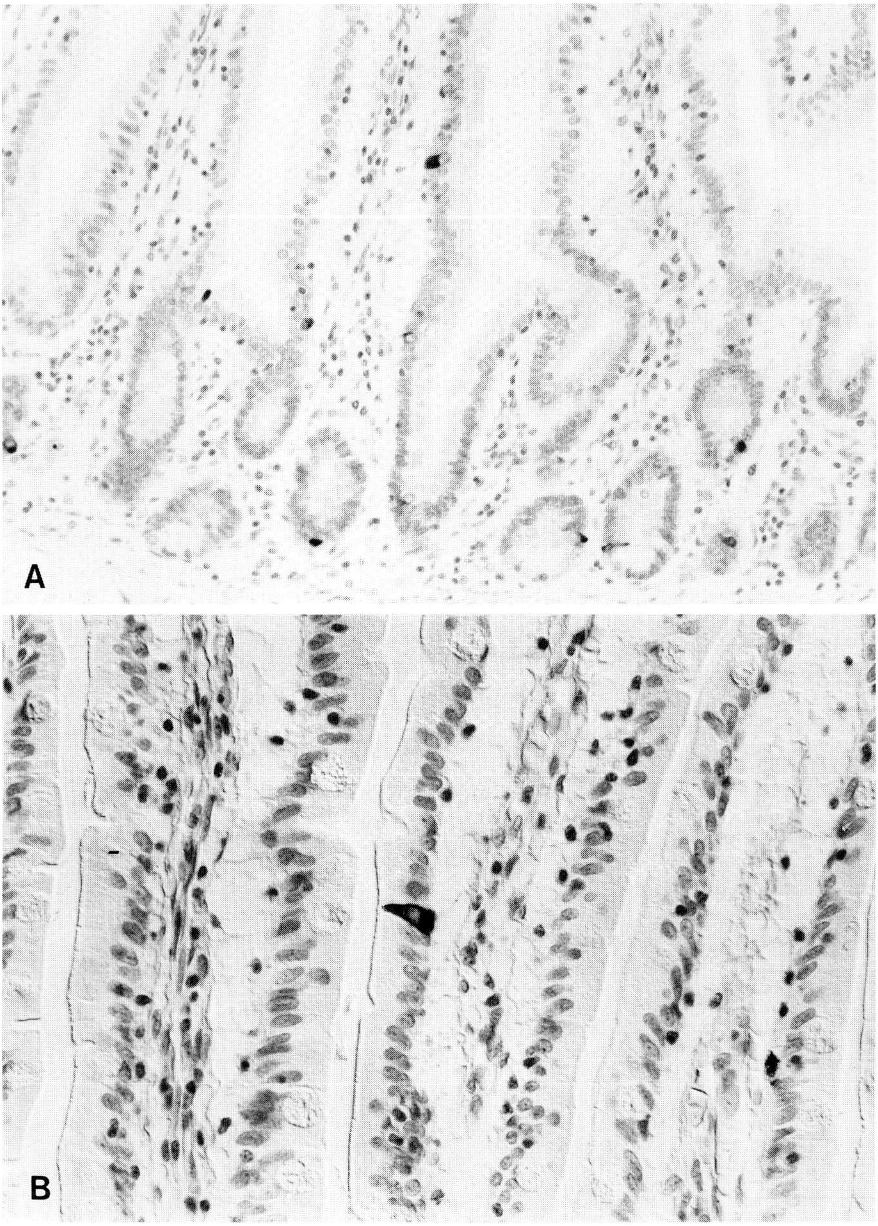

Fig. 1. A Scattered CCK cells immunostained in the villi and crypts of human duodenum using the peroxidase anti-peroxidase method. The section was counterstained with haematoxylin. **B** High-power micrograph of a CCK-immunoreactive cell in the human duodenum showing its characteristic flask shape and lumenal connection

the common C-terminal tetrapeptide amine of CCK and gastrin, has also been described as a separate entity and appears to be produced by both the gastrointestinal and nervous systems [28,45].

Endocrine Cells

The first localization of CCK to gut endocrine cells was reported in the mid-1970s [5,41]. The cells were immunostained using antibodies to natural CCK-33 in duodenum (Fig. 1) and jejunum of man, dog and pig. Electron microscopy [41] identified the CCK-immunoreactive cells as the I cells of the modified Wiesbaden classification [55] (Fig. 2). However, these initial studies were not wholly satisfactory as some cross-reaction of the anti-CCK sera with G cells was observed. This problem of cross-reactivity was resolved when the central 9–20 dodecapeptide sequence of CCK was synthesized and antibodies to it became available. Subsequent light [42] and electron [3] microscopical studies made with these antibodies successfully confirmed the original circumstantial evidence that the I cell produces CCK. Conversely, the production of gastrin by an intestinal cell type completely separate from I cells was demonstrated using a series of antibodies to distinct regions of the gastrin-34 molecule [4].

More recently, in situ hybridization has been used to study the cells producing gastrin and CCK in the human gut. Using biotinylated DNA

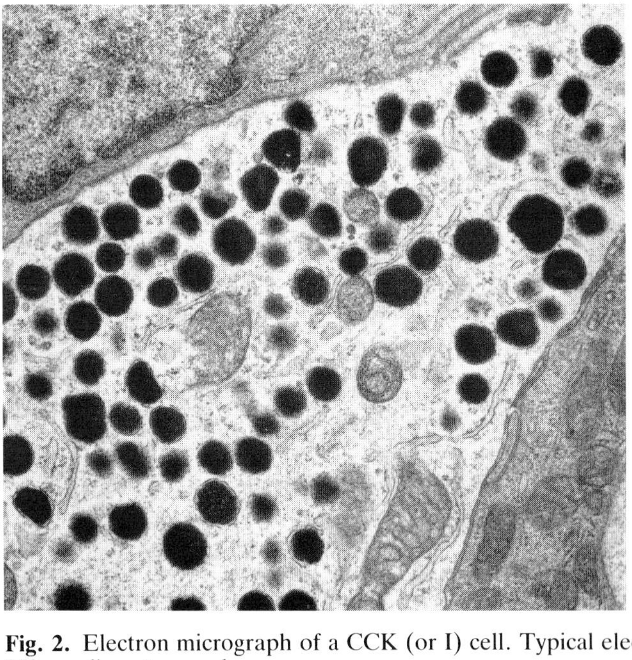

Fig. 2. Electron micrograph of a CCK (or I) cell. Typical electron-dense granules of 250 nm diameter can be seen

probes it was possible to show that cells with CCK mRNA are confined to the small intestine and do not contain gastrin mRNA [61].

Nerves

The first suggestion of a neural origin for a CCK-related peptide came in 1975 when Vanderhaegen and co-workers described the exstence of a brain peptide which reacted with antibodies raised to gastrin. Subsequent investigations revealed that CCK is present in very high concentrations in several regions of the brain, particularly the cerebral cortex, hippocampus, amygdala and hypothalamus [10,32,46,48] (Fig. 3). CCK-immunoreactive nerve cell bodies and fibres are abundant in all areas shown to have a high CCK concentration [21,29,31,36]. CCK-like immunoreactivity has been found to co-exist in the brain with other transmitters; it is present in dopaminergic neurons of the ventral mesencephalon of several mammals including man, and in the serotoninergic neurons of the medulla oblongata of rat, and it is co-stored with gamma-aminobutyric acid (GABA) in cortex and hippocampus of cat, monkey and rat [see 19].

Abundant CCK immunoreactivity has also been found in the dorsal horn of the spinal cord, in fibres corresponding to the central branches of primary sensory neurons [7,15,23] (Fig. 4) and the peptide is colocalized with substance P in cells of the dorsal root ganglia [7]. CCK immunoreactivity has been reported in large cell bodies in the ventral spinal cord but this

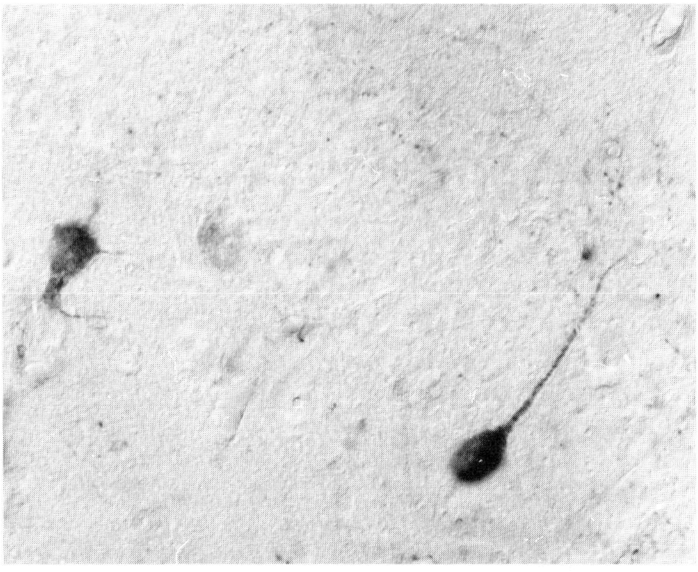

Fig. 3. CCK-immunoreactive neurons and nerve terminals in the pyramidal cell layer of rat hippocampus

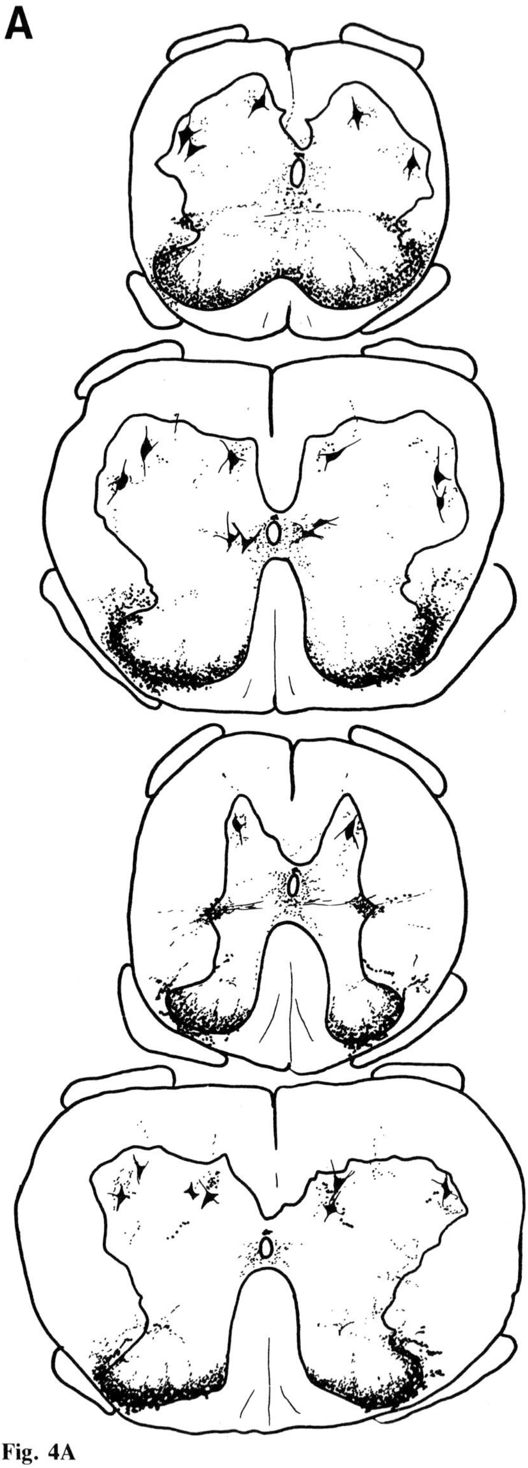

Fig. 4A

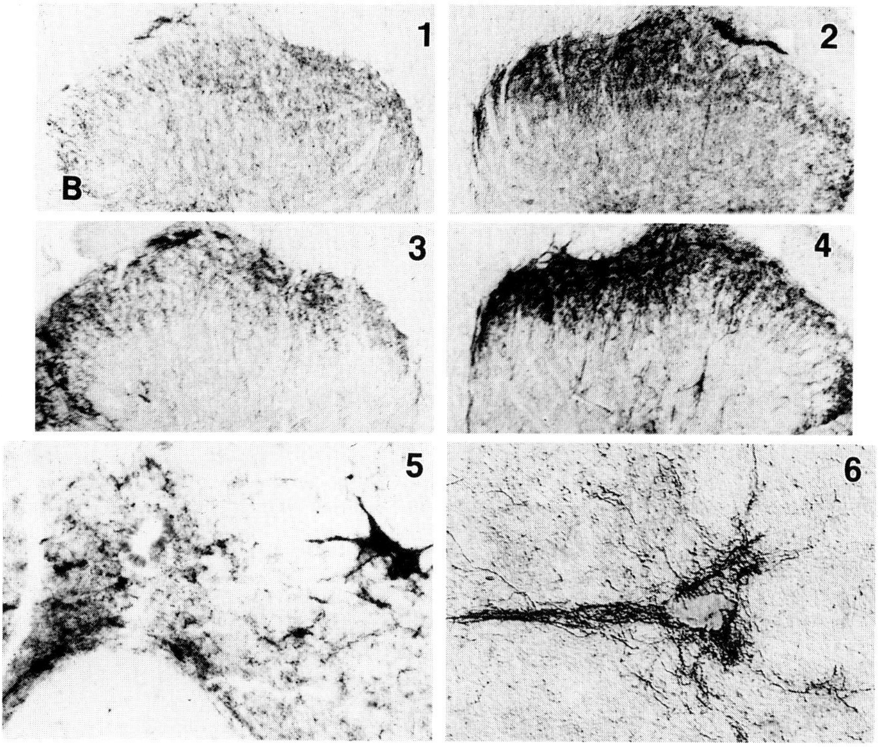

Fig. 4. **A** The distribution of CCK-immunoreactive fibres and cell bodies in (from *top* to *bottom*) cervical, thoracic, lumbar and sacral segments of rat spinal cord. **B** CCK-immunoreactive fibres in the dorsal spinal cord of the L_4 segment of the rat spinal cord 14 days following application of capsaicin to one sciatic nerve (1,2). There is a marked loss of immunoreactivity from the ipsilateral side (*1*) compared with the intact (*2*) side of the spinal cord. This provides evidence that a major component of CCK immunoreactivity in the spinal cord derives from primary sensory neurones located in the dorsal root ganglia. A similar loss of substance P immunoreactivity occurs in the L_4 dorsal spinal cord after local application of capsaicin to one sciatic nerve: ipislateral (*3*) contralateral dorsal horn (*4*). Note similar distributions of CCK and substance P immunoreactivities in the spinal cord and in the dorsal root ganglia immunoreactivities for these two peptides often occur in the same subpopulation of neurones. CCK-immunoreactive fibres and multipolar, magnocellular cell bodies in lamina X, the area around the central canal in rat spinal cord (*5*). CCK-immunoreactive fibres concentrated around preganglionic neurones in the intermediolateral cell column of the rat thoracic spinal cord (*6*)

finding has been shown recently to be the result of cross-reactivity between antisera to CCK and calcitonin gene-related peptide in the cells [60]. Cell bodies located around the central canal represent authentic CCK-producing cells.

A neuronal localization of gastrointestinal CCK was first revealed in 1979 [29,46]. As in brain, the CCK-8 form predominates in gut nerves, and the concentration of CCK immunoreactivity in the myenteric plexus and longitudinal muscle of guinea pig jejunum has been reported to be about 15% of that in the mucosa [10]. The most detailed studies of the distribution of CCK-immunoreactive gut nerves have been made in the rat and guinea pig [30,53]. Some CCK nerves in the gut are supplied by afferent vagal fibres. Intrinsic neurons lie in the submucous plexus from where they project to the mucosa and the myenteric plexus. The latter neurons project in several direction: along the myenteric plexus in an anal direction to other ganglia, to the Submucous plexus, to the mucosa and to preverteabral ganglia. Early studies [53] showed that, in the proximal colon of guinea pig, CCK immunoreactivity is co-localized with somatostatin in neuronal cell bodies of the submucous plexus. More recently, it has been demonstrated that CCK in the submucosa occurs in nerves which also contain not only somatostatin but also neuropeptide Y, calcitonin gene-related peptide and choline acetyltransferase, which synthesizes acetylcholine. Some neurons showing this pattern of transmitter co-localization can be found in the myenteric plexus, where they show a Dogiel Type III morphology. CCK also occurs in this plexus in neurons with the appearance of Dogiel Type I cells, and these also contain vasoactive intestinal polypeptide, dynorphin, enkephalin and gastrin-releasing peptide.

Other Localizations

Although in most mammals CCK is produced in gut, by both endocrine cells and nerves, and in the CNS, cell types in other organs have been reported to produce it. Nerves containing immunoreactivity for the common C-terminal tetrapeptide of CCK and gastrin have been described in the pancreatic islets of pig, cat and hamster [47]. These nerves were also found in pancreatic ganglia, surrounding non-immunoreactive neuronal cell bodies. The CCK-immunoreactive nerves in islets showed a beaded appearance, suggestive of axon terminals. These findings, along with the observation that CCK-4 is a more potent stimulator of insulin release than larger gastrin and CCK molecules [44], were taken to suggest that the peptide mediates neural control of islet hormone secretion. The parafollicular cells of the rat thyroid were found, at light and electron microscopical levels to contain immunoreactivity for the C-terminal tetrapeptide of CCK/gastrin [1,27], although antibodies to other regions of the CCK molecule did not immunostain cells. Likewise, a CCK-like peptide has been localized to A-cells of the human and rat pancreas [16], cells which are notorious for causing nonspecific adherence of antibodies.

CCK can sometimes be found outside the brain-gut axis in nerves which appear to be sensory in nature. For example, a CCK-like peptide is present in ocular nerves originating from the trigeminal ganglion [2,24]. An unusual localization of CCK is in monkey spermatozoa, where immunoreactivity is found in the acrosome [34,35]. In addition, low concentrations of CCK have been detected in feline nasal mucosa and lung [37] and, although the endocrine cell or nerve of origin has not yet been identified, CCK octapeptide has been shown to cause contractile responses in guinea pig trachea and human bronchus [57].

In Vitro Autoradiography of CCK Binding Sites

Numerous studies have been made using isolated cell or membrane preparations on the interaction of CCK with receptors in the brain, and pancreas (see Miller this volume, for review). However, information on the anatomical distribution of these receptors in intact tissues is limited. In addition, it is possible that the process of cell/membrane isolation may affect peptide binding characteristics. We now describe previous reports on the use of in vitro autoradiography to map CCK binding sites and give the previously unpublished results of a study of CCK receptors in guinea pig lung.

Gut and Pancreas

As part of its satiety effect, CCK inhibits gastric emptying at physiological doses [14]. The exact sites where the peptide mediates this action in rat gut have been revealed by in vitro autoradiography using ^{125}I-labelled CCK-33 [54]. Sections of all areas of rat gut were incubated with the radiolabelled peptide but the localization of receptors was restricted to the circular muscle of the pyloric sphincter. The relative affinity of these receptors for gastrin was not established. CCK is known to contract pyloric sphincter [18] and, thus, it appears that a direct effect of CCK on the muscle delays gastric emptying. Examination of CCK-33 binding sites using a similar approach in the developing rat upper gastrointestinal tract showed that the pyloric CCK binding occurred from the earliest stage examined (day 17 of gestation) [49]. Additional binding of radiolabelled CCK-33 was seen in the mucosa and antral muscle but this disappeared during post-natal development.

The advantages of using in vitro autoradiography were highlighted in a recent study which compares CCK receptors on gall bladder muscle with those on pancreatic acinar cells. Although much work has been done on pancreatic acinar cells, the problems of obtaining adequate material from small animals meant that binding studies on gall bladder were limited to bovine membrane preparations. With in vitro autoradiography, using ^{125}I-labelled CCK-8, it was possible to localize and characterize CCK receptors in guinea pig gall bladder and pancreatic acini under identical conditions [59]. The results showed that CCK receptors were present on the smooth muscle of the gall bladder and spread diffusely on pancreatic acinar cells, and that binding sites in both tissues have similar affinites for various agonists and antagonists.

Two studies have used combined electron and light microscopy and autoradiography to examine in detail the distribution of CCK-receptors in endocrine and exocrine components of the rat pancreas. Saturable CCK binding sites were identified in islet cells of isolated pancreas perfused with ^{125}I-labelled Bolton Hunter-CCK-33 [52]. Binding was also seen to acinar cells and ducts. In islets, the densest binding was seen to β (insulin-producing) cells, which accounted for 69% of the total specific binding. In the other study [51], only acinar cells were examined, and electron microscope autoradiographs localized binding of the same ligand to the basolateral plasmalemma of the cells. It was estimated that each acinar cell possessed between 5000 and 10000 CCK binding sites. In vitro autoradiography of ^{125}I-labelled CCK-33 in the developing rat pancreas failed to demonstrate binding until between 3 and 10 days of post-natal development [49].

Brain

In view of the difficulty of obtaining homogenates of specific brain nuclei, in vitro autoradiography has been a major aid to the anatomical study of central receptors. Thus, many studies have used this technique to localize and characterize CCK binding sites in the brain. CCK receptors are widely distributed in the CNS, with the highest densities of binding being found in cortical, olfactory, visual and limbic systems [see 12,22]. In the cortex, binding sites show a laminar distribution, with the densest binding being seen in layers II-IV and VI. CCK-immunoreactive neurons are also found in layers II and III, where cortical association neurons occur, suggesting that CCK acts in the processing of cortical-cortical information. In vitro autoradiography shows that, within the olfactory and visual systems, the receptors occur on axons and may mediate pre-synaptic modification of the sensory input to the CNS. In the limbic system, CCK receptors appear to act in the modulation of emotions and are concentrated in mammillary nuclei, the hippocampus and the amygdala.

Lung

The work described in this section was carried out in collaboration with Dr. M.K. Church, Clinical Pharmacology Group, Southampton General Hospital, Southampton, UK. Recent studies have questioned the role of CCK-8 in the physiology of trachea in both normal and sensitized guinea pigs [57]. CCK is a potent constrictor of the trachea in normal guinea pigs, and the effect is significantly enhanced in animals that have been sensitized to ovalbumin. The precise localization of binding sites in the respiratory tract of guinea pig is uncertain; thus binding sites were localized in tissue sections from guinea pig respiratory tract using in vitro autoradiography to determine the sites of action of CCK. The results were compared with the morphology of the tissues demonstrated by various histological techniques, including haematoxylin and eosin staining, toluidine blue staining and electron microscopy, in order to identify the labelled cell type. Guinea pigs with acute respiratory infection were compared with normal controls. The trachea and lungs were dissected out of all animals and unfixed cryostat sections were incubated with ^{125}I-labelled CCK-8 in the absence or presence

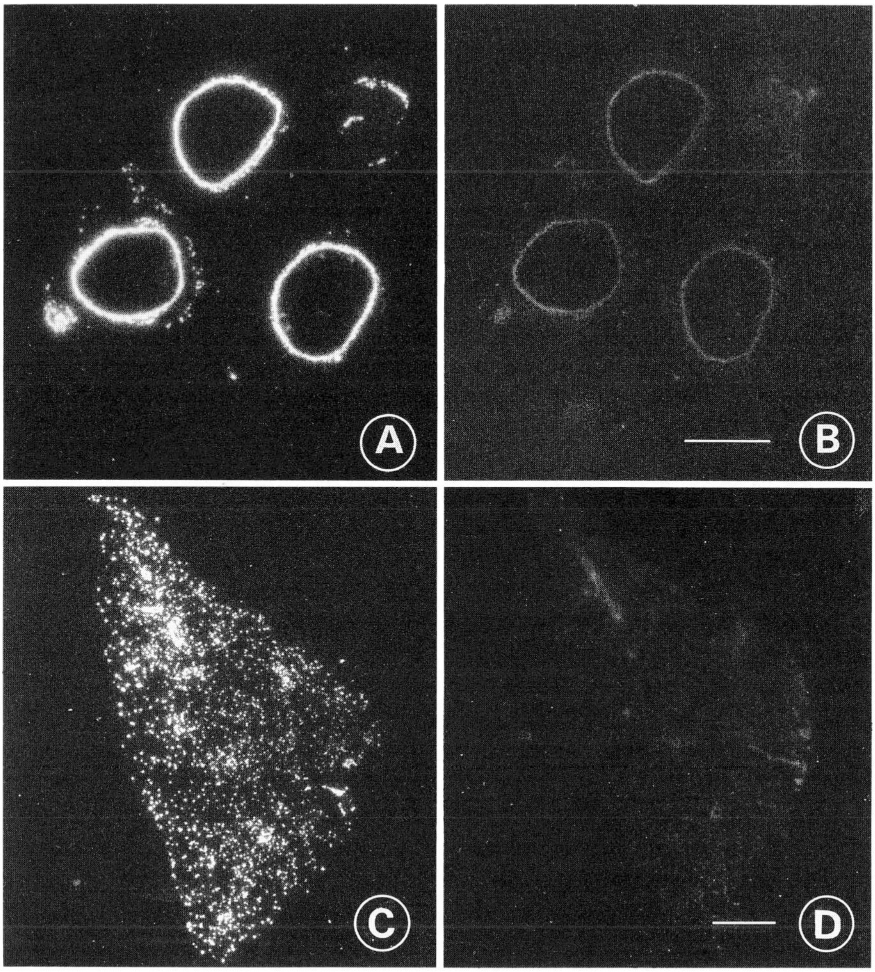

Fig. 5A-D. ^{125}I-labelled CCK-8 binding to guinea pig trachea and lung. **A** Cryostat section (10 μm) of guinea pig trachea incubated with ^{125}-labelled CCK-8 alone and exposed to Hyperfilm-^{3}H. **B** Specific binding is observed on the epithelium and submucosa that is inhibited competitively in the presence of unlabelled peptide. **C** Section of guinea pig lung showing binding of ^{125}I-labelled CCK-8 to scattered regions of lung parenchyma. **D** The labelling is also inhibited in the presence of excess unlabelled peptide. *Bar* = 1 mm

of excess unlabelled CCK-8 (nonsulphated form). Autoradiographs were generated either on film or by dipping the slides in photographic emulsion. The characteristics of the CCK-8 binding sites were determined using computerized image analysis of the generated autoradiographs (IBAS, Kontron). The inflammatory response in the animals with respiratory infections consisted of eosinophilic cell infiltration in the trachea and lung. The eosinophil

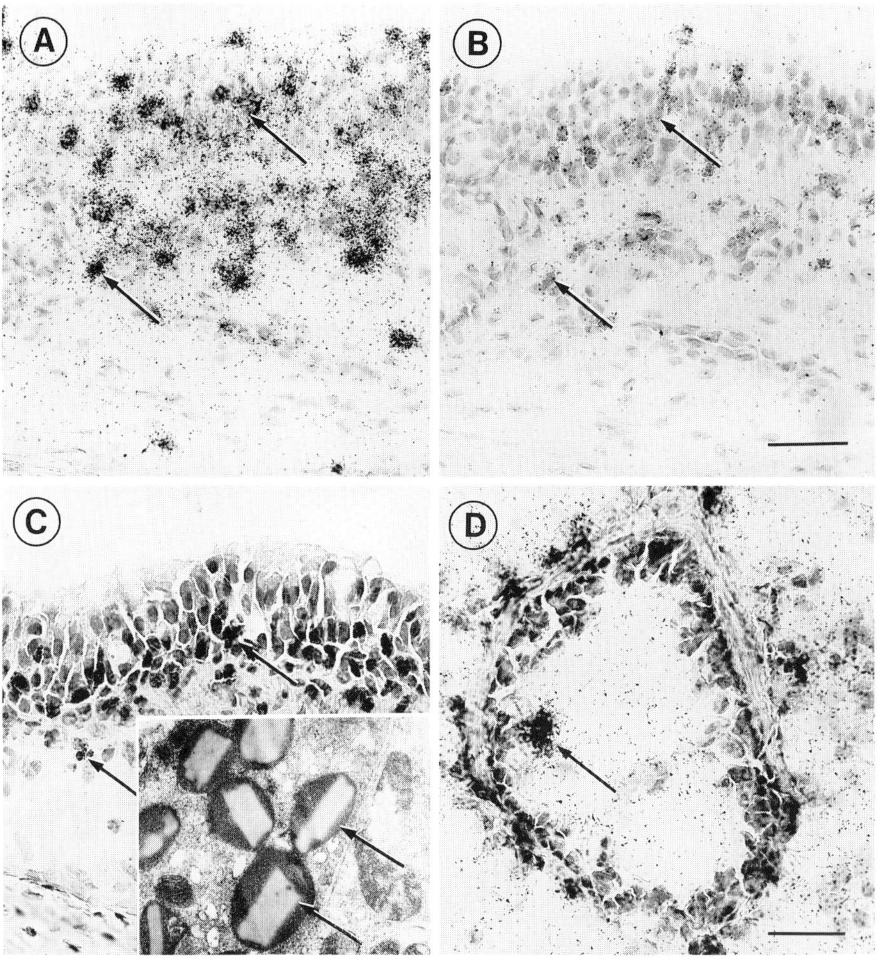

Fig. 6A-D. Emulsion-dipped sections of guinea pig trachea showing (**A**) localization of binding sites to scattered cells in the epithelium (*arrows* in **A** and **B**). **B** Serial section showing that the labelling is inhibited by co-incubation with an excess of unlabelled CCK-8. **C** Haematoxylin and eosin-stained section of guinea pig trachea. Scattered eosinophilic cells are seen in the epithelium (*arrow*). (*Bar* 50 μm). *Inset electron micrograph* shows cytoplasmic granules (*arrows*) with dense, crystalloid cores characteristic of eosinophils. **D** Localization of ^{125}I-labelled CCK binding sites to scattered cells (*arrows*) in bronchioles

migration was observed in epithelium and basement membrane of the epithelium and surrounding connective tissues of the trachea, bronchi, and bronchioles. This was also seen in the alveoli and pulmonary vascular bed.

Examination of autoradiographs of normal guinea pig lung showed no evidence of ^{125}I-labelled CCK-8 binding sites. In infected lung, labelling was seen over the epithelium, submucosa and connective tissues around cartilage and small blood vessels of trachea, the airway septa and bronchioles of lung (Fig. 5). Analysis of the autoradiographs showed that the binding of ^{125}I-labelled CCK-8 to tissue sections was rapid and saturable with an IC_{50} of 0.5 $\times$ 10^{-7} for trachea and lung. Scatchard analysis showed the affinity of binding sites with a maximum binding capacity (B_{max}) of 53.3 amol/mm^2 and a binding constant (K_d) of 44.2 nM. Microscopical examination of emulsion-dipped slides of respiratory tract showed the silver grains clustering on the eosinophilic cells located on the epithelial basement membrane, submucosa and small blood vessels around trachea and bronchi (Fig. 6). Ultrastructural analysis of these cells showed that they possessed specific granules containing dense crystalloid structures parallel to the long axis of the granules and were thus identified as eosinophils. The binding obtained could only be displaced by CCK-8 in a nonsulphated form. These results suggest that CCK-8 binding sites may be involved in the regulation of synthesis and release of eosinophil products which cause epithelial damage and bronchoconstriction in the lung. CCK-8 may thus play a crucial role in the pathogenesis of various respiratory tract diseases.

Conclusions

In the 15 years since CCK was first localized to a specific cell type, morphological techniques have provided crucial information on the distribution and sites of action of the various molecular forms of this peptide. The advent of new technology, in the form of molecular biological methods, will no doubt continue to maintain the important role of histology in CCK research.

References

1. Arias J, Scopsi L, Fischer JA, Larsson LI (1989) Light- and electron-microscopical localization of calcitonin, calcitonin gene-related peptide, somatostatin and C-terminal gastrin CCK immunoreactivities in rat thyroid. Histochemistry 91:265–272
2. Bjorklund H, Fahrenkrug J, Sieger A, Vanderhaeghen JV, Olson L (1985) On the origin and distribution of vasoactive intestinal polypeptide-, peptide HI- and cholecystockinin-like-immunoreactive nerve fibres in the rat iris. Cell Tissue Res 242:1–7
3. Buchan AMJ, Polak JM, Solcia E, Capella C, Hudson D, Pearse AGE (1978) Electron immunohistochemical evidence for the human intestinal I cell as the source of CCK. Gut 19:403–407

4. Buchan AMJ, Polak JM, Solcia E, Pearse AGE (1979) Localization of intestinal gastrin in a distinct endocrine cell type. Nature 277:138–140
5. Buffa R, Solcia E, Go VLW (1976) Immunohistochemical identification of the cholecystokinin cell in the intestinal mucosa. Gastroenterolopy 70:528–532
6. Coons AH, Leduc EH, Connolly JM (1955) Studies on antibody production. I.A method for the histochemical demonstration of specific antibody and its application to study of the hyperimmune rabbit. J Exp Med 102:42–60
7. Dalsgaard CJ, Vincent SR, Hokfelt T, Lundberg JM, Dahlstrom A, Schultzberg M, Dockray GJ, Cuello AC (1982) Coexistence of cholecystokinin- and substance P-like peptides in neurons of the dorsal root ganglia of the rat. Neurosci Lett 33:159–163
8. Dalsgaard CJ, Hokfelt T, Schultzberg M, Lundberg JM, Terenius L, Dockray GJ, Goldstein M (1983) Origin of peptide-containing fibers in the inferior mesenteric ganglion of the guinea pig: immunocytochemical studies with antisera to substance P, enkephalin, vasoactive intestinal peptide, cholecystokinin and bombesin. Neuroscience 9:191–211
9. De Mey J, Moeremans M, Geuens G, Nuydens R, de Brabander M (1981) High resolution light and electron microscopic localization of tubulin with the IGS (immunogold staining) method. Cell Biol Int Rep 5:889–899
10. Dockray GJ (1980) Cholecystokinin. In: Bloom SR, Polak JM (eds) Gut hormones. Livingstone, Edinburgh, pp 229–239
11. Dockray GJ, Gregory RA, Hutchinson JB (1978) Isolation, structure and biological activity of two cholecystokinin octapeptides from sheep brain. Nature 274:711–713
12. Gaudreau P, St-Pierre S, Pert CB, Quirian R (1985) Cholecystokinin receptors in mammalian brain. Ann NY Acad Sci 448:198–219
13. Gaulton VN, Green MI (1986) Idiotypic mimicking of biological receptors. Am Rev Immunol 4:253–280
14. Gibbs J, Young RC, Smith GP (1975) Cholecystokinin elicits satiety in rats with open gastric fistulas. J Comp Physiol Psychol 84:448–495
15. Gibson SJ, Polak JM, Bloom SR, Wall PD (1981) The distribution of nine peptides in rat spinal cord with special emphasis on the substantia gelatinosa and on the area around the central canal (lamina X). J Comp Neurol 201:65–79
16. Grube D, Maier V, Raptis S, Schelgel W (1978) Immunoreactivity of the endocrine pancreas. Evidence for the presence of cholecystokinin-pancreozymin within the A-cell. Histochemistry 56:13–35
17. Gulber U, Chua AO, Hoffman BJ, Collier KJ (1984) Cloned cDNA to cholecystokinin mRNA predicts an identical pre-pro-cholecystokinin in pig brain and gut. Proc Natl Acad Sci USA 81:4307–4310
18. Harvey RF (1975) Hormonal control of gastrointestinal motility. Am J Dig Dis 20:523–539
19. Hokfelt T, Skirboll L, Everitt B, Meister B, Brownstein M, Jacobs T, Faden A, Kuga S, Goldstein M, Markstein R, Dockray GJ, Rehfeld JF (1985) Distribution of cholecystokinin-like immunoreactivity in the nervous system. Ann NY Acad Sci 448:255–274
20. Hsu SM, Raine L, Fanger H (1981) Use of avidin-biotin-peroxidase complex (ABC) in immunoperoxidase techniques: a comparison between ABC and unlabelled antibody (PAP) procedures. J Histochem Cytochem 29:1196–1204
21. Innis RB, Correa FMA, Uhl GR, Schemder B, Snyder SH (1979) Cholecystokinin octapeptide-like immunoreactivity: histochemical localizaltion in rat brain. Proc Natl Acad Sci USA 76:521–526
22. Innis RB, Aghajanian GK (1985) Integrated anatomical and physiological studies of neuronal cholecystokinin receptors. Ann NY Acad Sci 448:188–197
23. Jancso G, Hokfelt T, Lundberg JM, Kiraly E, Halasz N, Nilsson G, Terenius L, Rehfeld J, Steinbusch H, Verhofstad A, Elde R, Said S, Brown M (1981) Immunohistochemical studies on the effect of capsaicin on peptide and mono-

amine neurons using antisera to substance P, gastrin/CCK, somatostatin, VIP, enkephalin, neurotensin and 5-hydroxytryptamine. J Neurocytol 10:963–980
24. Kuwayama Y, Stone RA (1986) Cholecystokinin-like immunoreactivity occurs in ocular sensory neurons and partially co-localizes with substance P. Brain Res 381:266–274
25. Lackie PM, Cuttitta F, Minna JD, Bloom SR, Polak JM (1984) Localization of receptors using a dimeric ligand and electron immunocytochemistry. Histochemistry 83:57–59
26. Larsson LI (1979) Simultaneous ultrastructural demonstration of multiple peptides in endocrine cells by a novel immunocytochemical methods. Nature 28:743–746
27. Larsson LI (1985) Differential changes in calcitonin-, somatostatin-, gastrin/cholecystokinin-like immunoreactivities in rat thyroid parafollicular cells during ontogeny. Histochemistry 82:121–130
28. Larsson LI, Rehfeld JF (1979) A peptide resembling the COOH-terminal tetrapeptide amide of gastrin in a new gastrointestinal endocrine cell type. Nature 277:575–578
29. Larsson LI, Rehfeld JF (1979) Localization and molecular heterogeneity of cholecystokinin in the central and peripheral nervous system. Brain Res 165: 201–218
30. Llewellyn-Smith IJ (1989) Neuropeptides and the microcircuitry of the enteric nervous sytem. In: Polak JM (ed) Regulatory peptides. Birkhauser, Basel, pp 247–265
31. Loren I, Alumets J, Hakanson R, Sundler F (1979) Distribution of gastrin and CCK-like peptides in rat brain. An immunocytochemical study. Histochemistry 59:249–257
32. Muller JE, Straus E, Yalow RS (1977) Cholecystokinin and its COOH-terminal octapeptide in the pig brain. Proc Natl Acad Sci 74:3035–3037
33. Mutt V, Jorpes JE (1968) Structure of porcine cholecystokinin pancreozymin. I. Cleavage with thrombin and with trypsin. Eur J Biochem 6:156–162
34. Pelto-Huikko M, Persson H, Schalling M, Rehfeld JF, Hokfelt T (1989) Immunocytochemical demonstration of cholecystokinin-like immunoreactivity in spermatozoa in monkey testis and epididymis. Acta Physiol Scand 137:456–466
35. Persson H, Ericsson A, Schalling M, Rehfeld JF, Hokfelt T (1988) Detection of cholecystokinin in spermatogenic cells. Acta Physiol Scand 134:565–566
36. Pirget M, Straus E, Yalow RS (1978) Localization of cholecystokinin-like immunoreactivity in isolated nerve terminals. Proc Natl Acad Sci USA 75: 6324–6326
37. Polak JM, Bloom SR (1982) Regulatory peptides and neuron-specific enolase in the respiratory tract of man and other mammals. Exp Lung Res 3:313–328
38. Polak JM, McGee JO'D (1990) In situ hybridization: principles and practice. Oxford University Press, Oxford
39. Polak JM, van Noorden S (1986) Immunocytochemistry: modern methods and applications. Wright, Bristol.
40. Polak JM, Pearse AGE, Heath CM (1975) Complete identification of endocrine cells in the gastrointestinal tract using semithin-thin sections to identify motilin cells in human and animal intestine. Gut 16:225–229
41. Polak JM, Pearse AGE, Bloom SR, Buchan AMJ, Rayford PC, Thompson JC (1975) Identification of cholecystokinin-secreting cells. Lancet 2:1016–1017
42. Polak JM, Pearse AGE, Szelke M, Bloom SR, Hudson D, Facer P, Buchan AMJ, Bryant MG, Christofides N, MacIntyre I (1977) Specific immunostaining of CCK cells by use of synthetic fragment antisera. Experientia 33:762–763
43. Power RF, Wharton J, Zhao Y, Bloom SR, Polak JM (1989) Autoradiographic localization of endothelin binding sites in the cardiovascular and respiratory systems. J Cardiovasc Pharmacol 13:550–556

44. Rehfeld JF (1971) Effect of gastrin and its C-terminal tetrapeptide on insulin secretion in man. Acta Endocrinol (Copenh) 66:169–176
45. Rehfeld JF, Goltermann NR (1979) Immunochemical evidence of cholecystokinin and tetrapeptides in hog brain. J Neurochem 32:1339–1341
46. Rehfeld JF, Goltermann N, Larsson LO, Emson PM, Lee CM (1979) Gastrin and cholecystokinin in central and peripheral neurons. Fed Proc 38:2325–2329
47. Rehfeld JF, Larsson LI, Goltermann NR, Schwartz TW, Holst JJ, Jensen SL, Morley JS (1980) Neural regulation of pancreatic hormone secretion by the C-terminal tetrapeptide of CCK. Nature 284:33–38
48. Robberecht PM, Deschodt-Lanckman M, Vanderhaegan JJ (1978) Demonstration of biological activity of brain gastrin-like peptide material in the human: its relationship with the COOH-terminal octapeptide of cholecystokinin. Proc Natl Acad Sci USA 75:524–528
49. Robinson PH, Moran TH, Goldrich M, McHugh PR (1987) Development of cholecystokinin binding sites in rat upper gastrointestinal tract. Am J Physiol 252:G529–G534
50. Romano EL, Romano M (1977) Staphyloccal protein A bound to colloidal gold: a useful reagent to label antigen-antibody sites in electron microscopy. Immunocytochemistry 14:711–715
51. Rosenzweig SA, Miller LI, Jamieson JD (1983) Identification and localization of cholecystokinin-binding sites on rat pancreatic plasma membranes and acinar cells: a biochemical and autoradiographic study. J Cell Biol 96:1288–1297
52. Sakamoto C, Goldfine ID, Roach E, Williams JA (1985) Localization of saturable CCK binding sites in rat pancreatic islets by light and electron microscope autoradiography. Diabetes 34:390–394
53. Schultzberg M, Hokfelt T, Nilsson G, Terenius L, Rehfeld JF, Brown M, Elder R, Goldstein M, Said S (1980) Distribution of peptide- and catecholamine-containing neurons in the gastrointestinal tract of rat and guinea-pig: immunohistochemical studies with antisera to substance P, vasoactive intestinal polypeptide, enkephalins, somatostatin, gastrin/cholecystokinin, neurotensin and dopamine-B-hydroxylase. Neuroscience 5:689–744
54. Smith GT, Moran TH, Coyle JT, Kuhar MJ O, Donohue TL, McHugh PR (1984) Anatomic localization of cholecystokinin receptors in pyloric sphincter. Am J Physiol 246:R127–R130
55. Solcia E, Pearse AGE, Grube D, Kobayashi S, Bussolatti G, Creutzfeldt W, Gepts W (1973) Revised Wiesbaden classification of gut endocrine cells. Rend Gastroenterol 5:13–16
56. Sternberger LA (1979) The unlabelled antibody enzyme peroxidase antiperoxidase (PAP) method. In: Sternberger LA (ed) Immunocytochemistry, Wiley, New York, pp 104–169
57. Stretton CD, Barnes PJ (1989) Cholecystokinin-octapeptide constricts guinea-pig and human airways. Br J Pharmacol 97:675–682
58. Vanderhaegen JJ, Signeau JC, Gepts W (1975) New peptide in the vertebrate CNS reacting with anti-gastrin antibodies. Nature 257:603–605
59. Von Schrenck T, Moran TH, Heinz-Erian P, Gardner JS, Jensen RT (1988) Cholecystokinin receptors on gall bladder muscle and pancreatic acinar cells: a comparative study. Am J Physiol 255:G512–G521
60. Williams RG, Dimaline R, Varro A, Isetta AM, Trizio D, Dockray GJ (1987) Cholecystokinin octapeptide in rat central nervous system. Immunocytochemical studies using a monoclonal antibody that does not cross react with CGRP. Neurochem Int 11:433–442
61. Yabu M, Himeno S, Kariya Y, Fujita H, Tarvi S (1989) Identification of gastrin and cholecystokinin cells in human gastrin antrum and duodenum using in situ hybridization techniques. Acta Histochem Cytochem 22:309–314
62. Young WS, Kuhar MJ (1979) A new method for receptor autoradiography: (3H) opioid receptors in rat brain. Brain Res 179:255–270

Heterogeneity of CCK Receptors: Classification and Characterization*

L.J. Miller[1]

Receptors which recognize cholecystokinin (CCK) peptides are particularly interesting and notable, both for their similarities and for their differences. There appear to be a family of such receptors which will likely be homologous, yet possess exquisite differences in their structural specficities.

Targets of CCK

There are a large number of cell types which are targets for this family of hormones (CCK and gastrin). These are much more widespread than the classical targets for CCK, the pancreatic acinar cell and gallbladder muscularis smooth muscle cell, and for gastrin, the parietal cell. Additional potential targets include the brain, spinal cord, peripheral neural structures including many areas of the enteric plexuses, smooth muscle along the gut from esophagus to colon, endocrine cells along the gut and pancreas, chief cells, and various tumors such as small cell carcinomas and carcinoids.

CCK Receptor Classification

If one were to accept all the observations from all the laboratories working on all these tissues from multiple species, noting absolute and relative potencies for biological activities, binding affinities of a series of agonists and antagonists, and biochemical characterization, there would be literally tens of different receptor types, or at least subtypes, for these hormones. Experience tells us that there are good reasons for apparent and even real differences in some of these paramenters, while still dealing with a single type of receptor. We believe that, at this time, we should approach this categorization cautiously. The most conservative such classification would suggest the presence of two or three major types of receptors for CCK and

* This work was supported by grants from the National Institutes of Health (DK32878 and DK34988) and the Chadwick Foundation.

[1] Center for Basic Research in Digestive Diseases, Mayo Clinic, Rochester, MN 55905, USA.

G. Adler and C. Beglinger (Eds.)
CCK Antagonists in Gastroenterology

gastrin. There are clearly distinguishable type A and B CCK receptors, and possibly a distinct gastrin receptor, which has many features in common with the B receptor.

The *type A receptor* is characterized by a basic minimal requirement for the C-terminal heptapeptide, including the tyrosine sulfate [8]. Further shortening of the peptide ligand shifts biological activity and binding curves several orders of magnitude to the right. It is typical for these receptors to have relative affinities for CCK-8 which are approximately 500 times that for desulfated CCK-8, and 10000 times that for CCK-4. This type of specificity is observed in receptors on the pancreatic acinar cell and islets, the gallbladder muscularis smooth muscle, pyloric smooth muscle, neurons in the lower esophageal sphincter and myenteric plexus, and certain brain nuclei including the interpeduncular nucleus, the area postrema, and the nucleus tractus solitarius.

The *type B receptor* is characterized by a basic minimal requirement for the C-terminal tetrapeptide [8]. It is typical for these receptors to have relative affinities for CCK-8 which are approximately ten times that for desulfated CCK-8, gastrin, and even CCK-4. This is clearly much less selective than the type A receptor. The typical target is the predominant brain receptor, widely distributed through the cerebral cortex. This type of specificity is also observed on some small cell carcinoma lines and on gastric and enteric smooth muscle from some species, while that in other species appears more like a gastrin receptor [16,17].

The typical *gastrin receptor* also has a basic minimal requirement for the C-terminal tetrapeptide [8]. It differs, however, in that it recognizes gastrin and CCK essentially identically. Here, too, the affinities for desulfated CCK peptides and for CCK-4 are lower than those for CCK-8 and gastrin. Desulfated CCK-8 has an afinity approximately 100 times less than CCK-8, and CCK-4 has an affinity approximately 600 times less than CCK-8. The classical target is the gastric parietal cell, but some gastric and enteric smooth muscle cells appear to have the same specificity. In addition, some cells with typical type A CCK receptors appear to have gastrin receptors as well [34]. This seems to be peculiar to some species. The methodology to adequately distinguish one type receptor from another, particularly when they are present in divergent numbers of sites, is just beginning to evolve.

Conformation of Ligands Recognized by CCK Receptors

Since most linear peptides are quite flexible, able to assume a large number of configurations, linear structure-activity data provide little about the recognition requirements of a particular receptor. Much more useful are conformationally restricted compounds, which might take the form of peptides with unnatural amino acids or cyclization or cross-bridges, and might be non-peptide molecules. There are now examples of both kinds of molecules which are capable of interacting with CCK receptors [3,5,7,25, 28]. Most of the agonists in this group are relatively selective for the type B receptor. These would seem to limit the peptides' ability to linearize – all would favor some kind of a bend in the peptide. In fact, several of the predicted structures using computer modeling would be consistent with this. It has been postulated that the peptide is folded while interacting with the type B receptor, and somewhat elongated while interacting with the type A receptor.

A selective type A CCK receptor agonist has recently been reported [12]. Replacement of the aspartate in position 32 of CCK with its *N*-methyl derivative makes this molecule 700 times more selective for type A receptors than type B receptors, while maintaining potency equal to that of native CCK-8. Unfortunately, this modification would not be expected to yield a conformationally restricted product, and therefore provides little insight into the structural requirements for activation of the type A receptor.

CCK-Receptor Antagonists

Notable insights have come from the much more rigid, non-peptide molecules which are antagonists. It would be particularly interesting if it were possible to modify one of these to yield a selective agonist, however, to date this has not been reported. The story of the development of antagonists for this family of hormones is quite extraordinary, and makes a particularly strong case for rational drug design. Since this is the focus of much of this volume, we will provide only a brief overview. Many compounds have been shown to antagonize CCK action. These may be grouped into several classes.

The first class described represents derivatives of cyclic nucleotides [23]. These are extremely weak antagonists, with Bt2cGMP being the most potent, having a K_i of 0.1 mM. The mechanism of action of these has never been clear. The second class includes amino acid derivatives, like proglumide, benzotript, and carbobenzoxy amino acids [8,15]. An extensive structure-activity series based on proglumide has been studied. One of the derivatives (lorglumide) has a K_i of 0.1 μM. The third class of antagonists represent C-terminal analogues of CCK, incorporating deletions and C-terminal modifications [8,15]. At a number of different receptors, it has been possible to uncouple binding from activation. The idea is to remove a group critical for biological activity while maintaining a reasonable binding affinity. This is true of CCK-27-32-amide, with a K_i of 2 μM. Another interesting analogue of CCK replaces the phenylalanine amide with a phenethyl ester, yielding a compound with a different shape of dose-response curve from that of native hormone [6].

Finally, a most interesting class of compounds represents benzodiazepine derivatives [5]. As part of a screening program of natural products, a fermentation product from *Aspergillus alliaceus* was found to have CCK-antagonistic properties. The active compound was purified and characterized, and named asperlicin. This was viewed as a 1,4-benzodiazepine with a large 3-substituent derived from tryptophan and leucine and a quinazolone fused to the 1,2 positions. At the time of discovery, this was the first antagonist to show selectivity for the CCK receptors from different tissues, thus confirming the presence of receptor subtypes. Through impressive insight, that group has been able to focus on the important component parts of this molecule to maintain activity, and, as a result of this, to develop a series of totally synthetic non-peptide CCK-receptor antagonists [2,5].

The benzodiazepine moiety in these molecules seems to represent only a vehicle for the placement of appropriate functional groups. A series of related antagonists has recently been built upon a benzolactam structure, which uses analogous functional groups [18]. Both of these structure-activity series have been helpful to identify the critical components for interaction with CCK receptors. In addition to the selectivity for type A CCK receptors of the antagonists first developed, there are now also members of these series of compounds which selectively antagonize type B CCK receptors [13].

CCK Receptor Characterization

Several of the CCK receptors described above have been characterized pharmacologically based on biological activity, functionally based on binding activity, morphologically to determine cellular and subcellular localization, and biochemically. Clearly resources are in place for the cDNAs for these receptors to be cloned and sequenced. It will be fascinating to finally be able to understand the structural basis for the varied specificities observed at these receptors.

Biochemical Characterization of CCK Receptors

The biochemical characterization of receptors for CCK has provided notable insight into the issue of homology and heterogeneity. This work has been quite difficult due to the absence of a target particularly rich in receptors. The most useful source for these receptors has been the healthy pancreatic acinar cell, with approximately 5000 copies per cell [26]. A powerful technique for the characterization of sparse receptors is affinity labeling. In this, receptors are identified on the basis of their specific binding to a high-affinity radiolabeled probe, usually based on a native ligand for that receptor. An important feature of such a probe is the ability to chemically attach it in place. In simple affinity labeling, a bifunctional chemical cross-linker is utilized, choosing it so that one end is appropriately reactive to bind to the ligand probe and the other end is reactive with nucleophilic groups likely to be on the receptor. Another alternative is the specialized case of photoaffinity labeling in which a photoreactive moiety is chosen for attachment to or inclusion within the ligand probe, such that upon photolysis a highly reactive intermediate is generated which can then react to form a covalent bond with adjacent molecules. After cross-linking, the membrane proteins are solubilized, separated on a sodium dodecyl sulfate-(SDS)-polyacrylamide gel, and the labeled proteins are visualized by autoradiography.

The obvious initial choice for a probe for affinity labeling the CCK receptor, given the requirements for high-affinity binding, high specific radioactivity, and ability to be cross-linked in place, is Bolton-Hunter-labeled CCK-33. Indeed, that was the first probe used to affinity label a pancreatic membrane protein of $M_r = 80\,000$ [26]. This was confirmed by a number of groups using the same probe (variably described as between $M_r = 76\,000$ and $M_r = 95\,000$) [4,14,29,33].

To attempt to confirm the identification of that molecule as the receptor, affinity labeling was attempted using shorter probes, in which the site of cross-linking might be closer to the receptor-binding domain [19,21,22]. A series of such probes was developed and applied to this question. Of note, the $M_r = 80\,000$ protein previously labeled by CCK-33-based probes was not the most prominent band specifically labeled using these probes. Instead, these probes labeled a band that migrated at $M_r = 85\,000 - 95\,000$. Carbohydrate characterization was performed to be certain that the two glycoproteins were not the same protein which was differentially glycosylated [20]. Indeed, the protein cores of these proteins were different, with the $M_r = 80\,000$ protein labeled by CCK-33 having a core of $M_r = 65\,000$ [27] and the $M_r = 85\,000 - 95\,000$ protein labeled by short probes having a core protein of $M_r = 42\,000$ [20]. Protease peptide mapping of these core proteins similarly demonstrated differences [10].

To gain insight into the identity of the hormone-binding subunit of this receptor, another type of affinity-labeling probe was developed. This represented probes with sites of covalent attachment located within the theoretical receptor-binding domain, called "intrinsic" probes [9,24]. To accomplish this, a photolabile residue was incorporated into that domain, such that receptor binding would not be disturbed excessively. Three probes of this type have been reported [9,24]. Positioning nitro or azido derivatives of phenylalanine in the position of Phe-33, or a nitrotryptophan in the position of Trp-30, provided probes that were photolabile and had high receptor binding affinities. Of note, all three "intrinsic" probes labeled the same $M_r = 85\,000 - 95\,000$ protein previously labeled by the "short" probes [9,19,20,24]. Deglycosylation and peptide mapping studies confirmed this. Thus, the evidence is reasonably strong that this represents the hormone-binding subunit of the receptor.

Analogous studies have been performed with type A CCK receptors on gallbladder muscularis smooth muscle from cow and man [30,32]. It is of interest that the apparent size of the bovine gallbladder receptor is smaller

(M_r = 70 000 – 85 000) than the rat pancreatic receptor (M_r = 85 000 – 95 000). Further, the human gallbladder receptor (M_r = 85 000 – 95 000) is a different apparent size than the bovine receptor on the same target tissue, but it is the same apparent size as the rat pancreatic receptor. Comparison of deglycosylation and protease peptide mapping data from each of these CCK targets has revealed that each of the two gallbladder receptors are differentially glycosylated, with protein cores which are similar in size and which map similarly to each other [31]. The gallbladder receptor protein cores appear to be slightly different from that of the rat pancreatic receptor [20,31]. This suggests that there is a family of proteins which represent type A CCK receptors, and that there are species and organ differences in glycosylation, and species and possibly organ differences in protein cores.

The type A CCK receptor on the CHP212 human neuroblastoma cell line [1] has recently further supported this hypothesis [11]. This provided an opportunity to study another human target and to compare it to the human gallbladder receptor. Of interest, it was differentially glycosylated, but had a protein core indistinguishable from that of the human gallbladder receptor. Thus, the protein cores of type A CCK receptors from different tissues of a single species appear to be well conserved.

The affinity labeling data available to date support the presence of a family of related receptor molecules which represent type A CCK receptors from different targets and different species. As similar data for type B receptors become available, and as the genes encoding these molecules are cloned and sequenced, it will be extremely interesting to define their structural similarities as well as their heterogeneity.

References

1. Barrett RW, Steffey ME, Wolfram CA (1989) Type-A cholecystokinin receptors in CHP212 neuroblastoma cells: evidence for association with G protein and activation of phosphoinositide hydrolysis. Mol Pharmacol 35:394–400
2. Chang RS, Chen TB, Bock MG, Freidinger RM, Chen R, Rosegay A, Lotti VJ (1989) Characterization of the binding of [^{3}H]L-365 260: a new potent and selective brain cholecystokinin (CCK-B) and gastrin receptor antagonist radioligand. Mol Pharmacol 35:803–808
3. Durieux C, Corringer PJ, Bergeron F, Roques BP (1989) [^{3}H]pBC 264, first highly potent and very selective radioligand for CCK-B receptors. Eur J Pharmacol 168:269–270
4. Fourmy D, Lopez P, Poirot S, Jimenez J, Dufresne M, Moroder L, Powers SP, Vaysse N (1989) A new probe for affinity labelling pancreatic cholecystokinin receptor with minor modification of its structure. Eur J Biochem 185:397–403
5. Freidinger RM (1989) Cholecystokinin and gastrin antagonists. Med Res Rev 9:271–290
6. Gaisano HY, Klueppelberg UG, Pinon DI, Pfenning MA, Powers SP, Miller LJ (1989) Novel tool for the study of cholecystokinin-stimulated pancreatic enzyme secretion. J Clin Invest 83:321–325
7. Hruby VJ, Fang S, Knapp R, Kazmierski W, Lui GK, Yamamura HI (1990) Cholecystokinin analogs with high affinity and selectivity for brain versus

peripheral membrane receptors. In: Rivier JE, Marshall GR (eds) Peptides: chemistry, structure and biology. ESCOM, Leiden, pp 53–55
8. Jensen RT, Wank SA, Rowley WH, Sato S, Gardner JD (1989) Interaction of CCK with pancreatic acinar cells. Trends Pharmacol Sci 10:418–423
9. Klueppelberg UG, Gaisano HY, Powers SP, Miller LJ (1989) Use of a nitrotryptophan-containing peptide for photoaffinity labeling the pancreatic cholecystokinin receptor. Biochemistry 28:3463–3468
10. Klueppelberg UG, Powers SP, Miller LJ (1989) Protease peptide mapping of affinity-labeled rat pancreatic cholecystokinin-binding proteins. Biochemistry 28:7124–7129
11. Klueppelberg UG, Molero X, Barrett RW, Miller LJ (1990) Biochemical characterization of the cholecystokinin receptor on CHP212 human neuroblastoma cells. Mol Pharmacol (in press)
12. Lin CW, Holladay MW, Witte DG, Miller TR, Wolfram CAW, Bianchi BR, Bennett MJ, Nadzan AM (1990) A71378: CCK agonist with high potency and selectivity for CCK- A receptors. Am J Physiol 258:G648–G651
13. Lotti VJ, Chang RS (1989) A new potent and selective non-peptide gastrin antagonist and brain cholecystokinin receptor (CCK-B) ligand: L-365 260. Eur J Pharmacol 162:273–280
14. Madison LD, Rosenzweig SA, Jamieson JD (1984) Use of the heterobifunctional cross-linker m-maleimidobenzoyl N-hydroxysuccinimide ester to affinity label cholecystokinin binding proteins on rat pancreatic plasma membranes. J Biol Chem 259:14818–14823
15. Maton PN, Jensen RT, Gardner JD (1986) Cholecystokinin antagonists. Horm Metab Res 18:2–9
16. Menozzi D, Gardner JD, Jensen RT, Maton PN (1989) Properties of receptors for gastrin and CCK on gastric smooth muscle cells. Am J Physiol 257:G73–G79
17. Miller LJ (1984) Characterization of cholecystokinin receptors on human gastric smooth muscle tumors. Am J Physiol 247:G402–G410
18. Parsons WH, Patchett AA, Holloway MK, Smith GM, Davidson JL, Lotti VJ, Chang RSL (1989) Cholecystokinin antagonists. Synthesis and biological evaluation of 3-substituted benzolactams. J Med Chem 32:1681–1685
19. Pearson RK, Miller LJ (1987) Affinity labeling of a novel cholecystokinin-binding protein in rat pancreatic plasmalemma using new short probes for the receptor. J Biol Chem 262:869–876
20. Pearson RK, Miller LJ, Hadac EM, Powers SP (1987) Analysis of the carbohydrate composition of the pancreatic plasmalemmal glycoprotein affinity labeled by short probes for the cholecystokinin receptor. J Biol Chem 262: 13850–13856
21. Pearson RK, Miller LJ, Powers SP, Hadac EM (1987) Biochemical characterization of the pancreatic cholecystokinin receptor using monofunctional photoactivatable probes. Pancreas 2:79–84
22. Pearson RK, Powers SP, Hadac EM, Gaisano H, Miller LJ (1987) Establishment of a new short, protease-resistant, affinity labeling reagent for the cholecystokinin receptor. Biochem Biophys Res Commun 147:346–353
23. Peikin SR, Costenbader CL, Gardner JD (1979) Actions of derivatives of cyclic nucleotides on dispersed acini from guinea pig pancreas. Discovery of a competitive antagonist of the action of cholecystokinin. J Biol Chem 254: 5321–5327
24. Powers SP, Fourmy D, Gaisano H, Miller LJ (1988) Intrinsic photoaffinity labeling probes for cholecystokinin (CCK)-gastrin family receptors D-Tyr-Gly-[$Nle^{28,31}$,pNO_2-Phe^{33})CCK-26-33). J Biol Chem 263:5295–5300
25. Rodriguez M, Lignon MF, Galas MC, Amblard M, Martinez J (1990) Highly selective cyclic cholecystokinin analogs for central receptors. In: Rivier JE, Marshall GR (eds) Peptides: chemistry, structure and biology. ESCOM, Leiden, pp 108–110

26. Rosenzweig SA, Miller LJ, Jamieson JD (1983) Identification and localization of cholecystokinin-binding sites on rat pancreatic plasma membranes and acinar cells: a biochemical and autoradiographic study. J Cell Biol 96:1288–1297
27. Rosenzweig SA, Madison LD, Jamieson JD (1984) Analysis of cholecystokinin-binding proteins using endo-beta-*N*-acetylglucosaminidase F. J Cell Biol 99: 1110–1116
28. Roy P, Charpentier B, Durieux C, Dor A, Roques BP (1990) Conformational behavior of cyclic CCK-related peptides determined by 400-MHz ^{1}H-NMR: relationships with affinity and selectivity for brain receptors. Biopolymers 28: 69–79
29. Sakamoto C, Goldfine ID, Williams JA (1984) Pancreatic CCK receptors: characterization of covalently labeled subunits. Biochem Biophys Res Commun 118:623–628
30. Schjoldager B, Molero X, Miller LJ (1989) Functional and biochemical characterization of the human gallbladder muscularis cholecystokinin receptor. Gastroenterology 96:1119–1125
31. Schjoldager B, Molero X, Miller LJ (1990) Gallbladder CCK receptors: species differences in glycosylation of similar protein cores. Regul Pept 28:265–272
32. Shaw MJ, Hadac EM, Miller LJ (1987) Preparation of enriched plasma membranes from bovine gallbladder muscularis for characterization of cholecystokinin receptors. J Biol Chem 262:14313–14318
33. Svoboda M, Lambert M, Furnelle J, Christophe J (1982) Specific photoaffinity crosslinking of [^{125}I]cholecystokinin to pancreatic plasma membranes. Evidence for a disulfide-linked M_r 76000 peptide in cholecystokinin receptors. Regul Pept 4:163–172
34. Yu D-H, Huang SC, Wank SA, Mantey S, Gardner JD, Jensen RT (1990) Pancreatic receptors for cholecystokinin: evidence fot three receptor classes. Am J Physiol 258:G86–G95

Biological Actions of CCK in the Gastrointestinal Tract

T.E. Solomon[1]

CCK was first described over 60 years ago as a putative hormone that caused gallbladder contraction in response to fat in the intestine [1]. Thirty-five years later, it was shown that CCK was chemically identical with pancreozymin [2], another putative hormone thought to cause pancreatic enzyme secretion in response to fat and protein in the intestine [3]. In the years since the discoveries of these two major actions, CCK has been found to have many additional effects in the gastrointestinal tract and other organ systems. Early progress consisted mainly of describing the effects of increasingly pure preparations of CCK (including synthetic forms) and determining responses of many target organs. These approaches provided a wealth of data on the potential effects of CCK and continue to do so today, but they do not define which of these many responses of the gastrointestinal tract to exogenous stimulation are in fact regulated by endogenous CCK. Table 1 summarizes many of the reported actions of exogenous CCK.

The last 15 years have seen an explosion of new information about this peptide, generated by methodological advances in peptide chemistry, measurement of CCK in blood and tissue, and the development of specific antagonists of CCK receptors. These new tools make it possible to define the quantitative role of CCK in gastrointestinal function with increasing certainty. At present, strong evidence supports CCK as a major regulator of its two classical target actions, gallbladder contraction and exocrine pancreatic secretion. CCK also appears to be important in regulating postprandial release of pancreatic polypeptide (PP). It is still controversial as to whether CCK plays a major role in regulating gastric emptying, insulin secretion, or gastric secretion. Other effects of CCK on gut motility, exocrine and endocrine secretion, cell growth and differentiation, and other responses have not been studied in sufficient detail to allow evaluation of their importance.

CCK is synthesized and released by specific populations of endocrine cells and neurons in the gastrointestinal tract, implying that CCK may act through endocrine and paracrine pathways and as a neurotransmitter to

[1]Kansas City, VA Medical Center, 4801 Linwood Blvd., Kansas City, MO 64068 USA.

G. Adler and C. Beglinger (Eds.)
CCK Antagonists in Gastroenterology

Table 1. Actions of exogenous CCK on gastrointestinal function

Target organ or function	Effect
Billiary tract	
Bile secretion	+
Gallbladder motility	+
Sphincter of Oddi motility	−
Exocrine pancreas	
Enzyme secretion	+
Bicarbonate secretion	+
Cell growth, enzyme synthesis	+
Endocrine pancreas	
Insulin secretion	+
Pancreatic polypeptide secretion	+
Stomach	
Acid secretion	+,−
Pepsinogen secretion	+
Somatostatin secretion	+
Emptying	−

+ indicates stimulation, − indicates inhibition. In addition, CCK administration affects motility of the esophagus, small intestine, and colon; mucosal growth; endocrine secretion of numerous peptides; and neuronal activity in the gut among many other responses.

regulate various gut functions. However, there is little information about any mechanism of action for CCK other than the classical endocrine pathway because of difficulties in studying paracrine and neurocrine mechanisms in the intact, conscious (i.e., unanesthetized) organism. Progress is being made in this area, and the near future should bring useful new findings about these other potential pathways.

Several guidelines can be used to evaluate the importance of CCK in endocrine regulation of a particular function of the gastrointestinal tract. These criteria are described below, and examples are given of the experimental approaches taken to satisfy each criterion. More detailed summaries of the effects of CCK on specific target organs are found in other chapters in this book.

First, CCK concentrations in the arterial supply of the responding organ should increase in concert with the response. Ingestion of food is a well-established stimulant of CCK release, and is, in fact, the only physiological event known to increase plasma CCK. Thus, a very broad interpretation of this criterion is that any physiologic response to a meal is potentially regulated by circulating CCK. The plasma CCK response to food ingestion is caused by the entry of protein, fat, and their digestion products into the upper small intestine [4]. While the intraluminal and cellular events that cause and modulate CCK release from intestinal endocrine cells are still being defined, it is a fact that plasma CCK increases in response to certain nutrients in the intestinal lumen. Thus, if CCK is thought to mediate a physiologic response, it should be reproduced by intestinal perfusion with these substances. It is reasonable to expect correlation between the magnitude of the physiologic response and the level of plasma CCK, which implies that temporal correlation will also be seen. However, strong quantitative or temporal correlation between plasma CCK levels and the physiologic response is not proof of causality. Neither does the lack of such correlation disprove a regulatory role for CCK, as there may be other inhibitory or stimulatory factors that interact with CCK to obscure these correlations. In studies on the relationship between food ingestion or intestinal perfusion with nutrients, plasma CCK changes, and a physiologic response, it is most enlightening if the meal is similar in amount, nutrient composition, and consistency to those eaten by real people in the real world (or by real dogs, rats, pigs, etc.) and if the concentrations, chemical forms, and load (amount per unit time) of intestinal perfusates are similar to those measured after a meal.

Second, exogenous infusion of CCK in doses reproducing plasma concentrations of the same molecular forms released by a meal or intestinal perfusion with nutrients should initiate part or all of the physiologic response. Administration of several doses of CCK usually provides a better picture of the relative potencies of exogenous versus endogenous CCK. However, this "copying criterion" is not as simple to fulfill as was once thought. It appears that multiple molecular forms of CCK exist in plasma [5,6]; CCK-58, the largest form characterized so far, appears to be the major component in humans and dogs. This CCK form has not been available in sufficient quantities to perform in vivo studies, and evidence suggests that use of other CCK forms may not be an adequate approach to this criterion. It has been reported recently that CCK-58 often has lower cross-reactivity in CCK radioimmunoassays as well as lower bioactivity in an in vitro bioassay system than do shorter mocular forms [7,8]. These observations suggest that most or all previous studies using radioimmunoassay or bioassay have resulted in underestimation of the true plasma concentrations of endogenous CCK. On the other hand, CCK-58 may indeed by inherently less bioactive than other forms [8]; thus, copying artifactually low endogenous plasma CCK levels by giving CCK forms of artifactually high bioactivity (compared to CCK-58) tends to offset these differences. When coupled with the possibility that the usual methods for collecting blood samples may produce almost instantaneous degradation of CCK-58 and variable conversion to more immunoreactive and bioactive shorter forms [5,6], it is highly likely that the available estimates of relative potencies of endogenous and exogenous CCK are tenuous at best. Until a reliable, relatively simple, and quantitative method for measuring all molecular forms of CCK in plasma becomes available, studies comparing responses to exogenous and endogenous CCK must be interpreted cautiously. Another consideration is that this criterion holds only when CCK is the sole or at least the predominant factor involved in regulation of a given response. Exogenous infusion of CCK in fasted subjects does not reproduce all of the regulatory events that occur postprandially. It is possible that these other meal-induced factors act additively or synergistically with CCK to increase its effectiveness or that inhibitory factors decrease the effectiveness of endogenous CCK. In both cases, exogenous infusion of CCK alone could lead to erroneous estimates of the importance of endogenous CCK. Other guidelines can be derived from this criterion. For example, a useful rule is that a physiologic response initiated by very low doses of exogenous CCK is likely to be regulated by endogenous CCK. A corollary is that the CCK dose- or concentration-response pattern of a potential target should be similar to that of a "known" CCK target such as gallbladder contraction or pancreatic enzyme secretion.

Third, preventing the release of intestinal CCK in response to a meal or other stimuli should also prevent or lower the physiologic response. CCK release could theoretically be prevented by administering a selective inhibitor of its secretion, but no such agent has been found. Selective removal of CCK-secreting endocrine cells is another theoretical possibility but one impossible to accomplish at present without effects on other regulatory cells.

Fourth, specific blockade of the binding of CCK to its receptor should lessen or abolish the physiologic response to endogenous stimulants thought to act through CCK. Immunoabsorption (administration of specific, high affinity anti-CCK antibodies) is one approach to this, but specific CCK-A receptor blockers are by far more commonly used. However, some caution is required in interpreting the results of studies with such antagonists in vivo, because many potential CCK targets may be blocked at one time, leading to indirect changes in organ function. For example, administration of CCK receptor antagonists may increase the rate of gastric emptying and alter the pattern of delivery of nutrients to the small intestine. While this might change the magnitude of some other secretory or motor response that depends on intestinal nutrient load, it would not be due to a direct effect of the CCK antagonist on the organ response being studied. Thus it is important to consider all the potential effects of a CCK antagonist in vivo and to measure or control as many as possible before making strong conclusions about the role of CCK in regulation of a particular function. This and other possible "nonspecific effects" of specific receptor antagonists are reasons to remember that a compound that is a potent, specific receptor antagonists when used in in vitro systems may not necessarily be as selective in the intact organism. Although it is not proof that the antagonist is indeed acting specifically, it is useful to demonstrate the typical pattern of competitive inhibition for each in vivo response system that is studied. A high level of suspicion is warranted when a CCK antagonist that produces competitive kinetics for inhibition of CCK in vitro is shown to produce noncompetitive kinetics for inhibition of the same response in vivo [9]. It is unlikely that any effects of such an antagonist on in vivo responses to food or intestinal nutrients can be ascribed to specific antagonism of endogenous CCK on the target organ.

A fifth criterion is that receptors for CCK are present on the presumed target tissue and that their sensitivity and specificity are appropriate for the action of CCK as a major regulator of that target. If such receptors are not present, it is possible that CCK acts indirectly by releasing other factors or by causing changes in other target responses that alter the response being studied. Conversely, the presence of specific CCK receptors on a target does not rule out an important role for such indirect effects of CCK.

Examples of experiments testing some of these criteria will be given for several actions of CCK. As a first approach, it is interesting to compare the effects of exogenous CCK and intestinal nutrients that release CCK on various potential targets. Many studies have shown that exogenous CCK (at least at some doses under some conditions) stimulates pancreatic enzyme secretion, gallbladder contraction, release of PP and insulin, and inhibits gastric emptying. The effects of intestinal fatty acids and amino acids should be similar. Intestinal perfusion with long chain fatty acids increases plasma CCK levels [4,10], stimulates pancreatic enzyme secretion [4] and gallbladder contraction [10], and inhibits gastric emptying [11]. Effects of intestinal fatty acids on PP release are variable, while insulin secretion after intestinal fatty acids has not been well characterized. The only amino acids that have been shown to release CCK during intestinal perfusion are phenylalanine in man [12] and tryptophan in dog [13]; other amino acids have not been studied, although methionine, valine, and tryptophan are also effective stimulants of pancreatic secretion in man [14] and both tryptophan and phenylalanine are effective in the dog [15]. Intestinal phenylalanine also causes gallbladder contraction and insulin secretion in man [12]. Intestinal tryptophan inhibits gastric emptying in dog but phenylalanine does not [16]. Thus, although the patterns of target responses to exogenous CCK and intestinal releasers of CCK are generally similar, there are gaps and contradictions in our knowledge. More information about the effects of specific amino acids on CCK release and comparison of their potencies for CCK release and target organ responses, for example, would be helpful in quantitating the role of CCK in their actions.

There are few direct comparisons of dose-response effects of exogenous CCK on two or more potential CCK target responses in the same subjects under similar experimental conditions. Most of these have shown that pancreatic enzyme secretion and gallbladder contraction have similar sensitivities to low doses of CCK-8 and CCK-33 [17–20]. One group of investigators has reported that similar low doses of CCK-8 contructed the gallbladder [10], slowed gastric emptying [21], and augmented insulin responses to intravenous amino acids [22] in different groups of subjects. Others have reported that low CCK-8 doses strongly contracted the gallbladder but had only slight effects on intestinal or colonic motility [23] and strongly stimulated both pancreatic enzyme secretion and PP release [20]. These types of studies indicate that the primary actions of CCK, based on administration of low doses of exogenous peptide, may include stimulation of gallbladder contraction, pancreatic enzyme secretion, PP release, insulin release by amino acids, and inhibition of gastric emptying. Based on technical ease and sensitivity to exogenous CCK, gallbladder contraction appears to be the physiologic response best suited to such comparative studies. Estimation of gallbladder contraction by sonographic methods is relatively simple, accurate, and sensitive (although it requires expensive equipment), and the gallbladder responds to very low doses of CCK [24].

There have been several studies that compare various gastrointestinal responses to exogenous and endogenous CCK at plasma levels measured after a meal or intestinal nutrients. In man, pancreatic enzyme responses are nearly identical when compared as a function of plasma CCK levels after endogenous release and exogenous infusion [20,25], but in dogs there is less response to exogenous CCK [4]. No explanation exists for this difference. Similar plasma CCK levels after endogenous release and exogenous administration also appear to cause equal degrees of gallbladder contraction [10] and inhibition of gastric emptying [21,26] in man. Administration of CCK-8 to fasting subjects at doses causing plasma CCK increases similar or slightly more than after a meal has no effect on fasting plasma insulin or glucagon, or on insulin responses to intravenous glucose [12,22]. PP levels are significantly increased, however, under the same conditions [20]. One group reported that physiologic doses of CCK-8 augmented the insulin and glucagon responses to intravenous arginine and the insulin responses to large amounts of mixed amino acids [22], but others could not reproduce these results [27]. Stimulatory effects of intraduodenal phenylalanine on insulin secretion do not appear to be mediated by CCK, but rather by the effects of absorbed phenylalanine itself [12]. Postprandial CCK levels may actually reduce the insulin response to orally ingested glucose by inhibiting gastric emptying and the rate of glucose delivery to the small intestine [11]. Overall, these types of studies indicate that the levels of CCK released by a meal or intestinal nutrients are a major factor regulating pancreatic enzyme secretion, PP secretion, gallbladder contraction, and gastric emptying. The role of endogenous CCK in regulating postprandial insulin secretion is less clear; it probably does not act directly on beta cells during normal meals, but it may lower insulin secretion by slowing the rate of delivery of nutrients by its inhibitory effects on gastric emptying.

The effects of CCK receptor antagonists have provided the most clear-cut data on the quantitative role of CCK in regulation of these target responses. This exciting area of research is still evolving, but there is already a substantial body of information that clarifies our concepts of the physiological role of CCK in gastrointestinal function. The CCK receptor antagonist loxiglumide abolishes gallbladder contraction in response to a meal in humans [28,29]. However, under similar experimental conditions, loxiglumide reduces pancreatic enzyme secretion only 40%–60% in response to intraduodenal nutrient perfusion [20] and even less in response to oral food ingestion (C. Beglinger, personal communication). This difference between gallbladder contraction and pancreatic enzyme secretion may be due to a greater dependence of the latter on cholinergic mechanisms (G. Adler and C. Beglinger, personal communication). The situation appears to differ in rats because the CCK antagonist L-364 718 (MK-329) abolishes pancreatic enzyme secretion after liquid meals [30] or intestinal perfusion with nutrients [31]. Loxiglumide and L-364 718 also strongly inhibit PP secretion in response to food in man [32,33] and dog [34]. Effects of these antagonists on gastric emptying are less clear; one group found a reduction in emptying of relatively large markers with loxiglumide [28], but another found no effect on liquid meal emptying with doses of L-364 718 that strongly reduced gallbladder contraction [35]. Finally, it has been reported that L-364 718 did not alter postprandial insulin or glucagon secretion in humans, although PP levels were reduced [33]. These types of studies, considered with the results of other experiments discussed above, clearly establish a prominent role for CCK in regulating meal-induced gallbladder contraction, pancreatic enzyme secretion, and PP secretion.

After 60 years, it is now possible to make definite statements about the quantitative importance of CCK as a regulator of gastrointestinal function. The next few years will be exciting ones for those interested in the physiology of CCK. It should also be possible now to dissect the role, if any, of CCK in various gastrointestinal diseases, either as a primary cause or a secondary mediator of pathophysiologic changes.

References

1. Ivy AC, Oldberg E (1928) A hormone mechanism for gallbladder contraction and evacuation. Am J Physiol 86:599–613
2. Jorpes E, Mutt V (1966) Cholecystokinin and pancreozymin, one single hormone? Acta Physiol Scand 66:196–202
3. Harper AA, Raper HS (1943) Pancreozymin, a stimulant of the secretion of pancreatic enzymes in extracts of the small intestine. J Physiol (Lond) 102: 115–125
4. Dale WE, Turkelson CM, Solomon TE (1989) Role of cholecystokinin in intestinal phase and meal-induced pancreatic secretion. Am J Physiol 257: G782–G790
5. Eysselein VE, Eberlein GA, Hesse WH, Singer MV, Goebell H, Reeve JR Jr (1987) Cholecystokinin-58 is the major circulating form of cholecystokinin in canine blood. J Biol Chem 262:214–217
6. Eberlein GA, Eysselein VE, Hesse WH, Goebell H, Schaefer M Reeve JR Jr (1987) Detection of cholecystokinin-58 in human blood by inhibition of degradation. Am J Physiol 253:G477–G482
7. Turkelson CM, Reeve JR Jr, Solomon TE (1990) Low immunoreactivity of canine cholecystokinin-58. Gastroenterology 99:646–651

8. Reeve JR Jr, Eysselein VE, Liddle RA (1988) CCK-8 is more potent than CCK-58 for pancreatic amylase release in vitro. Gastroenterology 94:A372
9. Konturek SJ, Tasler J, Cieszkowski M, Szewczyk K, Hladij M (1988) Effect of cholecystokinin receptor antagonist on pancreatic responses to exogenous gastrin and cholecystokinin and to meal stimuli. Gastroenterology 94:1014–1023
10. Liddle RA, Goldfine ID, Rosen MS, Taplitz RA, Williams JA (1985) Cholecystokinin bioactivity in human plasma. Molecular forms, responses to feeding, and relationship to gallbladder contraction. J Clin Invest 75:1144–1152
11. Liddle RA, Rushakoff RJ, Morita ET, Beccaria L, Carter JD, Goldfine ID (1988) Physiological role for cholecystokinin in reducing postprandial hyperglycemia in humans. J Clin Invest 81:1675–1681
12. Reimers J, Nauck M, Creutzfeldt W, Strietzel J, Ebert R, Cantor P, Hoffmann G (1988) Lack of insulinotropic effect of endogenous and exogenous cholecystokinin in man. Diabetologia 14:271–280
13. Singer MV, Niebel W, Jansen JBMJ (1989) Pancreatic secretory response to intravenous caerulein and intraduodenal tryptophan: studies before and after stepwise removal of the extrinsic nerves of the pancreas in dogs. Gastroenterology 96:925–934
14. Go VLW, Hofmann AF, Summerskill WHJ (1970) Pancreozymin bioassay in man based on pancreatic enzyme secretion: potency of specific amino acids and other digestive products. J Clin Invest 49:1558–1564
15. Meyer JH, Kelly GA, Spingola LJ, Jones RS (1976) Canine gut receptors mediating pancreatic responses to luminal L-amino acids. Am J Physiol 231: 669–677
16. Stephens JR, Woolson RF, Cooke AR (1975) Effects of essential and non-essential amino acids on gastric emptying in the dog. Gastroenterology 69: 920–927
17. MacGragor IL, Knill JR, Meyer JH (1976) Similar sensitivities of pancreatic and biliary secretion to cholecystokinin plus secretin infusion. Am J Dig Dis 21: 641–644
18. Kerstens PJSM, Lamers CBHW, Jansen JBMJ, de Jong AJL, Hessels M, Hafkenscheid JCM (1985) Physiological plasma concentrations of cholecystokinin stimulate pancreatic enzyme secretion and gallbladder contraction in man. Life Sci 36:565–569
19. Cantor P, Petronijevic L, Pedersen JF, Worning H (1986) Cholecystokinin and pancreozymic effect of O-sulfated gastrin compared with nonsulfated gastrin and cholecystokinin. Gastroenterology 91:1154–1163
20. Hildebrand P, Beglinger C, Gyr K, Jansen JBMJ, Rovati LC, Zuercher M, Lamers CBHW, Setnikar I, Stalder GA (1990) Effects of a cholecystokinin receptor antagonist on intestinal phase of pancreatic and biliary responses in man. J Clin Invest 85:640–646
21. Liddle RA, Morita ET, Conrad CK, Williams JA (1986) Regulation of gastric emptying in humans by cholecystokinin. J Clin Invest 77:992–996
22. Rushakoff RJ, Goldfine ID, Carter JD, Liddle RA (1987) Physiological concentrations of cholecystokinin stimulate amino acid-induced insulin release in humans. J Clin Endocrinol Metab 65:395–401
23. Kellow JE, Miller LJ, Phillips SF, Haddad AC, Zinsmeister AR, Charboneau JW (1987) Sensitivities of human jejunum, ileum, proximal colon, and gallbladder to cholecystokinin octapeptide. Am J Physiol 252:G345–G356
24. Hopman WPM, Kerstens PJSM, Jansen JBMJ, Rosenbusch G, Lamers CBHW (1985) Effect of graded physiologic doses of cholecystokinin on gallbladder contraction measured by ultrasonography. Determination of threshold, dose-response relationships and comparison with intraduodenal bilirubin output. Gastroenterology 89:1242–1247
25. Beglinger C, Fried M, Whitehouse I, Jansen JB, Lamers CB Gyr K (1985) Pancreatic enzyme response to a liquid meal and to hormonal stimulation.

Correlation with plasma secretin and cholecystokinin levels. J Clin Invest 75: 1471–1476

26. Kleibeuker JH, Beekhuis H, Jansen JBMJ, Piers DA, Lamers CBHW (1988) Cholecystokinin is a physiological hormonal mediator of fat-induced inhibition of gastric emptying in man. Eur J Clin Invest 18:173–177
27. Schmid R, Schusdziarra V, Schulte-Frohlinde E, Maier V, Classen M (1989) Effect of CCK on insulin, glucagon, and pancreatic polypeptide levels in humans. Pancreas 4:653–661
28. Meyer BM, Werth BA, Beglinger C, Hildebrand P, Jansen JBMJ, Zach D, Rovati L, Stalder GA (1989) Role of cholecystokinin in regulation of gastrointestinal motor functions. Lancet 2:12–15
29. Malesci A, de Fazio C, Festorazzi S, Bonato C, Valentini A, Tacconi M, Rovati L, Setnikar I (1990) Effect of loxiglumide on gallbladder contractile response to cerulein and food in humans. Gastroenterology 98:1307–1310
30. O'Rourke MF, Reidelberger RD, Solomon TE (1990) Effect of CCK antagonist L-364718 on meal-induced pancreatic secretion in rats. Am J Physiol 258: G179–G184
31. Chariot J, Nagain C, Hugonet F, Tsocas A, Roze C (1990) Control of interdigestive and intraduodenal meal-stimulated pancreatic secretion in rats. Am J Physiol 259:G198–G204
32. Meier R, Hildebrand P, Thumshirn M, Albrecht C, Studer B, Gyr K, Beglinger C (1990) Effect of loxiglumide, a cholecystokinin antagonist, on pancreatic polypeptide release in humans. Gastroenterology 99:1757–1762
33. Liddle RA, Gertz BJ, Kanayama S, Beccaria L, Gettys TW, Taylor IL, Rushakoff RJ, Williams VC, Coker LD (1990) Regulation of pancreatic endocrine function by cholecystokinin: studies with MK-329, a nonpeptide cholecystokinin receptor antagonist. J Clin Endocrinol Metab 70:1312–1318
34. Hosotani R, Chowdhury P, Rayford PL (1989) L-364718, a new CCK antagonist, inhibits postprandial pancreatic secretion and PP release in dogs. Dig. Dis. Sci. 34:462–467
35. Liddle RA, Gertz BJ, Kanayama S, Beccaria L, Coker LD, Turnbull TA, Morita ET (1989) Effects of a novel cholecystokinin (CCK) receptor antagonist, MK-329, on gallbladder contraction and gastric emptying in humans. Implications for the physiology of CCK. J Clin Invest 84:1220–1225

Biological Actions of CCK in the Central Nervous System*

R.Y. Wang and C.R. Ashby, Jr.[1]

Molecular Forms of CCK Present in the Brain

Cholecystokinin (CCK), a gastrointestinal hormone [37], mediates digestive functions and feeding behaviors. Vanderhaeghen et al. [67] demonstrated the presence of gastrin-like immunoreactivity in mammalian brain, and subsequent studies indicate that the majority of this immunoreactivity could be attributed to CCK. Although a large peptide containing 58 amino acid (CCK58) is the major circulating form of CCK in humans and dogs [21,23], the predominant molecular form of CCK in the brain is CCK_8 (CCK_{26-33}, the eight amino acids at the C terminus of CCK), which contains a sulfated tyrosine residue [14,54]. However, the unsulfated form (CCK_{8US}) has been detected, in addition to CCK_4 [54]. Overall, CCK_{33} is only present in the brain in small (2%–5% of CCK immunoreactivity) amounts [54].

Pharmacological Characterization and Localization of Central CCK Receptors

In 1980, radioligand binding studies demonstrated the existence of binding sites for CCK in the brain using ^{125}I-labeled Bolton-Hunter-CCK [36,58], and that there was a distinct difference between CCK receptors in the brain compared to the periphery regarding their pharmacological profiles [36,58]. It has been shown that the brain and pancreatic CCK receptors represent structurally distinct entities [59]. Subsequently, it was suggested that CCK receptors localized primarily in the gastrointestinal tract be designated as CCK_A (alimentary) receptors, whereas those in the central nervous system be referred to as CCK_B [46]. CCK_A receptors have a high affinity for CCK_{8S}, which is three to four orders of magnitude more potent than CCK_{8US} and CCK_4 in displacing ^{125}I-labeled CCK_{33} binding in the pancreas [36,58]. Binding studies, using the CCK_A receptor radioligand ^{3}H-devazepide, indi-

* The research was supported by USPHS Grants MH-41440 and MH-00378 to RYW. CRA was supported by NRSA MH-09791.

[1] Department of Psychiatry and Behavioral Science State University of New York at Stony Brook Putnam Hall, South Campus Stony Brook, NY 11794-8790, USA.

G. Adler and C. Beglinger (Eds.)
CCK Antagonists in Gastroenterology

cate that CCK_A receptors are located predominantly in the periphery, although CCK_A receptors are found in discrete brain regions such as the medial nucleus tractus solitarius, interpeduncular nucleus, area postrema, and anterior nucleus accumbens [32,46]. In contrast, CCK_B receptors display no or only a 10-fold difference in affinity for CCK_{8S}, CCK_{8US} and CCK_4 [36]. The highest concentrations of CCK_B receptors are found in the brain in discrete areas such as the cerebral cortex, nucleus accumbens, amygdala, hippocampus and olfactory bulbs [31]. The brain CCK_B receptors more closely resemble gastrin receptors than pancreatic CCK_A receptors. Studies in peripheral tissues indicate that CCK_A receptors are positively coupled to phosphoinositide hydrolysis [26]. However, the second messenger system coupled to CCK_B receptors remains to be elucidated, although it has been suggested that CCK_B receptors may be linked to adenylate cyclase via an inhibitory G protein [65]. Wennogle et al. [71] have reported that central CCK receptors may be linked to nucleotide regulatory proteins. However, the isolation and reconstitution of the appropriate components must be achieved to support the linkage of CCK receptors to nucleotide regulatory proteins.

CCK_A Receptor Agonists and Antagonists

The first CCK antagonist to be developed was dibutyryl cyclic guanosine monophosphate (cGMP) [53], which competitively antagonized CCK-induced secretion from guinea pig pancreatic acini, However, this compound is a relatively weak CCK antagonist, with an IC_{50} value of 100 μM to inhibit the binding of ^{125}I-labeled CCK to pancreatic acini [2]. Proglumide, a glutaramic acid derivative, and benzotript, a derivative of tryptophan, inhibited CCK binding in rat pancreatic acini, but both were slightly less potent than dibutyrl cGMP [27,29]. Makovec et al. [43] reported the synthesis of lorglumide (CR-1409), a 4-benzamido-*N*, *N*-dialkyl-glutaramic acid derivative, which was three to four orders of magnitude more potent than proglumide in inhibiting the binding of ^{125}I-labeled CCK to rat pancreatic acini. Furthermore, this compound displayed low affinity for CCK_B receptors [75]. Chang et al. [8] reported the isolation of the compound asperlicin, a 5-phenyl-l-benzodiazepine derivative, from a strain of *Aspergillus iliaceus*, which demonstrated high affinity for CCK_A receptors [8]. This compound did not display partial agonists properties and had low affinity for CCK_B receptors [8]. However, this compound displayed poor bioavailability, thereby limiting its possible therapeutic effectiveness. This limitation was overcome by the development of devazepide (L-364 718), which displayed good bioavailability [7]. This compound also displayed a high affinity and selectivity for CCK_A receptors.

A recent study has reported the synthesis and characterization of a novel series of tetrapeptide derivatives that display agonistic action at CCK_A

receptors [62]. One derivative, A 71623, potently stimulates amylase secretion and this effect is blocked by the CCK_A receptor antagonist devazepide. Furthermore, this compound has a high selectivity for CCK_A compared to CCK_B receptors.

The Development of Compounds Selective for CCK_B/Gastrin Receptors

Over the last 4–5 years, a number of peptide and nonpeptide compounds have been developed based on the rationale that the presence of distinct binding sites for CCK in the brain and periphery indicates that it must adopt different biological conformations [57]. Subsequent chemical studies demonstrated that CCK_8 exists in folded conformations characterized by both N- and C-terminal turns. A series of derivatives, mimicking this folding, were synthesized, possessing a cyclized structure between the NH_2 group of D-Lys^{29} residue and the alpha-carboxyl group of (L or D) Asp^{26} or (L or D) Glu^{26} [9]. These derivatives display a 1000- to 2000-fold greater affinity for CCK_B than for CCK_A receptors. The combination of cyclization and the replacement of Met and Gly with *N*-isoleucine produces a compound that has a 4500-fold higher affinity for CCK_B receptors compared to CCK_A receptors [9]. The most selective CCK_B receptor compounds synthesized to date are cyclic CCK analogues of the C-terminal hepta- and hexapeptides of CCK in which position 28 and 31 have been replaced by lysine residues and whose side chains are connected by a succinic moiety [56]. Overall, cyclization and modification of the C-terminal of CCK_8 produces a conformation that is unfavorable for peripheral CCK_A receptors but can interact favorably with central CCK_B receptors. Although the compounds mentioned above display high affinity and selectivity for CCK_B receptors, their classification as agonists or antagonists is uncertain in most cases since only binding data was obtained. However, the stimulation of cell firing in hippocampal slices [3,4] by CCK_{8S}, which is mediated by CCK_B receptors, may serve as a useful bioassay. Thus, the compound BC 264, (retro-inverso bond at Nle-Gly and N-Me-Nle^{31}) is 50 times more potent than CCK_{8US} in stimulating the firing of rat CA hippocampal neurones [12]. Furthermore, the stereotaxic injection of BC 264 into the ventral tegmental area potentiates dopamine-induced hypolocomotion, which is possibly mediated by CCK_B receptors [10]. These results suggest that BC 264 is a potent and selective CCK_B receptor agonist.

Recently, two nonpeptide derivatives for CCK receptors have been synthesized. L-365260, a benzodiazepine derivative, displays a 100-fold higher affinity for cortical than for pancreatic receptors [22,42]. L-365260 has been characterized as a highly potent and selective antagonist for gastrin receptors, compared with CCK_A receptors [42]. Hughes et al. [35] have reported that two nonpeptide derivatives, PD 134308 and PD 135158, have a 1600- and 500-fold higher affinity for CCK_B receptors, respectively. The

Table 1. Selective CCK agonists and antagonists for CCK_A and CCK_B receptors

	CCK_A	CCK_B
Selective agonists	A 71378 [41] A 71623 [62]	BC 264 [12] CCK_{8US} [36] CCK_4 [36]
Selective antagonists	Lorglumide [43] Devazepide [7] L 365031 [32] A 64718 [48]	L 365260 [22] PD 134308 [35]

compound PD 134308 potently blocks the effect of CCK_{8S} on ventromedial hypothalamic neurons, an effect mediated by CCK_B receptor [35]. In addition to L-365260 and PD 134308, it has also been demonstrated that dipeptoid derivatives of CCK, particularly those containing an α-methyl-Trp moiety, exhibit a 500- to 2500-fold higher affinity for CCK_B than for CCK_A receptors; they are potentially selective CCK_B receptor antagonists [34]. The specific agonists and antagonists for CCK_A and CCK_B receptors are summarized in Table 1.

Species and Molecular Heterogeneity of Central CCK Receptors

Recent radioligand binding studies indicate that there are species differences regarding CCK receptors [20,61,73]. Furthermore, it has been shown that subtypes of CCK_B may be present in the guinea pig brain [20]. Durieux et al. [19] have reported that using $[^3H]$ Boc $(diNle_{28,31})$ CCK_{27-33}, two different sites were present in cortical tissue. These sites displayed differential sensitivity to sodium, had disparate K_D and B_{max} values and radioligand binding was altered differentially by CCK_8, CCK_4, and various CCK-related compounds at these sites. These findings may explain some of the biphasic behavioral response observed after microinjection of CCK_8 into the brain [11,74]. However, until the detection of specific genes or DNA sequences that code for these subtypes is demonstrated, the absolute acceptance of the presence of CCK subtypes in the brain should be viewed with caution.

CCK Receptors and Satiety

Gibbs et al. [28] first reported that exogenous CCK decreases food intake in rats. Subsequently, this finding has been extended to a large number of animal species including humans. In addition, CCK elicits the sequence of behavior that characterized the onset of postprandial satiety [63]. The inhibitory action of CCK on food intake could be mediated by its action on brain feeding centers [13] or by a peripheral action mediated by abdominal vagal afferents [64]. The discovery of selective antagonists has opened doors for further examining the respective roles of these receptor types in mediating CCK-induced satiety.

The selective CCK_A receptor antagonists lorglumide and devazepide [16,55,60], but not the CCK_B receptor antagonist L-365 260, dose dependently blocked or reversed CCK-induced inhibition of food intake. In addition, it has been shown that both devazepide [55,60] and L-365 260 [17] increase food intake and postpone the onset of satiety in satiated rats. L-365 260 was two orders of magnitude more potent than devazepide in preventing satiety [17]. These finding suggest that whereas CCK_B receptors are involved in mediating CCK receptor antagonists-induced food intake, CCK_A receptors are responsible for exogenous CCK-induced inhibition of feeding.

CCK and Dopamine Interactions

In 1980, using the technique of immunohistocytochemistry, it was shown that CCK coexists with dopamine (DA) in a subset of midbrain DA neurons primarily in the ventral tegmental area (VTA or A10), which projects to various limbic structures [33]. Since the DA hypothesis of schizophrenia postulates hyperactive DA neurotransmission as an etiological factor in schizophrenic symptomatology [44], the coexistence of CCK with DA suggests that CCK may have a role in pathophysiology of schizophrenia and in the therapeutic action of antipsychotic drugs. Accordingly, over the past decade, numerous studies have been conducted regarding the interaction of CCK and DA using electrophysiological, behavioral and biochemical approachesin in vitro and in vivo preparations in a variety of animals. Overall, ample evidence indicates that CCK and DA closely interacts at both presynaptic DA/CCK terminals and postsynaptic DA/CCK target neurons (see [69] for review). However, due to the lack of potent and selective CCK receptor antagonists, the results of the initial studies have proved somewhat mixed or inconclusive regarding the nature of the CCK-DA interaction (see [66,69] for review).

Recent studies, using more specific CCK antagonists, have aided in the interpretation of the CCK-DA interaction in the CNS. For example, Wang et al. [70] demonstrated that CCK receptors located in the nucleus accumbens resemble type A because the CCK receptor-mediated responses are highly sulfate dependent and blocked by selective CCK_A receptor antagonist lorglumide. Vickroy et al. [68] have reported that the increase in DA release from the rat nucleus accumbens is antagonized by the selective CCK_A antagonist A 65 186. Jiang et al. [38] have shown that the microinjection of lorglumide into the medial nucleus accumbens, but not in the caudate putamen or lateral nucleus accumbens, reverses the depolarization inactivation of A10 DA cells produced by the chronic administration of haloperidol in rats. Recently, it has been reported that the i.v. administration of CCK_A antagonist devazepide, but not the CCK_B antagonist L-365 260 (2 μg/kg), reverses the chronic haloperidol- and chronic clozapine-induced decrease in the number of spontaneously active A10 DA cells [45]. These results suggest that CCK receptors in the nucleus accumbens have an important role in mediating or maintaining the therapeutic action of antipsychotic drugs. In addition, it is suggested that CCK_A agonists may be effective antipsychotic agents.

CCK and CCK Analogues as Neuroleptics

Early studies with CCK and various analogues in the treatment of schizophrenia showed some positive results [47,49]. In contrast to the results obtained from open clinical trials, subsequent double-blind studies have shown largely negative results (see [69] for review). However, failure to observe a therapeutic effect for CCK_{8S} or cerulein could simply be due to insufficient amounts of these peptides passing the blood-brain barrier. Therefore, the development of enzyme-resistant, selective CCK receptor agonists that readily cross the blood-brain barrier may prove useful in determining the utility of CCK in the treatment of schizophrenia.

CCK and Anxiety

Currently, only a few studies have been published regarding CCK and its possible role in anxiety. Cerulein administration has an anxiogenic-like effect on the exploratory behavior of mice in the elevated plus-maze test [30]. Bradwejn and De Montigny [5,6] have shown that the CCK_{8S}-induced activation of hippocampal neurons is antagonized by the acute administration of benzodiazepines, which may be related to their anxiolytic action. Thus, it is predicted that CCK receptor antagonists may be effective anxiolytic agents. A recent report, using the CCK_B receptor antagonist PD 134 308, provides support for this concept [35]. The systemic administration of PD 134 308 (0.001–30 mg/kg) was effective in tests indicative of anxiolytic activity in rats, mice, and marmosets. This compound was also effective in preventing withdrawal anxiogenesis from chronic diazepam administration. Furthermore, PD 134 308 did not produce ataxia or sedation and there was no development of tolerance to its anxiolytic action. Although further studies with other CCK_B receptor antagonists must be conducted, these results suggest that CCK_B antagonists may be efficacious in the pharmacotherapy of anxiety.

Involvement of CCK in Analgesia

The systemic administration of CCK produces a biphasic effect of pain threshold in rodent. Whereas doses over 50 µg/kg elicit analgesia and sedation [1,32,39], lower doses (5–20 µg/kg) antagonize morphine and β-endorphin-induced analgesia [15,25,50]. It has been shown that CCK may antagonize the physiological effects of opiates [24,25]. Initial studies using the nonselective and weak CCK receptor antagonists proglumide and benzotript have shown that these compounds potentiate β-endorphin and morphine analgesia [40,52]. Currently, the mechanism of action by which CCK and CCK receptor antagonists modulate opiate-induced analgesia is unknown. However, it has been hypothesized that CCK and opiates may interact with neurons in the spinal cord and periaqueductal gray area, as both are known to be involved in the transmission of nociceptive stimuli [1]. In addition, both contain a high concentration of opioid peptides and CCK as well as a high density of CCK and opioid receptors.

The development of selective CCK receptor antagonists has allowed for the characterization of the CCK receptor subtypes involved in the mediation of CCK's action on opioid-induced analgesia. Hill and Woodruff [31] have shown that the primate and rat spinal cord primarily contain CCK_A and CCK_B receptors, respectively. Consistent with this finding, it has been reported that L-365 260 enhances morphine analgesia and blocks tolerance to morphine after systemic administration in rodents [18] and this compound is 5 and 40 times more potent than the CCK_A receptor antagonists devazepide and L-365 031, respectively, in potentiating morphine analgesia. Like L-365 260, PD 134 308 has also been shown to significantly potentiate the antinocipeptive effect of morphine as well as its depressive effect on the flexor reflex in the rat [72]. However, in the squirrel monkey, the systemic administration of either the CCK_B receptor antagonist L-365 260 or the CCK_A receptor antagonist devazepide potentiates morphine-induced analgesia [51]. Thus, the sites and mechanisms of CCK receptor-mediated effect on opioid annalgesia remain to be elucidated. Again, the development of selective CCK_A and CCK_B agonists that penetrate the blood-brain barrier would prove useful in the further elucidation of the role of CCK_A and CCK_B receptors in opioid-induced analgesia.

Conclusions

In conclusion, since the detection of CCK in the CNS, numerous reports have been published regarding the pharmacology and physiology of CCK receptors. At the present time, data from animal studies suggest that CCK receptor antagonists might prove useful in the pharmacotherapy of pain, appetite, and anxiety disorders. However, in order to substantiate this claim, data from double-blind, placebo-controlled trials in humans must be obtained. Although the role of CCK in the symptomatology of schizophrenia remains to be elucidated, initial studies in rats suggest that CCK_A receptor agonists may prove potentially useful in treating schizophrenia. At any rate, the development of enzyme-resistant agonists that cross the blood-brain barrier and are CCK receptor subtype selective would further facilitate research in this area. Without any doubt, CCK may mediate additional physiological processes in the CNS and ongoing studies may yield new and exciting information.

Acknowledgement. We thank Joyce Shepherd for the manuscript preparation.

References

1. Baber NS, Dourish CT, Hill DR (1989) The role of CCK caerulein, and CCK antagonists in nociception. Pain 39:307–328
2. Barlas N, Jensen RI, Beinfeld MC, Gardner JD (1982) Cyclic nucleotide antagonists of the cholecystokinin: structural requirements for interaction with the cholecystokinin receptor. Am J Physiol 242:G161–G167
3. Bohme GA, Stutzmann JM, Blanchard JC (1988) Excitatory effects of cholecystokinin in rat hippocampus: pharmacological response compatible with central or B-type receptors. Brain Res 451:309–318
4. Bohme GA, Durieux C, Stutzmann JM, Charpentier B, Rogues BP, Blanchard JC (1989) Electrophysiological studies with new CCK-analogs: correlation with binding affinity of B-type receptors. Peptides 10:407–414
5. Bradwejn J, DeMontigny C (1984) Benzodiazepines antagonize cholecystokinin-induced activation of rat hippocampal neurons. Nature 312:363–364
6. Bradwejn J, DeMontigny C (1985) Effects of PK 8165, a partial benzodiazepine receptor agonist on cholecystokinin-induced activation of hippocampal pyramidal neurons: a microiontophoretic study in the rat. Eur J Pharmacol 112: 415–417
7. Chang RSL, Lotti VJ (1986) Biochemical and pharmacological characterization of an extremely potent and selective nonpeptide cholecystokinin antagonist, Proc Natl Acad Sci USA 83:4923–4926
8. Chang RSL, Lotti VJ, Monaghan RL, Birnbaum J, Stapley EO, Goetz MA, Albers-Schonberg G, Patchett AA, Liesch JM, Hensens OD, Springer VJ (1985) A potent nonpeptide cholecystokinin antagonist selective of peripheral tissues isolated from *Aspergillus alliaceus*. Science 230:177–179
9. Charpentier B, Dor A, Roy P, England P, Pham H, Durieux C, Roques BP (1989) Synthesis and binding affinities of cyclic and related linear analogues of CCK_8 selective for central receptors. J Med Chem 32:1184–1190
10. Crawley JN (1989) Microinjection of cholecystokinin into the rat ventral tegmental area potentiates dopamine-induced hypolocomotion. Synapse 3:346–355
11. Crawley JN, Hommer DW, Skirboll LR (1984) Behavioral and neurophysiological evidence for a facilitatory interaction between co-existing transmitters: cholecystokinin and dopamine. Neurochem Int 6:755–760
12. Dauge V, Bohme GA, Crawley JN, Durieux C, Stutzmann JM, Feger J, Blanchard JC, Roques BP (1990) Investigation of behavioral and electrophysiological response induced by selective stimulation of CCK B receptors by using a new highly potent CCK analog, BC 264, Synapse 6:73–80
13. Della-Fera MA, Baile CA (1979) Cholecystokinin octapeptide: continuous picomole injections into the cerebral ventricles suppress feeding. Science 206: 471–473

14. Dockray GJ(1976) Immunohistochemical evidence of cholecystokinin-like peptides in the brain. Nature 264:568–570
15. Dourish CT, Coughlan J, Hawley D, Clark ML, Iversen SD (1988) Blockade of CCK-induced hypophagia and prevention of morphine tolerance by the CCK antagonist L-364718. In: Wang RY, Schoenfeld R (eds) Cholecystokinin antagonists. Liss, New York, pp 307–325
16. Dourish CT, Ruckert AC, Tattersall FD, Iversen SD (1989a) Evidence that decreased feeding induced by systemic injection of cholecystokinin is mediated by CCK-A receptors. Eur J Pharmacol 173:233–234
17. Dourish CT, Rycroft W, Iversen SD (1989b) Postponement of satiety by blockade of brain cholecytokinin (CCK_B) receptors. Science 245:1509–1511
18. Dourish CT, O'Neill MF, Coughlan J, Kitchener SJ, Hawley D, Iversen SD (1990) The selective CCK-B receptor antagonist L-365260 enhances morphine analgesia and prevents morphine tolerance in the rat. Eur J Pharmacol 176: 35–44
19. Durieux C, Coppey M, Zajac JM, Rogues BP (1986) Occurrence of two cholecystokinin binding sites in guinea pig brain cortex. Biochem Biophys Res Commun 137:1167–1173
20. Durieux C, Pham H, Charpentier B, Roques BP (1988) Discrimination between CCK receptors of guinea-pig and rat brain by cyclic CCK8 analogues. Biochem Biophys Res Commun 154:1301–1307
21. Eberlein GA, Eysselein JR, Hesse WH, Goebell H, Schaefer M, Reeve JR (1987) Detection of cholecystokinin-58 in human blood by inhibition of degradation. Am J Physiol 253:G477–G482
22. Evans BE, Bock MG, Rittle KE, Dipardo RM, Whitter WL, Veber DF, Anderson PS, Freidinger RM (1986) Design of potent, orally effective, nonpeptidal antagonists of the peptide hormone cholecystokinin. Proc Acad Natl Sci USA 83:4918–4922
23. Eysselein VE, Eberlein GA, Hesse WH, Singer MV, Goebell H, Reeve JR (1987) Cholecystokinin-58 is the major circulating form of cholecystokinin in canine blood. J Biol Chem 262:214–217
24. Faris PL (1985) Opiate antagonistic function of cholecystokinin in analgesia and energy balance systems. Ann NY Acad Sci 448:437–447
25. Faris PL, Komisarau BR, Watkins LR, Mayer DJ (1983) Evidence for neuropeptide cholecystokinin as an antagonist of opioid analgesia. Science 219:310–312
26. Florholmen J, Malm D, Vonen B, Burhol PG (1989) Effect of cholecystokinin on the accumulation of inositol phosphates in isolated pancreatic islets. Am J Physiol 257:G865–G870
27. Gardner JD, Jensen RT (1984) Cholecystokinin receptor antagonists. Am J Physiol 246:G471–G476
28. Gibbs J, Young RC, Smith GP (1973) Cholecystokinin decreases food intake in rats. J Comp Physiol Psychol 84:488–495
29. Hahne WF, Jensen RT, Lemp GF, Gardner JD (1981) Proglumide and benzotript: members of a different class of cholecystokinin receptor antagonists. Proc Natl Acad Sci USA 78:6304–6308
30. Harro J, Lang A, Vasar E (1990) Long term diazepam treatment produces changes in cholecystokinin receptor binding in rat brain. Eur J Pharmacol 180: 77–83
31. Hill DR, Woodruff GN (1990) Differentiation of central cholecystokinin receptor binding sites using the non-peptide antagonists MK-329 and L-365260. Brain Res 526:276–283
32. Hill DR, Campbell NJ, Shaw TM, Woodruff GN (1987) Autoradiographic localization and biochemical characterization of peripheral type CCK receptors in the rat CNS using highly selective non-peptide CCK antagonists. J Neurosci 7:2967–2976

33. Hokfelt T, Skirboll L, Rehfeld JF, Goldstein M, Markey K, Danno O (1980) A subpopulation of mesencephalic dopamine neurons projecting to limbic areas contains a cholecystokinin-like peptide: evidence from immunohistochemistry combined with retrograde tracing. Neurosci 5:2093–2124
34. Horwell DC, Hughes J, Hunter JC, Pritchard MC, Richardson RS, Roberts E, Woodruff GN (1991) Rationally designed "dipeptoid" analogues of CCK α-methyltryptophan derivatives as highly selective and orally active gastrin and CCK_B antagonists with potent anxiolytic properties. J Med Chem 34:404–419
35. Hughes J, Boden P, Costall B, Domeney A, Kelly E, Horwell DC, Hunter JC, Pinnock RD, Woodruff GN (1990) Development of a class of selective cholecystokinin type B receptor antagonists having potent anxiolytic activity. Proc Natl Acad Sci USA 87:6728–6732
36. Innis RB, Snyder S (1980) Distinct cholecystokinin receptors in brain and pancreas. Proc Natl Acad Sci USA 77:6917–6921
37. Ivy AC, Oldberg E (1928) A hormone mechanism for gallbladder contraction and evacuation. Amer J Physiol 86:599–613
38. Jiang LH, Kasser RJ, Wang RY (1988) Cholecystokinin antagonist lorglumide reverses chronic haloperidol-induced effects on doamine neurons. Brain Res 473:165–168
39. Jurna I, Zetler G (1981) Antinociceptive effect of centrally administered caerulein and cholecystokinin (CCK). Eur J Pharm 73:323–331
40. Katsuura G, Itoh S (1985) Potentiation of β-endorphin effects by proglumide in rats. Eur J Pharmacol 107:363–366
41. Lin CW, Hollaway MW, Witte DG, Miller TR, Wolfram CAW, Bianchi BR, Bennett MJ, Nadzan AM (1990) A71378: a CCK agonist with high potency and selectivity for CCK-A receptors. Am J Physiol 258:G648–G651
42. Lotti VJ, Chang RSL (1989) A new potent and selective non-peptide gastrin antagonist and brain CCK receptor (CCK-B) ligand: L-365260. Eur J Pharmacol 162:273–280
43. Makovec FR, Christe M, Bani MA, Pacini I, Setnikar I, Rovati LA (1985) New glutaramic acid derivatives with competitive and specific cholecystokinin-antagonist activity. Arzneirnttelforschung 35:1048–1051
44. Matthysse S (1973) Antipsychotic drug actions: a clue to the neuropathology of schizophrenia. Fed Proc 32:200–205
45. Minabe Y, Ashby CR Jr, Wang RY (1991) The systemic administration of the CCK_A receptor antagonist devazepide but not the CCK_B receptor antagonists L-365260 reverses the effects of chronic haloperidol and clozapine on midbrain dopamine neurons in the rat. Brain Res 549:151–154
46. Moran TH, Robinson PH, Goldrich MS, McHugh PR (1986) Two brain cholecystokinin receptors: implications for behavioral actions. Brain Res 362: 175–179
47. Moroji T, Watanaben, Aoki N, Itoh S (1982) Antipsychotic effect of caerulein, a decapeptide chemically related to cholecystokinin octapeptide, on schizophrenia. Int Pharmacopsychiat 17:255–273
48. Nadzan AM, Kerwin JF Jr, Kopecka H, Lin CW, Miller T, Witte D, Burt S (1988) Structural and functional relationships among CCK antagonists. In: Wang RY, Schoenfeld R (eds) Cholecystokinin antagonists. Liss, New York, pp 93–103
49. Nair NPV, Bloom DM, Nestoros JN (1982) Cholecystokinin appear to have antipsychotic properties. Prog Neuropsychopharmacol Biol Psychiat 6:509–512
50. O'Neill MF, Dourish CT, Iverson SD (1989) Morphine-induced analgesia in the rat paw pressure test is attenuated by CCK and enhanced by the CCK antagonist MK 329. Neuropharmacol 28:243–247
51. O'Neill MF, Dourish CT, Tye SJ, Iversen SD (1990) Blockade of CCK-B receptors by L-365260 induces analgesia in the squirrel monkey. Brain Res 534:287–290

52. Panerai AE, Rouati LC, Cocco E, Sacerdot P, Mantegazza P (1987) Dissociation of tolerance and dependence to morphine: a possible role for cholecystokinin. Brain Res 410:52–60
53. Peikin SR, Costenbader CL, Gardner JD (1979) Action of derivatives of cyclic nucleotides on dispersed acini from guinea pig pancreas. Discovery of a competitive antagonist of the action of cholecystokinin. J Biol Chem 254:321–327
54. Rehfeld JF (1978) Immunochemical studies on cholecystokinin. II. Distribution and molecular heterogeneity in the central nervous system. J Biol Chem 253: 4022–4030
55. Reidelberger RD, O'Rouke MF (1989) Potent cholecystokinin antagonist L-364 718 stimulated food intake in rats. Am J Physiol 257:R1512–R1518
56. Rodriguez M, Amblard M, Galas MC, Lignon MF, Aumelas A, Martinez J (1990) Synthesis of cyclic analogues of cholecystokinin highly selective for central receptors. Int Peptide Protein Res 35:441–451
57. Roques BP, Charpentier B, Marseigne I, Durieux C, Fournie-Zaluski MC, Dauge V, Feger J, Bohme A, Stutzman JM, Blanchard JC (1989) Development of selective CCK-related compounds as probes for biochemical and pharmacological characterization of CCK binding site heterogeneity. In: Hughes J, Dockray G, Woodruff G (eds) The neuropeptide cholecystokinin (CCK). Horwood, Chichester, pp 133–142
58. Saito AH, Sankaran H, Goldfine ID, Williams JA (1980) Cholecystokinin receptors in the brain: characterization and distribution. Science 208:1155–1156
59. Sakamoto C, Williams JA, Goldfine ID (1984) Brain CCK receptors are structurally distinct from pancreas CCK receptors. Biochem Biophys Res Comm 124:497–502
60. Schneider LH, Murphy RB, Gibbs J, Smith GP (1988) Comparative potencies of CCK antagonists for the reversal of the satiating effect of cholecystokinin. In: Wang RY, Schoenfeld R (eds) Cholecystokinin antagonists. Liss, New York, pp 263–284
61. Sekiguchi R, Moroji T (1986) A comparative study on characterizaton and distribution of cholecystokinin binding sites among the rat, mouse and guinea-pig brain. Brain Res 399:271–281
62. Shiosaki K, Lin CW, Kopecka H, Craig R, Wagenaar FL, Bianchi B, Miller T, Witte D, Nadzan AM (1990) Development of CCK-tetrapeptide analogues as potent and selective CCK-A receptor agonists. J Med Chem 33:2950–2952
63. Smith GP, Gibbs J (1985) The satiety effect of cholecystokinin: recent progress and current problems. Ann NY Acad Sci 448:417–423
64. Smith GP, Jerome C, Cushin BJ, Eterno R, Simansky KJ (1981) Abdominal vagotomy blocks the satiety effect of cholecystokinin in the rat. Science 213: 1036–1037
65. Studler JM, Reibaud M, Herve D, Blanc J, Glowinski J, Tassin JP (1986) Opposite effects of sulfated cholecystokinin on DA-sensitive adenylate cyclase in two areas of the rat nucleus accumbens. Eur J Pharmacol 126:125–128
66. Vanderhaeghen JJ, Crawley JN (eds) (1985) Neuronal cholecystokinin. The New York Academy of Sciences, New York
67. Vanderhaeghen JJ, Signeau JC, Gepts W (1975) New peptides in vertebrate CNS reacting with antigastrin antibodies. Nature 257:604–605
68. Vickroy TW, Bianchi BR (1989) Pharmacological and mechanistic studies of cholecystokinin-facilitated ^{3}H-dopamine efflux from rat nucleus accumbens. Neuropeptide 13:43–50
69. Wang RY (1988) Cholecystokinin, dopamine and schizophrenia: recent progress and current problems. Ann NY Acad Sci 537:362–379
70. Wang RY, Kasser RJ, Hu XT (1988) Cholecystokinin receptor subtypes in the rat nucleus accumbens. In: Wang RY, Schoenfeld R (eds) Cholecystokinin antagonists. Liss, New York, pp 199–216

71. Wennogle LP, Wysowkyj H, Steel DJ, Petrack B (1988) Regulation of central cholecystokinin by guanyl nucleotides. J Neurochem 50:954–959
72. Wiesenfeld-Hallin Z, Xu XJ, Hughes J, Horwell DC, Hokfelt T (1990) PD 134308, a selective antagonist of cholecystokinin type B receptor, enhances the analgesic effect of morphine and synergistically interacts with intrathecal galanin to depress spinal nociceptive reflexes. Proc Natl Acad Sci USA 87:7105–7109
73. Williams JA, Gryson KA, McChesney DJ (1986) Brain CCK receptors: species differences in regional distribution and selectivity. Peptides 7:293–296
74. Worms PJ, Martinez C, Briet B, Castro B, Biziere K (1986) Evidence for a dopaminomimetic effect of intrastriatally injected cholecystokinin in mice. Eur J Pharmacol 121:395–401
75. Yasuhiko I, Ritsuko Y, Takeshi K (1987) CR 1409: a potent inhibitor of cholecystokinin-stimulated amylase release and cholecystokinin binding in rat pancreatic acini. Pancreas 12:85–90

Vagally Mediated Actions of CCK

G.J. Dockray[1]

Introduction

The possibility that the vagus nerve might mediate some of the actions of CCK was first suggested by Smith et al. [27]. They showed that the inhibition of food intake by i.p. CCK was reduced in rats after selective lesioning of the gastric branches of the vagus. There are three possible mechanisms that might account for these findings: first, CCK might act directly on vagal afferents; second, it might act indirectly via changes in smooth muscle tone or some other variable that influences afferent discharge; third, it could act by a mechanism that requires a passive input provided by the intact vagus. These possibilities are by no means mutually exclusive; there is now, however, a compelling body of evidence to support the first possibility, namely that CCK exerts direct actions on vagal afferents. This mechanism probably accounts for the satiety effect exerted by i.p. CCK, but it is also likely to be physiologically important in mediating the action of CCK on inhibition of gastric emptying [3,4]. The relevant evidence will be reviewed here, together with the significance of this pathway for the physiology of circulating CCK.

The Evidence that CCK Acts on Vagal Fibres

Two types of experimental approach (autoradiography and electrophysiology) have provided evidence for the idea that CCK acts on the vagus. Zarbin et al. [31] first showed that following ligation of the cervical vagus in the rat there is an accumulation of CCK binding sites on the central side of the ligature. This indicates that CCK binding sites are transported down the vagus towards the periphery. Moran et al. [18] subsequently showed that this pathway could be traced to sub-diaphragmatic vagal fibres including those that serve the stomach. They also made the important observation that these sites had a specificity resembling that of the pancreatic or gall

[1] MRC Secretory Control Research Group, Department of Physiology, University of Liverpool, Liverpool, UK.

G. Adler and C. Beglinger (Eds.)
CCK Antagonists in Gastroenterology

bladder type of receptor (CCK-A) and distinct from the major CNS receptor type (CCK-B). It seems likely that afferent neurons with their cell bodies in the nodose ganglia synthesize CCK-A-type receptors that are then transported intra-axonally to both peripheral and central terminals. The central terminals of the afferents are found in the nucleus tractus solitarius (NTS) and numerous CCK-A receptors have been localized here by autoradiography [10]. At present the function of the NTS receptors is unclear. There is, however, clear electrophysiological evidence to suggest that CCK acts at the peripheral terminals of vagal afferents.

In order to examine the possible mechanisms by which circulating CCK might influence neuronal activity in the dorsomedial medulla, Raybould et al. [21] made recordings of extracellular unit activity in NTS and related structures in urethane-anaesthetized rats. It was found that neurons in the dorsomedial medulla that responded to passive gastric distension also responded to i.v. injections of CCK. These cells are therefore on the pathway by which signals of gastric volume are transmitted to the brain. Two types of response occurred: about 60% of the cells identified were excited by gastric distension and 40% were inhibited. The responses to CCK were always in the same direction as those to gastric distension. This observation suggests that CCK and gastric distension might be activating a common pathway. The site of action of CCK was localized to the splanchnic bed, because close-arterial injections of CCK to the coeliac artery produced the same responses as intravenous injection of CCK, except that the range of doses required for an effect was approximately 100 times lower. It was thought unlikely that CCK acted via changes in gastric motility, because the motility response to CCK is a fall in intragastric pressure (which is itself probably a consequence of activation of vago-vagal reflexes; see below), whereas passive distension of the stomach produced an increase in intragastric pressure. The responses to both CCK and gastric distension were blocked by vagotomy, but not by coeliac ganglionectomy, or by antrectomy [23]. The conclusions drawn from recording dorsomedial medullary neuron discharges have subsequently been confirmed by recordings from single vagal fibres [1]. Thus, in the rat, CCK and gastric distension appear to excite a single population of vagal afferent fibres. There are no primary afferent fibres that are inhibited by CCK, so that the medullary neurons that are depressed by CCK and gastric distension are presumably at least one inhibitory synapse downstream of the first order interneurone.

Vagally Dependent Actions of CCK

The original finding of Smith et al. [27] that the satiety effect of i.p. CCK was blocked by gastric vagotomy has been confirmed several times [16,19], and has been extended by showing that intact vagal afferent rather than efferent fibres are required for the action of CCK [28]. In addition, a number of other central effects evoked by exogenous CCK and related peptides have been reported to be abolished by vagotomy. These include enhancement of memory retention in mice, release of prolactin, release of oxytocin, inhibition of somatic reflexes, stimulation of dopaminergic neurons and release of dopamine in rats [5,9,11–13,25]. At least some of these actions can also be produced by passive gastric distension, e.g. inhibition of food intake and stimulation of oxytocin neurons [25].

It has been recognized for many years that stimulation of gastric mechanoreceptors by gastric distension activates vago-vagal reflexes. Two reflex responses are well known; one is the inhibition of gastric motility that occurs following gastric distension; this is the basis for the receptive relaxation which occurs early in digestion. The other is the stimulation of gastric acid secretion. If CCK and gastric distension activate a common afferent pathway one might anticipate that CCK would reproduce these reflexes. It has been difficult to determine whether CCK influences acid secretion by this route, since it plainly influences acid secretion at several other sites, e.g. direct stimulation of parietal cells, but also inhibition via release of somatostatin, and more work will be needed to discriminate between the possible mechanisms of action in intact animals. There is now, however, good evidence that CCK works via the vagus to modify gastric motility. Injection of CCK in anaesthetized rats produces a prompt relaxation of the body of the stomach [22]. In part the effects seen in the anaesthetized rat can be attributed to release of noradrenaline, but more importantly these effects are also strongly inhibited by vagotomy. The importance of vagal afferents for this and other vagally mediated actions of CCK is demonstrated by the fact that local application to the vagus of the sensory neurotoxin capsaicin inhibits the effect of CCK [17,20,29]. It is worth noting that the action of CCK on gastric motility in vivo is different to that in vitro. CCK is a direct stimulant of gastric smooth muscle in vitro; the relaxation in vivo presumably reflects the fact that the reflex inhibition mentioned above overrides the direct excitatory effects.

Physiological Role of Vagal CCK Receptors

The primary physiological role of circulating CCK can be considered as the integration of upper gastrointestinal function to regulate protein and fat digestion in the small intestine. On the one hand this is achieved by stimulation (mostly by direct action) of pancreatic secretion and gall bladder contraction and on the other hand by inhibition of gastric emptying and of food intake. In this way CCK acts to ensure that the delivery of pancreatic enzymes and bile salts to the small intestine is matched to the delivery of nutrients from the stomach. There is now good evidence from the use of CCK antagonists that in at least some circumstances, the satiety effect is a physiological one [24]. Similarly, the use of CCK antagonists has extended the findings from several other experimental approaches which indicate that regulation of gastric emptying by CCK is a physiological effect [2,8,14,15]. There are several factors that regulate rates of gastric emptying, i.e. changes in pressure in the body of the stomach and duodenum and resistance to flow across the pylorus, and there is evidence that CCK influences each of them [7,26,30]. The vagally mediated effects of CCK are probably only of relevance for control of pressure in the body of the stomach. In the present context it is therefore relevant to ask what importance can be attached to the latter component of the action of CCK, and whether CCK released from gut endocrine cells (as opposed say to CNS or peripheral neurons) is capable of influencing gastric emptying by this route.

Protein and the protease inhibitor FOY-305 (which acts as a specific releaser of CCK from intestinal endocrine cells) inhibit gastric emptying in the rat by mechanisms sensitive to the CCK-A antagonist L-364 718, and both require access to at least the distal duodenum in order to exert these effects [7,8]. This provides direct evidence, then, that CCK released from intestinal endocrine cells controls gastric emptying. The effects of both peptone and FOY-305 are inhibited by previous treatment of rats with capsaicin which lesions small diameter afferents, supporting the idea that CCK activates a visceral reflex. The possibility that CCK acts locally in the small intestine on afferent terminals (vagal or splanchnic) in the immediate vicinity of the CCK cell can be excluded: both vagal and splanchnic afferents serving the small intestine pass though the coeliac ganglion, and removal of the coeliac ganglion does not impair the action of CCK-releasing meals on gastric emptying. Coeliac ganglionectomy does, however, impair the action of hyperosmolal solutions in delaying gastric emptying, indicating that different meal types regulate upper gastrointestinal tract motility in different ways. Pyloroplasty does not change the rate of emptying of CCK-releasing solutions so that the pylorus is not an important target for CCK in this context. As a whole then, these data support the idea that CCK controls gastric emptying by a vagal reflex that regulates pressure in the body of the stomach. There are two possible efferent mechanisms by which CCK-evoked reflexes might control pressure in the body of the stomach. First, reflex inhibition of a tonically active cholinergic excitatory pathway (the preganglionic cell could correspond to the population of medullary neurons inhibited by gastric distension), and second, by stimulation of a vagal efferent inhibitory pathway. The final transmitter involved in the latter case is probably vasoactive intestinal polypeptide (VIP), since it has been shown recently that VIP antibodies depress the effect of peptone in inhibiting gastric emptying in the rat [6].

Overview

The evidence reviewed above supports the idea that CCK is able to act on vagal gastric afferents to exert a number of effects. At least two, inhibition of gastric emptying and of food intake, appear to be physiologically

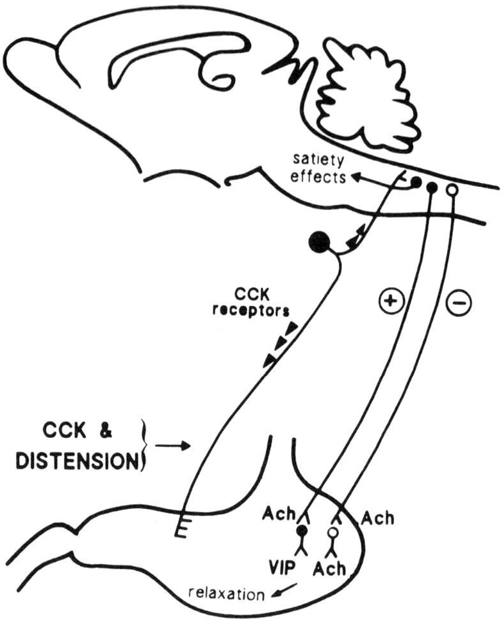

Fig. 1. Schematic representation of the action of CCK on vagal afferents. CCK-A-type receptors on gastric vagal mechanoreceptor afferents are proposed to stimulate afferent discharge with at least two consequences of potential physiological importance: inhibition of food intake, and inhibition of gastric motility leading to delayed gastric emptying. The latter effect may be a consequence of reflex inhibition, (⊖) of tonically active cholinergic excitatory pathways, and reflex stimulation (⊕) of a VIP-mediated inhibition of gastric motility. *Ach*, acetylcholine; *VIP*, vasoactive intestinal polypeptide

important. The particular importance of this site of action lies in the fact that it allows integration of at least two visceral signals namely the presence of nutrient in small intestine (represented by plasma CCK) and the volume of gastric contents (represented by intragastric pressure), with CNS and other autonomic information (Fig. 1). Thus, by acting on the vagus, CCK can be seen as part of the mechanism by which information on nutrient status in the lumen of the small intestine is conveyed to the brain in order to modulate both behaviour and the autonomic control of the digestive tract. In the future it will be worthwhile examining the possibility (a) that other gut peptides act by similar mechanisms, and (b) that the vago-vagal actions of CCK influence other gastrointestinal functions.

Acknowledgement. The help of Christine Carter in preparing this manuscript is gratefully acknowledged.

References

1. Davison JS, Clark GD (1988) Mechanical properties and sensitivity to CCK of vagal gastric slowly adapting mechanoreceptors. Am J Physiol 255:G55–G61
2. Debas HT, Farooq O, Grossman MI (1975) Inhibition of gastric emptying is a physiological action of cholecystokinin. Gastroenterology 68:1211–1217
3. Dockray GJ (1989) The integrative functions of CCK in the upper gastrointestinal tract. In: Hughes J, Dockray G, Woodruff G (eds) The neuropeptide cholecystokinin (CCK). Horwood, Chichester, pp 232–239
4. Dockray GJ (1990) Neuronal actions of cholecystokinin. In: Thompson JC (eds) Gastrointestinal endocrinology: receptors and post-receptor mechanisms. Academic, San Diego, pp 321–332
5. Flood JF, Smith GE, Morley JE (1987) Modulation of memory processing by cholecystokinin: dependence on vagus nerve. Science 236:832–834
6. Forster ER (1990) The role of vasoactive intestinal polypeptide in the control of gastric emptying in the rat. J Physiol (Lond) 424:12P
7. Forster ER, Green T, Elliot M, Bremner A, Dockray GJ (1990) Gastric emptying in rats: role of afferent neurons and cholecystokinin. Am J Physiol 258: G552–G556
8. Green T, Dimaline R, Peikin S, Dockray GJ (1988) Action of the cholecystokinin antagonist L-364718 on gastric emptying in the rat. Am J Physiol 255:G685–G689
9. Hamamura T, Kazahaya, Otsuki S (1989) Ceruletide suppresses endogenous dopamine release via vagal afferent system, studied by in vivo intracerebral dialysis. Brain Res 483:78–83
10. Hill DR, Campbell NJ, Shaw TM, Woodruff GN (1987) Autoradiographic localization and biochemical characterization of peripheral type CCK receptors in rat CNS using highly selective nonpeptide CCK antagonists. J Neurosci 7:2967–2976
11. Hodson CA, Burden HW, Lawrence IE Jr (1986) Intraperitoneal cholecystokinin administration inhibits prolactin release: an effect prevented by vagotomy. IRCS Med Sci 14:551
12. Hommer DW, Palkovits M, Crawley JN, Paul SM, Skirbol LR (1985) Cholecystokinin-induced excitation in the substantia nigra: evidence for peripheral and central components. J Neurosci 5:1387–1392
13. Kawasaki K, Kodama M, Matsushita A (1983) Caerulein, a cholecystokinin-related peptide, depresses somatic function via the vagal afferent system. Life Sci 33:1045–1050
14. Kleibeuker JH, Beekhuis H, Jansen JBMJ, Piers DA, Lamer CBHW (1988) Cholecystokinin is a physiological hormonal mediator of fat-induced inhibition of gastric emptying in man. Eur J Clin Invest 18:173–177
15. Liddle RA, Morita ET, Conrad CK, Williams JA (1986) Regulation of gastric emptying in humans by cholecystokinin. J Clin Invest 77:992–996
16. Lorenz DN, Goldman SA (1982) Vagal mediation of the cholecystokinin satiety effect in rats. Physiol Behav 29:599–604
17. McCann MJ, Verbalis JG, Stricker EM (1988) Capsaicin-treatment attenuates multiple responses to cholecystokinin in rats. J Auton Nerv Syst 23:265–272
18. Moran TH, Smith GP, Hostetler AM, McHugh PR (1987) Transport of cholecystokinin (CCK) binding sites in subdiaphragmatic vagal branches. Brain Res 415:149–152
19. Morley JE, Levine AS, Kneip J, Grace M (1982) The effect of vagotomy on the satiety effects of neuropeptides and nalaxone. Life Sci 30:1943–1947
20. Raybould HE, Tache Y (1988) Cholecystokinin inhibits gastric motility and emptying via a capsaicin-sensitive vagal pathway in rats. Am J Physiol 255: G242–G246

21. Raybould HE, Gayton RJ, Dockray GJ (1985) CNS effects of circulating CCK-8: involvement of brainstem neurones responding to gastric distension. Brain Res 342:187–190
22. Raybould HE, Roberts ME, Dockray GJ (1987) Reflex decreases in intragastric pressure in response to cholecystokinin in rats. Am J Physiol 253:G165–G170
23. Raybould HE, Gayton RJ, Dockray GJ (1988) Mechanisms of action of peripherally administered cholecystokinin octapeptide on brain stem neurons in the rat. J Neurosci 8:3018–3024
24. Reidelberger RD, O'Rourke MF (1989) Potent cholecystokinin antagonist L-364718 stimulates food intake in rats. Am J Physiol 257:R1512–R1518
25. Renaud LP, Tang M, McCann MJ, Stricker EM, Verbalis JG (1987) Cholecystokinin and gastric distension activate oxytocinergic cells in rat hypothalamus. Am J Physiol 253:R661–R665
26. Shillabeer G, Davison JS (1987) Proglumide, a cholecystokinin antagonist, increases gastric emptying in rats. Am J Physiol 252:R353–R360
27. Smith GP, Jerome C, Cushin BJ, Eterno R, Simansky KJ (1981) Abdominal vagotomy blocks the satiety effect of cholecystokinin in the rat. Science 213:1036–1037
28. Smith GP, Jerome C, Norgren R (1985) Afferent axons in abdominal vagus mediate satiety effect of cholecystokinin in rats. Am J Physiol 249:R638–R641
29. South E, Ritter RC (1988) Capsaicin application to central or peripheral vagal fibres attenuates CCK satiety. Peptides 9:601–612
30. Yamagishi T, Debas HT (1978) Cholecystokinin inhibits gastric emptying by acting on both proximal stomach and pylorus. Am J Physiol 234:E375–E378
31. Zarbin MA, Wamsley JK, Innis RB, Kuhar MJ (1981) Cholecystokinin receptors: presence and axonal flow in the rat vagus nerve. Life Sci 29:697–705

Part II: Chemistry of CCK Antagonists

Pentanoic Acid Derivatives

L.C. Rovati[1]

Introduction

During the 1960s at Rotta Research Laboratorium, Rovati [1] developed a gastrin receptor antagonist named proglumide, i.e., DL-4-benzamido-*N*, *N*-dipropyl-glutaramic acid. Proglumide has been used for several years for the treatment of peptic ulcer.

The similarities between gastrin and cholecystokinin (CCK), the two peptides sharing the same COOH-terminal pentapeptide amide, were such that it was foreseeable that proglumide would also be able to antagonize the interaction of CCK with its receptors. Actually, Hahne et al. [2] demonstrated that proglumide was able to competitively antagonize CCK-stimulated amylase secretion from guinea pig dispersed pancreatic acini, in close correlation with its ability to inhibit binding of ^{125}I-labeled CCK to its receptors on the same preparation.

Since the potency of proglumide was only in the millimolar range, we tried to develop new molecular entities that could be more potent and specific antagonists of CCK, especially for the separation of the activity on the CCK receptor from that on the gastrin receptor.

Synthesis and Characterization

The successful elaboration that led to compounds such as CR 1409 (lorglumide) and CR 1505 (loxiglumide), consisted in chemical manipulations of the structure of proglumide, as summarized in Fig. 1.

About 200 4-benzamido-5-oxo-pentanoic acid derivatives were synthesized [3]. Their biological activity was screened through their capacity to antagonize the contraction of isolated guinea pig gallbladder longitudinal strips, induced by a fixed concentration of 5 ng/ml of CCK-8. It soon became apparent that all three substitutions (R_1, R_2 and R_3 in Fig. 1) were equally important for the CCK-antagonistic activity.

[1] Department of Clinical Pharmacology, Rotta Research Laboratorium, 20052 Monza (Milano), Italy

G. Adler and C. Beglinger (Eds.)
CCK Antagonists in Gastroenterology

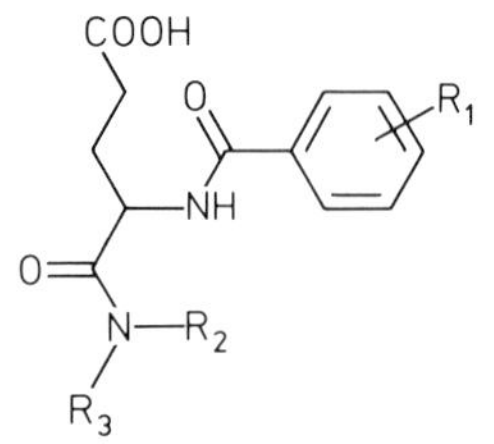

Compound	R_1	R_2	R_3
Proglumide	H	propyl	propyl
Lorglumide	3,4-dichloro	pentyl	pentyl
Loxiglumide	3,4-dichloro	pentyl	methoxypropyl

Fig. 1. Chemical structure of proglumide, lorglumide and loxiglumide. Molecular weights for the three compounds are 334.42, 459.41 and 461.38, respectively

Regarding the substitutions on the amide group (R_2 and R_3), the activity was optimized by the dipentyl group, while longer or shorter side chains produced a 100-fold decrease of anti-CCK activity. Likewise, the low activity exhibited by secondary and cyclic amides supported the hypothesis that both the two alkylic chains of the 4-benzamido-5-oxo-pentanoic acid derivatives could bind to two complementary hydrophobic pockets of the receptor surface with suitable dimensions (about 5 Å) for these lipophilic groups.

Regarding the substitutions on the aromatic ring (R_1) of 5-(dipentylamino)-pentanoic acid derivatives, the best results in this series were obtained with the 3,4-dichloro group: the resulting compound (CR 1409, lorglumide) showed an IC_{50} of 0.06 μg/ml (compared to 340 μg/ml for proglumide) on the above reported gallbladder contraction model, and caused a concentration-dependent rightward shift of the cumulative concentration-response curves to the agonist, without decreasing the maximum effect [4]. The Schild plot in the latter experiment was linear and the slope did not significantly differ from unity, suggesting a competitive antagonism, with a pA_2 value of 7.19.

The steric effect of this chemical substitution seemed to be important, because, for example, the same substitution in position two (instead of three) of the aromatic ring, as well as the introduction of bulky groups such as 4-propyl, produced a strong reduction of activity. The electronic effect seemed to be less crucial, since other electron-withdrawing groups, such as nitro or cyano, or electron-donor groups, such as amino or methoxy, were less biologically effective.

Unfortunately, lorglumide has a relatively poor local tolerability when parenterally given in concentrated solutions: in fact it has the chemical structure of a tensioactive substance, carrying a carboxylic group attached to a lipophilic moiety, that can disrupt the double layered phospholipid surface of the cell membrane in a concentration-dependent fashion. The substitution of one of the two pentyl groups with the 3-methoxypropyl group, i.e., a more hydrophilic group, led to the synthesis of a new molecule (CR 1505, loxiglumide), which is much safer in this respect. Conversely, loxiglumide has pharmacological properties that are not substantially different from those exhibited by the parent compound, lorglumide, and loxiglumide's IC_{50} on the guinea pig gallbladder strip model was 0.47 μg/ml, with a pA_2 value of 6.3 in the concentration-response curves to the agonist [5].

Binding studies demonstrated that both lorglumide and loxiglumide are selective ligands for the "peripheral" type CCK receptors present on rat pancreatic acini (IC_{50} 1.3×10^{-7} and 3.3×10^{-7} mol/l, for lorglumide and loxiglumide, respectively) and have an affinity for "cerebral" type CCK receptors present on mouse cerebral cortex membrane at least two orders of magnitude lower [5,6]. A similarly lower affinity was reported for gastrin receptors [7].

The analysis of the spatial structure of loxiglumide and lorglumide by X-ray crystallography and of the structure-activity relationships of the series further suggest the possible model for the site of the peripheral CCK-receptor to which the pentanoic acid derivatives bind. This site could consist of three hydrophobic pockets, large enough in size to receive bulky groups such as pentyl-, or aryl- and carrying a positively charged group which could bind the carboxylic radical.

Lorglumide and loxiglumide specificity of action was further tested on isolated tissue preparations and neither interactions with other mediators nor intrinsic activities were found. [4,5,7]. Thereafter, we fully characterized the two compounds in animal pharmacodynamic experiments. In view of the possible clinical activity of the CCK antagonists, studies were mainly conducted on biliary and gastrointestinal motility [8–11], satiety [12] and experimental pancreatitis [13,14]. These and other aspects of CCK physiology were then carefully studied by other authors and are dealt with in other chapters of this book.

It is important to note that both lorglumide and loxiglumide are a racemic mixture. In order to establish whether their CCK-antagonistic properties were stereospecific, we synthesized their two enantiomers, starting from D- or L-glutamic acid and using a stereoconservative method of synthesis. The D-enantiomers of both compounds were found to be between five and ten times more potent than their L-enantiomers, depending on the experimental model used. The difference in activity between the two enantiomers confirms the hypothesis that the peripheral CCK receptors are more sensitive to steric effects than to electronic effects or to hydrophobicity.

Pharmacokinetics of Loxiglumide

Because of its favorable pharmacological and toxicological profile, loxiglumide was chosen for further development in humans. Its pharmacokinetic pattern and tolerance were studied after single intravenous and oral administration [15], or repeated oral doses [16] in healthy volunteers.

Loxiglumide can be easily assayed in plasma and urine by a HPLC method. After either intravenous infusion or single oral administration, the plasma levels of loxiglumide fit with a two-compartment open model. The absolute bioavailability from the gastrointestinal tract is over 95%, and the compound is rapidly absorbed, appearing in blood only 15 min after oral administration and reaching the peak concentrations at between about 30 and 90 min after oral ingestion of an aqueous solution or a tablet formulation, respectively. The tablet formulation used has an over 80% relative bioavailability.

The elimination half-life of loxiglumide is about 6 h.

The urinary excretion of loxiglumide and its metabolites accounts for about 20% of the administered dose, so this is not the major excretory route: probably these substances are largely excreted by the biliary route and it is also likely that they have an enterohepatic recirculation.

After repeated oral doses there is a small accumulation of loxiglumide in plasma which is compatible with this administration course, and the steady state is reached after about 48 h. There is no retention of loxiglumide or related substances in the human body.

Loxiglumide was always well tolerated, except for the possible occurrence of episodes of loose stools in some subjects, probably due to the accelerating effects of the compound on colonic transit [17].

Conclusions

The new pentanoic acid derivatives are potent, selective, competitive and reversible antagonists of the peripheral CCK receptor.

Loxiglumide is currently used in humans in order to investigate new insights in digestive physiology and pathophysiology. Such studies are favored by the possibility of using constant intravenous infusions.

Furthermore, the existence of readily bioavailable oral formulations and the good tolerability of the compound render possible its use in the search for possible therapeutic indications.

Acknowledgements. The author wishes to thank Dr. F. Makovec for helpful discussions and advice.

References

1. Rovati AL (1968) The relationship between chemical structure of a new dicarboxylic amino-acid derivative and antigastrin activity in the rat. Br J Pharmacol 34:677–682
2. Hahne WF, Jensen RT, Lemp GF, Gardner JD (1981) Proglumide and benzotript: members of a different class of cholecystokinin receptor antagonists. Proc Natl Acad Sci USA 78:6304–6308
3. Makovec F, Chistè R, Bani M, Revel L, Setnikar I, Rovati AL (1986) New glutamic and aspartic derivatives with potent CCK-antagonistic activity. Eur J Med Chem 21:9–20
4. Makovec F, Chistè R, Bani M, Pacini MA, Setnikar I, Rovati LA (1985) New glutaramic acid derivatives with potent, competitive and specific, cholecystokinin-antagonistic activity. Arzneimittelforschung 35:1048–1051
5. Setnikar I, Bani M, Cereda R, Chistè R, Makovec F, Pacini MA, Revel L, Rovati LC, Rovati LA (1987) Pharmacological characterization of a new potent and specific nonpolypeptidic cholecystokinin antagonist. Arzneimittelforschung 37:703–707
6. Makovec F, Bani M, Chistè R, Revel L, Rovati LC, Rovati LA (1986) Differentiation of central and peripheral cholecystokinin receptors by new glutaramic acid derivatives with cholecystokinin-antagonistic activity. Arzneimittelforschung 36:98–102
7. Jensen RT, Zhon ZC, Murphy RB, Jones SW, Setnikar I, Rovati LA, Gardner JD (1986) Structural features of various proglumide-related cholecystokinin receptor antagonists. Am J Physiol 251:G839–G846
8. Makovec F, Bani M, Cereda R, Chistè R, Pacini MA, Revel L, Rovati LC (1987) Antispasmodic activity on the gallbladder of the mouse of CR 1409 (lorglumide) a potent antagonist of peripheral CCK. Pharmacol Res Commun 19:41–51
9. Makovec F, Bani M, Cereda R, Chistè R, Pacini MA, Revel L, Rovati LA, Rovati LC, Setnikar I (1987) Pharmacological properties of lorglumide as a member of a new class of cholecystokinin antagonists. Arzneimittelforschung 37:1265–1268
10. Setnikar I, Bani M, Cereda R, Chistè R, Makovec F, Pacini MA, Revel L (1987) Anticholecystokinin activities of loxiglumide. Arzneimittelforschung 37: 1168–1171
11. Rovati LC, Bani M, Makovec F, Revel L, Setnikar I (1987) Lorglumide and loxiglumide: two potent and specific antagonists of peripheral CCK. Excerpta Med Int Congr Ser 766:45–48
12. Makovec F, Bani M, Chistè R, Revel L, Rovati LC, Setnikar I (1986) Different peripheral and central antagonistic activity of new glutaramic acid derivatives on satiety induced by cholecystokinin in rats. Regul Pept 16:281–290
13. Makovec F, Bani M, Cereda R, Chistè R, Revel L, Rovati LC, Setnikar I, Rovati LA (1986) Protective effect of CR 1409 (cholecystokinin antagonist) on experimental pancreatitis in rats and mice. Peptides 7:1159–1164
14. Setnikar I, Bani M, Cereda R, Chistè R, Pacini MA, Revel L (1987) Loxiglumide protects against experimental pancreatitis. Arzneimittelforschung 37:1172–1174
15. Setnikar I, Chistè R, Makovec F, Rovati LC, Warrington SJ (1988) Pharmacokinetics of loxiglumide after single intravenous or oral doses in man. Arzneimittelforschung 38:716–720
16. Setnikar I, Chistè R, Giacovelli G, Rovati LC (1989) Pharmacokinetics and tolerance of repeated oral doses of loxiglumide. Arzneimittelforschung 39: 1454–1459
17. Meyer BM, Werth BA, Beglinger C, Hildebrand P, Jansen JBMJ, Zach D, Rovati LC, Stalder GA (1989) Role of cholecystokinin in regulation of gastrointestinal motor functions. Lancet 2:12–15

Characterization of MK-329

R.G. Berlin and R.M. Freidinger[1]

Introduction

Benzodiazepine derivative CCK antagonists originated from the discovery at Merck, by receptor-based screening, of a novel benzodiazepine-like fermentation product from Aspergillus alliaceus [1], asperlicin. Its lack of oral activity and the need for greater potency stimulated the design of improved antagonists. On the basis of structural relationships between asperlicin and the molecules diazepam and D-tryptophan, an indolylmethyl benzodiazepine was designed and synthesized [2]. This simpler compound proved to be comparable in potency and selectivity to asperlicin as a CCK antagonist. Structure-activity studies based on this lead produced a series of compounds with marked increases in potency and selectivity [3,4]. One optimized antagonist, devazepide (MK-329 or L-364 718, Fig. 1) [5], binds to the CCK-A (peripheral) receptor with an affinity comparable to CCK-8 (IC_{50} 0.08 n*M*) and shows greater than 1000-fold selectivity over the CCK-B receptor [6].

Benzodiazepine derivatives that are selective ligands of gastrin and CCK-B receptors have also been designed [7]. Several key structural modifications of devazepide-type structures resulted in a series of 3-arylurea-1,4-benzodiazepines typified by L-365 260 (Fig. 1). This antagonist has high affinity for gastrin and CCK-B receptors (IC_{50} 1 n*M*), which is over 100-fold greater than its CCK-A receptor affinity [8]. Pentagastrin-stimulated acid secretion is potently and competitively inhibited by L-365 260 [8].

Devazepide and L-365 260 are readily synthesized on a kilogram scale using similar processes [9,10]. The two compounds derive from opposite enantiomers of 3-aminobenzodiazepine and are hydrophobic molecules with very low water solubility.

Devazepide has been shown to be a competitive antagonist in vitro and is active at low dose levels by several routes of administration in a number of animal species [11]. In agreement with receptor binding studies, much

[1] Merck Sharp & Dohme Research Laboratories, Departments of Clinical Research (RGB) and Medicinal Chemistry (RMF), West Point, PA 19486, USA.

G. Adler and C. Beglinger (Eds.)
CCK Antagonists in Gastroenterology

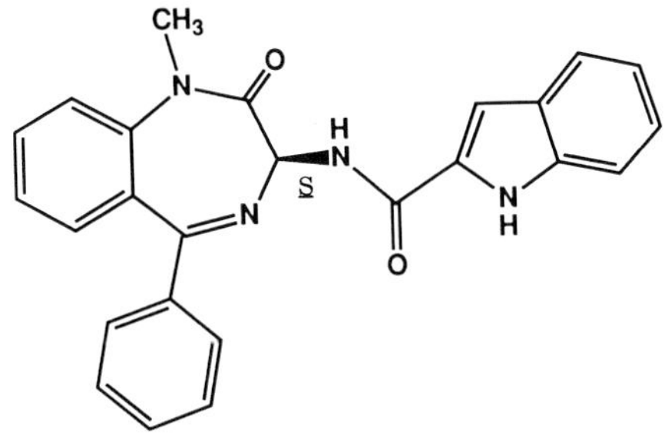

Devazepide

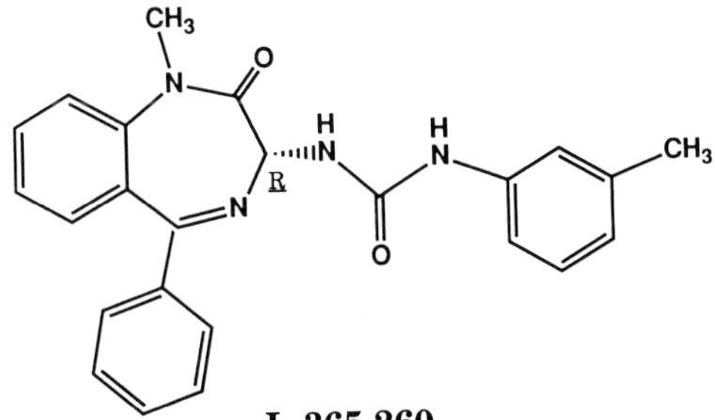

L-365,260

Fig. 1. Selective CCK antagonists

higher concentrations (μM) are required to inhibit gastrin-stimulated acid secretion. No effects on processes mediated by motilin, secretin, acetylcholine, or histamine were observed. No agonist activity has been observed in any of these studies at concentrations in the micromolar range, and the compound efficiently penetrates the blood-brain barrier [12].

Toxicity

MK-329 administered orally or i.p. to mice and hamsters has low acute toxicity; by either route the lethal dose for 50% of a group (LD_{50}) is approximately 1000 mg/kg. Subacute toxicity studies with oral dosing of up to 40 mg/kg per day in hamsters and up to 45 mg/kg per day in rhesus monkeys for 14 weeks showed that the no-effect dose was 20 and 15 mg/kg per day, respectively. In monkeys, a dose-dependent decrease in total serum cholesterol was observed at the two highest doses (30% at 45 mg/kg per day and 21% at 15 mg/kg per day), but no alterations occurred in total triglycerides and only minor effects on HDL cholesterol were noted. A study in baboons (45 mg/kg per day) failed to demonstrate a similar effect on plasma cholesterol concentrations.

Devazepide was administered orally to rats at doses of up to 100 mg/kg per day for 1 year. At a 6-month interim necropsy, changes were confined to increases in hepatic, adrenal, thyroid, and ovarian weight with a no-effect dose of 10 mg/kg per day except for thyroid (2 mg/kg per day) and ovarian weight changes; a no-effect level for the latter change was not established. At oral doses of up to 100 mg/kg per day in baboons, the only treatment-related physical sign was pale feces. A 6-month interim necropsy showed a nondose-dependent increase (50%–70%) in mean bile volume. Slight increases in serum bile acids and ALT and a slight decrease in serum cholesterol were noted. At 12 months small cholesterol-containing gallstones, 1–2 mm in diameter, were noted with a maximum nondose-dependent incidence of 2%.

MK-329 was evaluated for mutagenic potential in a microbial mutagenesis test system using mutant strains of *Salmonella typhimurium* and *Escherichia coli.* with and without a microsomal enzyme activation system prepared from the rat liver. MK-329 was not detectably mutagenic in these-assays.

Studies in rats and rabbits assessed the effects of MK-329 on reproductive performance, including mating and fertility, as well as the embryonal/fetal toxicity and teratogenic potential of the compound. These studies have shown no contraindication to clinical trials in women of childbearing potential.

Pharmacokinetics and Bioavailability

There was substantial species and intersubject variation in the pharmacokinetic parameters after oral dosing. At a dose of 5 mg/kg po, the dog showed a mean oral bioavailability of 20.3 ± 8.6% with $t_{1/2} = 28.2 \pm 12.3$ h, $T_{max} = 1.3 \pm 1.3$ h, and $C_{max} = 135 \pm 46$ ng/ml; the monkey showed an oral bioavailability of 5.5 ± 6.6%, $t_{1/2} = 5.1 \pm 2.7$ h, $T_{max} = 0.9 \pm 0.3$ h, and $C_{max} = 38 \pm 41$ ng/ml (means ± S.D.).

MK-329 undergoes first-pass metabolism. Analysis of metabolites in the bile in monkeys revealed that some possessed CCK-receptor binding activity (10%–20%, as compared to parent compound). No active metabolites were found in dog bile.

After i.v. administration to dogs of ^{14}C-labeled MK-329, 83% of the radioactivity was recovered in the feces and 10% in the urine within 144h; orally, 85% was recovered in the feces and 5% in the urine. Radioactivity in the feces was derived from biliary excretion; only trace amounts of parent compound were detectable in the bile.

In rats, after 4 weeks of oral doses of up to 500 mg/kg per day, mean plasma drug levels measured 24 h after the last dose increased two- to six-fold compared to those measured after a single dose. These increases were not dose proportional, suggesting possible saturation during absorption or saturation of the enzymes of the metabolic pathway and/or a possible induction of metabolizing processes. In baboons dosed orally with 3, 30, 90, and 270 mg/kg per day, there was a dose-proportional response in both AUC and C_{max} following the 3 and 30 mg/kg per day dosing, but these parameters were disproportionately lower at higher doses. The apparent $t_{1/2}$ was approximately 4 h and the T_{max} occurred at 1–2 h.

Equilibrium dialysis revealed MK-329 to be highly bound (>97%) to plasma proteins, using pooled dog, hamster, and human plasma over a wide range of concentrations (200–50 000 ng/ml).

In man, plasma devazepide levels were assayed utilizing a radio-receptor assay. Peak plasma levels occurred 2–4 h after an oral dose with marked interindividual variability. Limited data show an approximately proportional increase in mean plasma levels over an oral dose range of 0.5–10 mg and an elimination half-life on the order of 6 to 12 h.

Animal and Human Studies

The development of potent specific CCK antagonists such as devazepide provides the opportunity to study the physiologic role of CCK in the gastrointestinal system and to explore the potential therapeutic utility of this agent. Direct empirical trials in humans are the only way to resolve the contribution of CCK in the pathogenesis of gastrointestinal disorders.

Biliary System

The most clearly established role for CCK is the stimulation of gallbladder contraction [13–15]. Intravenous devazepide effectively antagonized the effect of CCK on gallbladder contraction in cats (ED_{50} = 210 μg/kg) [11] and guinea pigs (0.1 mg/kg) [6]. To explore the role of CCK on gallbladder emptying in humans and to determine the effect of orally administered devazepide, two series of experiments were carried out. In a double-blind, four-period crossover study, eight subjects received single doses of placebo or 0.5, 2, or 10 mg devazepide, followed by an intravenous infusion of CCK-8 (30 pmol/kg min). In subjects receiving placebo, the 2-h CCK infusion decreased gallbladder volume, determined ultrasonographically, by an average of 43%. Doses of devazepide of 10 mg and 2 mg significantly reduced gallbladder emptying by approximately, 100% and 36 ± 6.1%, respectively, but the 0.5 mg dose did not modify the response to CCK [16]. Gallbladder contraction was also measured after a mixed meal (614 kcal breakfast; 66.8 g carbohydrate, 29.4 g fat, and 20 g protein) in a two-period crossover study in which subjects received either 10 mg devazepide or placebo 2 h before eating. Gallbladder contraction was completely inhibited by devazepide [16]. Similarly, single, oral 10 mg doses of devazepide have been shown to inhibit CCK-8-stimulated biliary output [17] and meal-stimulated biliary output [18]. Dosing for up to 10 days with 1–5 mg bid devazepide orally resulted in persistent significant inhibition of meal-induced gallbladder emptying, indicating no tachyphylaxis [19]. These results demonstrate that devazepide is a potent, orally active CCK antagonist in humans and that CCK is a major regulator of post-prandial gallbladder contraction.

Pancreas

Exogenous CCK has been shown to stimulate pancreatic exocrine secretion in a dose-dependent manner in man [20,21] but the relative contribution of CCK versus other humoral (secretin) and neural (cholinergic) influences has not been defined. In animals, devazepide effectively blocks CCK-8-stimulated and blunts meal-stimulated pancreatic exocrine output [11,22–26]. In man, single oral doses of 10 mg of devazepide have been shown to effectively antagonize CCK-8-induced pancreatic exocrine secretion [17] and to slightly decrease postprandial trypsin output during the first 45 min following meal ingestion [18]. In three of four patients with chronic pancreatitis, a single 10 mg oral dose of devazepide suppressed meal-stimulated output of amylase (74%), lipase (81%) and trypsin (82%) and suppressed output of amylase (68%), lipase (82%), and trypsin (80%) in two patients perfused with phenylalanine (10 n*M*) intraduodenally [27]. CCK blockade with devazepide may be of use in treating the pain associated with chronic pancreatitis, although this remains to be studied.

Evidence supports negative feedback regulation of pancreatic enzyme secretion by intraduodenal trypsin and bile acids in animals and humans [28,29]. Interestingly, administration of devazepide to healthy volunteers resulted in a marked increase in postprandial CCK levels measured by RIA [16,18,27]. These results support the concept of negative feedback regulation of CCK secretion in humans. Devazepide did not alter CCK-8 clearance [16], supporting the role of increased CCK secretion as the mechanism for the observed potentiation of postprandial CCK concentrations after oral devazepide.

CCK is also a physiologically important regulator of growth of the exocrine pancreas, based on studies in rodents [30–32]. Indirect elevation of endogenous CCK levels by chronically feeding rats the protease inhibitor camostate results in pancreatic hypertrophy and hyperplasia which is blocked by devazepide [33]. A similar trophic effect of CCK on growth of pancreatic carcinoma has also been suggested. Cerulein (a structural analogue of CCK) and secretin stimulated growth of hamster pancreatic cancer cells (H-2-T) transplanted in cheek pouches of Syrian golden hamsters [34]. Growth of five human pancreatic cancer cell lines (SW-1990, PANC-1, MIA PaCa-2, BxPC-3, and RWP-2) in serum-free medium was increased 32%–45% in vitro by incubation with CCK-9 [35]. The presence of CCK receptors has been demonstrated in the human pancreatic cancer cell line SKI, but not CAV; and growth of only the former was stimulated by cerulein and inhibited by proglumide (a weak CCK antagonist) [36]. Growth of implants of the CCK receptor positive human pancreatic cancer cell line SKI in athymic nude mice was significantly inhibited by asperlicin [37]. Significant reduction in growth of the CCK receptor positive human pancreatic adenocarcinoma cell line PGER and SW-1990 xenografted to nude mice resulted from administration of devazepide [38,39]. A pilot trial in patients with pancreatic adenocarcinoma treated with devazepide for up to 12 weeks at doses up to 10 mg bid did not demonstrate any measurable regression of disease [40].

The role of CCK in the regulation of pancreatic endocrine function has been investigated [41]. CCK receptor blockade with devazepide, 10 mg, does not alter plasma insulin, glucagon, or glucose response to a mixed meal. However, the finding that CCK receptor blockade selectivity attenuates the postprandial increase in plasma PP concentrations supports a physiological role for CCK in regulating PP secretion.

Stomach

In animals, infustion of CCK-8 delays gastric emptying, and devazepide is capable of reversing this CCK-induced delay [11,32,42]. Devazepide has accelerated gastric emptying of meals in animals [43–45]. As opposed to the results in animals, in patient studies a single, oral, 10 mg dose of devazepide did not accelerate the gastric emptying of liquids or solids in a dual-labeled "typical" meal, despite total inhibition of meal-stimulated gallbladder contraction [16]. In contrast, in another study a meal with a solid food marker (1106 KJ, fat 45%, protein 17%, carbohydrate 38%) emptied significantly faster during the initial 25 min after 10 mg devazepide, but the time for 50% emptying did not differ from placebo [17].

Bowel Motility

CCK may play an important role in the humoral control of intestinal motility [46,47]. In dogs, devazepide did not alter motor or secretory components of the migrating myoelectric complexes (MMC) but did reduce the postprandial spike activity without restoring the fasted pattern [48]. In man, CCK-8 increases small bowel motility [49] as well as colonic motor and myoelectric response [46]. However, a CCK-8 infusion that produced physiologic postprandial CCK levels as measured by RIA did not lead to an increase in motor and myoelectric response of a magnitude typical of the normal postprandial gastrocolic response (W.J. Snape personal communication). In healthy subjects, 10 mg of devazepide produced no changes in the MMC pattern during fasting nor postprandially in either the gastric antrum or duodenum (P. Cantor, personal communication). An exploratory study of the effect of devazepide on postprandial colonic motility and spike activity in patients with irritable bowel is in progress.

Adverse Experience Profile

Devazepide has been generally well tolerated with toxicity primarily manifest as gastrointestinal side effects, particularly cramps or discomfort, and loose stools or frank diarrhea. The frequency and severity of these symptoms appears dose related at doses of 25 mg or above, but not at doses under 10 mg, where the frequency of such symptoms was nearly equivalent to placebo. Headache was more frequent at doses of 25 mg or above. Mild fecal fat elevations were seen in two subjects in the period 24–48 h following a 50-mg dose. A slight decrease in serum cholesterol was noted, but without a clear dose relationship, and it was not observed after 10 d of dosing with up to 5 mg bid.

Summary

Devazepide is a potent, nonpeptidal, peripheral (type A) CCK antagonist essentially devoid of agonist activity. Baboons develop cholesterol gallstones at 1 year, probably reflecting gallbladder stasis. In man, devazepide blocks gallbladder contraction induced by exogenous or endogenous (postprandial) CCK. In normal subjects, devazepide inhibits CCK-8-stimulated pancreatic secretion but has little or no effect on meal-stimulated pancreatic secretion, gastric emptying, or upper gut motility. In patients with chronic pancreatitis, a more pronounced effect may be seen on pancreatic output. Devazepide administration augments postprandial CCK levels, supporting a proposed feedback inhibition of CCK release. Even at high doses, no effect of CCK blockade on pancreatic adenocarcinoma has been seen. Devazepide is helping to elucidate the physiologic role of CCK in man, but preliminary studies suggest that CCK receptor blockade will produce limited advances for the therapy of gastrointestinal disorders.

References

1. Chang RSL, Lotti VJ, Monaghan RL, Birnbaum J, Stapley EO, Goetz MA, Albers-Schonberg G, Patchett AA, Liesch JM, Hensens OD, Springer JP (1985) A potent nonpeptide cholecystokinin antagonist selective for peripheral tissues isolated from *Aspergillus alliaceus*. Science 230:177–179
2. Evans BE, Bock MG, Rittle KE, DiPardo RM, Whitter WL, Veber DF, Anderson PS, Freidinger RM (1986) Design of potent orally effective non-

peptidal antagonists of the peptide hormone cholecystokinin. Proc Natl Acad Sci USA 83:4918–4922

3. Evans BE, Rittle KE, Bock MG, DiPardo RM, Freidinger RM, Whitter WL, Gould NP, Lundell GF, Homnick CF, Veber DF, Anderson PS, Chang RSL, Lotti VJ, Cerino DJ, Chen TB, Kling PJ, Kunkel KA, Springer JP, Hirschfield J (1987) Design of nonpeptidal ligands for a peptide receptor: cholecystokinin. J Med Chem 30:1229–1239.
4. Evans BE, Rittle KE, Bock MG, DiPardo RM, Freidinger RM, Whitter WL, Lundell GF, Veber DF, Anderson PS, Chang RSL, Lotti VJ, Cerino DJ, Chen TB, Kling PJ, Kunkel KA, Springer JP, Hirschfield J (1988) Methods for drug discovery: development of potent selective orally effective cholecystokinin antagonists. J Med Chem 31:2235–2246.
5. Freidinger RM, Berlin RG (1989) MK-329. Drugs Future 14:862–866
6. Chang RSL, Lotti VJ (1986) Biochemical and pharmacological characterization of an extremely potent and selective nonpeptide cholecystokinin antagonist. Proc Natl Acad Sci USA 83:4923–4926
7. Bock MG, DiPardo RM, Evans BE, Rittle KE, Whitter WL, Veber DF, Anderson PS, Freidinger RM (1989) Benzodiazepine gastrin and brain cholecystokinin receptor ligands: L-365 260. J Med Chem 32:13–16
8. Lotti VJ, Chang RSL (1989) A new potent and selective non-peptide gastrin antagonist and brain cholecystokinin receptor (CCK B) ligand: L-365 260. Eur J Pharmacol 162:273–280
9. Bock MG, DiPardo RM, Evans BE, Rittle KE, Veber DF, Freidinger RM, Hirshfield J, Springer JP (1987) Synthesis and resolution of 3-amino-1,3-dihydro-5-phenyl-2H-1,4-benzodiazepine-ones. J Org Chem 52:3232–3239
10. Reider PJ, Davis P, Hughes DL, Grabowski EJJ (1987) Crystallization-induced asymmetric transformation: stereospecific synthesis of a potent peripheral CCK antagonist. J Org Chem 52:955–957
11. Lotti VJ, Pendelton RG, Gould RJ, Hanson HM, Chang RSL, Clineschmidt BV (1987) In vivo pharmacology of L-364 718, a new potent nonpeptide peripheral cholecystokinin antagonist. J Pharmacol Exp Ther 241:103–109
12. Pullen RGL, Hodgson OJ (1987) Penetration of diazepam and the nonpeptide CCK antagonist, L-364 718, into rat brain. J Pharm Pharmacol 39:863–864
13. Lin TM (1975) Actions of gastrointestinal hormones and related peptides on motor function of the biliary tract. Gastroenterology 69:1006–1022
14. Ryan JP (1981) Motility of the gallbladder and biliary tree. In: Johnson LR (ed) Physiology of the gastrointestinal tract. Raven, New York, pp 473–494
15. Solomon TE, Yamada T, Elashoff J, Wood J, Beglinger C (1984) Bioactivity of cholecystokinin analogues: CCK-8 is not more potent than CCK-33. Am J Physiol 247:G105–G111
16. Liddle RA, Gertz BJ, Kanayama S, Beccaria L, Coker LD, Turnbull TA, Mortia ET (1989) Effects of a novel cholecystokinin (CCK) receptor antagonist, MK-329, on gallbladder contraction and gastric emptying in humans. J Clin Invest 84:1220–1225
17. Cantor P, Olsen O, Gertz BJ, Gjorup I, Worning H, Turnbull TA (1989) Inhibition of cholecystokinin (CCK)-induced pancreatic exocrine and biliary secretion by the CCK-receptor antagonist, MK-329. Gastroenterology 96: A73
18. Cantor P, Mortensen PE, Gjorup I, Myhre J, Worning H (1989) Effect of the cholecystokinin antagonist MK-329 on meal-stimulated pancreatic secretion in man. Digestion 43:134
19. Verpooten GA, Giuliano RA, Buntinx AP, Blockx P, Stahl E, Gertz B, DeBroe ME (1989) Dose related inhibition of gallbladder contraction by the cholecystokinin inhibitor MK-329. Eur J Clin Pharmacol [Suppl] 36:PP02.41
20. Beglinger C, Fried J, Whitehouse I, Jansen JB, Lamers CB, Gyr K (1985) Pancreatic enzyme response to a liquid meal and to hormonal stimulation. J Clin Invest 75:1471–1476

21. Cantor P, Petronijevic L, Pedersen JF, Worning H (1986) Cholecystokinetic and pancreozymic effect of O-sulfated gastrin compared with nonsulfated gastrin and cholecystokinin. Gastroenterology 91:1154–1163
22. O'Rourke MF, Reidelberger RD, Solomon TE (1990) Effect of CCK antagonist L-364718 on meal-induced pancreatic secretion in rats. Am J Physiol 258: G179–G184
23. Nakamura T, Fujii M, Okabayashi Y, Tani S, Fujisawa T, Koide M, Otsuki M (1990) Effects of L-364718 on pancreatic exocrine and endocrine secretion in the rat. Pancreas 5:216–221
24. Rosewicz S, Lewis LD, Wang XY, Liddle RA, Logsdon CD (1989) Pancreatic digestive enzyme gene expression effects of CCK and soybean trypsin inhibitor. Am J Physiol 256:G733–G738
25. Konturek SJ, Tasler J, Konturek JW, Cieskowski M, Szewczyk K, Hladij M, Anderson PS (1989) Effects of non-peptidal CCK receptor antagonist L-364718 on pancreatic response to cholecystokinin, gastrin, bombesin and meat feeding in dogs. Gut 30:110–117
26. Hosotani R, Chowdhury P, Rayford PL (1989) L-364718, a new CCK antagonist inhibits postprandial pancreatic secretion and PP release in dogs. Dig Dis Sci 34:462–467
27. Toskes P, Curington C, Cintron M, Liddle R, Berlin R (1990) Oral administration of the CCK antagonist MK-329 substantiates feedback control of pancreatic secretion in chronic pancreatitis patients. Gastroenterology 98:A237
28. Folsch UR, Cantor P, Wilms HM, Schafmayer A, Becker HD, Creutzfeldt W (1987) Role of cholecystokinin in the negative feedback control of pancreatic enzyme secretion in conscious rats. Gastroenterology 92:449–458
29. Owyang C, May D, Louie DS (1986) Trypsin suppression of pancreatic enzyme secretion: differential effect on cholecystokinin release and the enteropancreatic reflex. Gastroenterology 91:637–643
30. Johnson LR, Guthrie P (1976) Effect of cholecystokinin and 16,16-dimethyl prostaglandin E_2 on RNA and DNA of gastric and duodenal mucosa. Gastroenterology 70:59–65
31. Dembinski AR, Johnson LR (1980) Stimulation of pancreatic growth by secretin, caerulein, and pentagastrin. Endocrinology 106:322–328
32. Folsch UR, Winckler K, Wormsley KG (1978) Influence of repeated administration of cholecystokinin and secretin on the pancreas of the rat. Scand J Gastroenterol 13:663–671
33. Wisner JR, McLaughlin RE, Rich KA, Renner IG, Ozawa S (1988) Effects of L-364718, a new cholecystokinin receptor antagonist on camostate induced growth of the rat pancreas. Gastroenterology 94:109–113
34. Townsend CM, Franklin RB, Watson LC, Glass EJ, Thompson JC (1981) Stimulation of pancreatic cancer growth by caerulein and secretin. Surg Forum 32:228–229
35. Smith JP, Barrett B, Solomon TE (1987) CCK stimulates growth of five human pancreatic cancer cell lines in serum-free medium. Gastroenterology 92(5): 1646
36. Upp JR, Singh P, Townsend CM, Thompson JC (1987) Predicting response to endocrine therapy in human pancreatic cancer with cholecystokinin receptors. Gastroenterology 92(5):1677
37. Alexander RW, Upp JR, Singh P, Hugh T, Poston GJ, Townsend CM, Thompson JC (1987) Asperlicin inhibits the growth of a xenografted human pancreatic carcinoma. Gastroenterology 92(5):1293
38. Maani R, Townsend CM, Gomez G, Thompson JC, Singh P (1988) A potent CCK receptor antagonist (L-364718) inhibits the growth of human pancreatic cancer in nude mice. Gastroenterology 94(5):A274
39. Smith JP, Kramer S, Bagheri S (1990) Effects of a high-fat diet and L-364718 on growth of human pancreas cancer. Dig Dis Sci 35:726–732

40. Abbruzzese J, Daugherty K, Larson E, DuBrow R, Gholson C, Berlin R, Levin B (1990) Evaluation of cholecystokinin (CCK) receptor antagonist (MK-329) in patients with advanced pancreatic adenocarcinoma. Pancreas 5:697
41. Liddle RA, Gertz BJ, Kanayama S, Beccaria L, Gettys TW, Taylor IL, Rushakoff RJ, Williams VC, Coker LD (1990) Regulation of pancreatic endocrine function by cholecystokinin: studies with MK-329, a nonpeptide cholecystokinin receptor antagonist. J Clin Endocrinol Metab 70:1312–1318
42. Green T, Dimaline R, Peikin S, Dockray GJ (1988) Action of the cholecystokinin antagonist L-364718 on gastric emptying in the rat. Am J Physiol 255: G685–G689
43. Gould RJ, Cook PG, Fioravanti C, Solomon HF (1987) L-364718, a cholecystokinin antagonist promotes gastric emptying in cats. Clin Res 35(3):A590
44. Baker BJ, Cooper SJ, Booth DA (1989) Effects of the cholecystokinin receptor antagonist MK-329 and (+)–fenfluramine on gastric emptying in the rat. Br J Pharmacol 98[Suppl]:937P
45. Decktor DL, Pendelton RG, Elnitsky AT, Jenkins AM, McDowell AP (1988) Effect of metoclopramide bethanechol and the cholecystokinin receptor antagonist L-364718 on gastric emptying in the rat. Eur J Pharmacol 147:313–316
46. Snape WJ, Matarazzo SA, Cohen S (1978) Effect of eating and gastrointestinal hormones on human colonic myoelectric and motor activity. Gastroenterology 75:373–378
47. Renny A, Snape WJ Jr, Sun EA, London R, Cohen S (1983) Role of cholecystokinin on the gastrocolonic response to a fat meal. Gastroenterology 85:17–21
48. Thor P Laskiewicz J, Konturek P, Konturek SJ (1988) Cholecystokinin in the regulation of intestinal motility and pancreatic secretion in dogs. Am J Physiol 255:G498–G504
49. Kellow JE, Miller LJ, Philips SF, Haddad AC, Zinsmeister AR, Charboneau JW (1987) Sensitivities of the human jejunum, ileum, proximal colon and gallbladder to cholecystokinin octapeptide. Am J Physiol 252:G345–G356

Boc-Tyr(SO_3H)-Nle-Gly-Trp-Nle-Asp-2-Phenylethyl Ester – JMV180: A Unique CCK Analogue with Different Actions on High- and Low-Affinity CCK Receptors

J. Martinez, M-C. Galas, M-F. Lignon, M. Rodriguez, and P. Fulcrand[1]

Introduction

During investigations into the structure activity relationships of cholecystokinin (CCK), it soon became apparent that the C-terminal portion of the CCK molecule, more particularly the C-terminal phenylalanine residue, was of crucial importance for the complete biological activity of CCK analogues, both in the peripheral system and in the CNS. Suppression of the C-terminal phenylalanine residue, e.g., Z-CCK-27-32-NH_2 [Z-Tyr(SO_3H)-Met-Gly-Trp-Met-Asp-NH_2], led to CCK antagonists both in the peripheral system [1] and in the CNS [2,3]. We report here on the modulations in activity which resulted from suppression of the C-terminal primary amide function of CCK, and on its pharmacological consequences.

Compound JMV180 and Analogues

Effects on Amylase Secretion

Earlier studies of the binding of labeled CCK to pancreatic acini of different species indicated two different classes of CCK binding sites with high and low affinity for CCK [4–7]. The dose-response curve for CCK-stimulated enzyme secretion is biphasic. With increasing concentrations of CCK the dose-response curve for enzyme secretion increases, reaches a maximum, and then decreases at higher concentrations. It has been proposed that the occupancy of high-affinity binding sites by low concentrations of CCK (usually less than 100 pM) correlates with stimulation of amylase secretion, and that occupancy of high affinity binding sites by higher CCK concentrations (usually greater than 100 pM) correlates with the inhibition of amylase

CCIPE, Facultè de Pharmacie, 15 Av. C. Flahault, 34060 Montpellier Cèdex, France

G. Adler and C. Beglinger (Eds.)
CCK Antagonists in Gastroenterology

secretion [4,6]. Recently, we have synthesized a new series of analogues of the C-terminal heptapeptide of CCK, in which the C-terminal primary amide function has been suppressed [8]. These analogues, although less potent than CCK, showed the unique property of possessing the same efficacy for amylase release from rat pancreatic acini as CCK-8, but without any inhibition of amylase release at supramaximal concentrations [9, 10]. Among these analogues, Boc-Tyr(SO_3H)-Nle-Gly-Trp-Nle-Asp-2-phenylethyl ester, named JMV180, was found the most potent and used in subsequent studies. It appears to interact with both low- and high-affinity binding sites, and functions as an agonist at the high-affinity CCK receptor, and as an antagonist at the low-affinity CCK receptor. However, in terms of binding, JMV180 is less effective than CCK-8 in discriminating between high-affinity CCK receptors and low-affinity CCK receptors [11–14]. Occupation of the low-affinity CCK binding site by compound JMV180 is accompanied by no change in stimulated amylase secretion, whereas occupation of the low-affinity CCK binding sites by CCK-8 is accompanied by a progressive inhibition of enzyme secretion. Compound JMV180 is able to reverse the inhibition of stimulated enzyme secretion caused by supramaximal concentrations of CCK-8 (concentrations of CCK-8 that occupy low-affinity CCK binding sites) and can cause a parallel rightward shift in the downstroke of the dose-response curve for CCK-8 stimulated enzyme secretion, indicating that this inhibition is competitive in nature [9,11] (Fig. 1).

Previously, it has been demonstrated that by first incubating dispersed pancreatic acini with CCK-8 and then washing the cells to remove CCK-8 a reduction was obtained in the subsequent stimulation of amylase secretion caused by CCK-8 and by all secretagogues that mobilize cellular calcium [15]. Using compound JMV180, which acts as an antagonist at the low affinity CCK binding site, Menozzi et al. [16] have suggested that CCK-8 causes desensitization of enzyme secretion by interacting with low-affinity CCK receptors.

An N-terminal extended molecule of compound JMV180 useful for labeling of sequence D-Tyr-Gly-Asp-Tyr(SO_3H)-Nle-Gly-Trp-Nle-Asp-2-phenylethyl ester showed the same interesting properties as compound JMV180 and confirmed the important role of the C-terminal primary amide function for full biological activity of CCK analogues on pancreatic acini [13].

The inhibitory effects of compound JMV180 at the low affinity CCK receptor can not only be explained by a competitive inhibition at the low-affinity binding site, but also by reducing the number of receptors in the low-affinity configuration. It has been postulated that there exists one type of CCK receptor molecule that can be converted between states showing a high- or a low-affinity for CCK under different conditions, these two states existing in reversible equilibrium. In normal conditions, most receptors are in the low-affinity configuration. CCK-8 would bind to both receptor states,

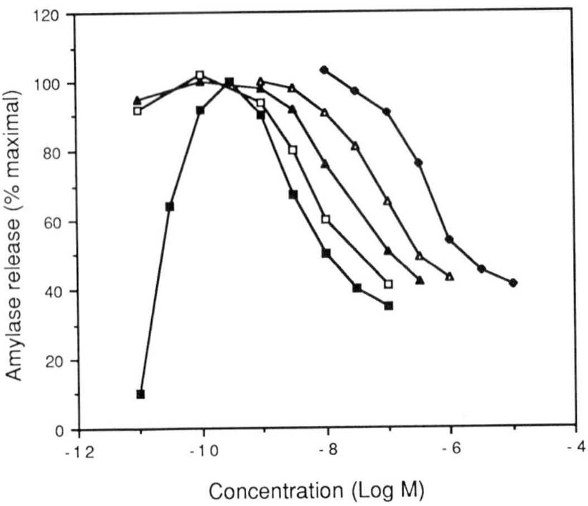

Fig. 1. Effects of compound JMV180 on amylase release from rat pancreatic acini stimulated by Boc-[Nle^{28},Nle^{31}]-CCK-7. Acini were incubated for 30 min at 37°C with various concentrations of Boc-[Nle^{28},Nle^{31}]-CCK-7 plus indicated concentrations of compound JMV180: (■) 0 μ*M*, (□) 0.1 m*M*, (▲) 1 μ*M*, (△) 5 μ*M*, (◆) 10 μ*M*. Results are expressed as a percentage of maximal stimulation obtained with Boc-[Nle^{28},Nle^{31}]-CCK-7 (40 ± 5% of the total amylase contained in the acini) minus the basal amylase secretion (10 ± 2% of the total amylase contained in the acini). In each experiment, each value was determined in duplicate and results given are means from at least five separate experiments

which would gradually become saturated as the concentration of CCK-8 is increased. By contrast, compound JMV180 would bind only to high-affinity binding sites. As the concentration of compound JMV180 increased, low-affinity binding sites would gradually convert into high-affinity binding sites as a result of the equilibrium between the two forms. Thus, compound JMV180 might act as a competitive inhibitor at the low-affinity binding site not by occupying the binding site, but by reducing the available number of these sites [12]. Recently, Molero et al. [14] reported that two affinity states of the CCK receptor exist in intact cells and membranes from bovine gallbladder, with the interconversion of these states, probably mediated by a G protein. Compound JMV180 showed equal affinity for both sites whereas CCK-8 interacted with the two sites with different affinities. However, further work is clearly needed to establish the precise biochemical differences between high- and low-affinity CCK binding sites [12,13].

By contrast, in mouse pancreatic acini, compound JMV180 interacts with, and occupies, high- and low-affinity CCK receptors with different affinities and acts as an agonist on both sites, thereby showing at supramaximal concentrations inhibition of amylase secretion and protein synthesis [12]. These results confirm species differences in CCK receptors which have already been reported.

These unique properties of JMV180 make its use particularly helpful in distinguishing actions mediated by occupation of high-affinity binding sites from actions mediated by occupation of low-affinity binding sites.

Inhibition of amino acid incorporation into proteins at supramaximal concentrations of CCK-8 is believed to be correlated to low-affinity CCK receptor [4]. In contrast to the CCK-8 biphasic effects on [^{3}H]leucine incorporation into proteins in rat acini, compound JMV180 increased [^{3}H]leucine incorporation but did not cause any decrease at high concentrations [12]. However, as with amylase secretion, JMV180 and analogues inhibited [^{3}H]leucine uptake in mouse pancreatic acini similar to the effects of CCK-8 [12].

Effects on Intracellular Mediators

Compound JMV180 is unique in that it can distinguish high-from low-affinity CCK receptors on the basis of its biological activity. It has been used to determine the relationships between occupation of each class of CCK binding sites and the accompanying changes in intracellular Ca^{2+}, phospholipid hydrolysis, and enzyme secretion and was compared to CCK-8.

Effects on Ca^{2+}

It is known that the stimulatory effect of CCK-8 on amylase secretion is mediated by the mobilization of intracellular Ca^{2+}, i.e., CCK-8 promotes phosphatidylinositol 4,5-biphosphate (PIP_2) hydrolysis [17,18] to produce both 1,2-diacylglycerol (DAG) and 1,4,5-inositol triphosphate (1,4,5-IP_3), the latter causing Ca^{2+} release from intracellular stores [19,20]. It has been proposed that DAG and Ca^{2+} mobilization, in activating protein kinase C, acts in a synergistic fashion in the stimulation of amylase secretion [20–23].

In terms of causing mobilization of Ca^{2+}, compound JMV180 is only 50%–60% as efficacious as CCK-8 or its potent analogue Boc-[Nle^{28},Nle^{31}]-CCK-7 [24–26] (Fig. 2). Compound JMV180 is also able to inhibit the mobilization of Ca^{2+} caused by a maximal effective dose of CCK-8, suggesting that CCK-8 and compound JMV180 interact with the same class of CCK receptors to promote intracellular Ca^{2+} mobilization [25]. It has been suggested that compound JMV180 produces mobilization of intracellular Ca^{2+} by interacting with the low-affinity CCK receptor [25]. From the studies of Matozaki et al. [12] it appears that both the actions of CCK-8 and compound JMV180 were dependent on an increase in Ca^{2+}, since these actions could be blocked by the Ca^{2+} chelator BAPTA loaded into acini. By using microspectrofluorometry of Fura-2 in individual acinar cells, low concentrations of CCK-8 that produce the upstroke in the dose-response curve of amylase secretion and compound JMV180 induced Ca^{2+} oscilla-

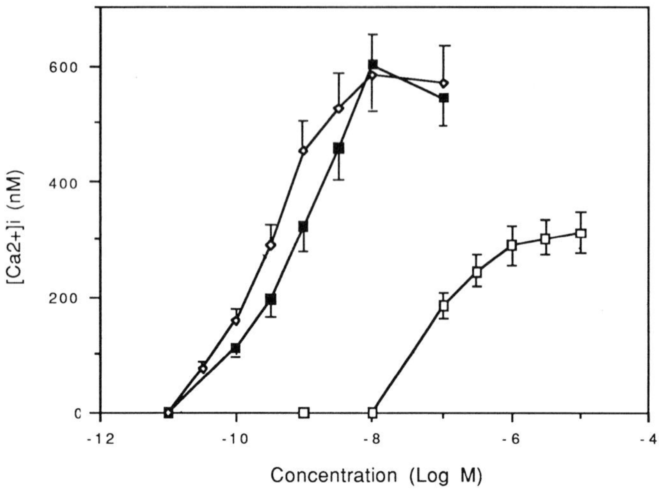

Fig. 2. Effects of CCK-8 (◇), Boc-[Nle[28],Nle[31]]-CCK-7 (■), and Boc-Tyr(SO_3H)-Nle-Gly-Trp-Nle-Asp-2-phenylethyl ester (compound JMV180) (□) on $[Ca^{2+}]_i$ in isolated rat pancreatic acini. Acini were pre-loaded with Fura-2 in the presence of 1.5 m*M* Ca^{2+}. Fluorescence was measured before and after addition of secretagogues in a 2 ml cell suspension aliquot, using a Perkin Elmer spectrofluorimeter set at 350 nm for excitation and 505 nm for emission. Results are the means (±SEM) of four to five separate experiments

tions [12,27]. By contrast, higher concentrations of CCK-8 (more than 100 p*M*) cause a large transient increase of intracellular Ca^{2+} followed by a small sustained increase of intracellular Ca^{2+} without oscillations. These results clearly indicated that low concentrations of CCK-8, or compound JMV180, induced Ca^{2+} oscillations probably responsible for amylase secretion, and have effects on intracellular Ca^{2+} different from those of high concentrations of CCK-8 [12].

Effects on Phospholipid Hydrolysis

The effects of compound JMV180 on phospholipid hydrolysis were examined and compared with those of CCK-8 and Boc-[Nle[28],Nle[31]]-CCK-7 [12,24, 28–30]. Compound JMV180 was almost ineffective in enhancing [^{3}H]inositol phosphate accumulation in rat pancreatic acini. Only a very small amount of [^{3}H]inositol phosphate accumulation was observed even at high concentrations. By contrast, high concentrations of CCK-8 or of the related analogue Boc-[Nle[28],Nle[31]]-CCK-7 produced a large increase in [^{3}H] inositol phosphate production, consistent with concentrations producing a transient large increase of intracellular Ca^{2+} and inhibition of amylase secretion [24]. Interestingly, compound JMV180 was also able to inhibit CCK-8 induced inositol phosphate accumulation, suggesting that the action of CCK-8 on inositol phosphate generation may be mediated by occupation of the low-affinity CCK binding site, and confirming that compound JMV180 acts as an antagonist at this binding site. Although is has been demonstrated that a guanine nucleotide-binding protein is involved in CCK-simulated PIP_2 hydrolysis to produce inositol phosphate in pancreatic acinar cells, the recent observation that the N-terminal extended form of compound JMV180 initiates a novel cascade not involving a guanine nucleotide-binding protein is consistent with these findings [13]. These results suggest that the mechanism for induction of Ca^{2+} oscillations, and subsequent amylase secretion, may be different from that for IP_3-induced large transient Ca^{2+} mobilization and subsequent amylase inhibition.

Effects on 1,2-Diacylglycerol

It has been demonstrated recently that the action of high concentrations of CCK-8 (10 n*M*) on isolated rat pancreatic acini resulted in a biphasic increase of DAG, consisting in an early peak at 5 s, coming from the hydrolysis of PIP_2, and a second, larger, gradual increase that was maximal by 15 min and coming from phosphatidylcholine hydrolysis, the latter contributing to the sustained generation of DAG and hence the maintained activation of protein kinase C. By comparison, a submaximal dose of CCK-8 (30 p*M*) for amylase secretion induced a monophasic increase of DAG sustained to 60 min, without an early peak [31]. Compound JMV180 caused a dose-dependent, monophasic and sustained stimulation of DAG without any early increase, in accordance with the limited effect of compound JMV180 on IP_3 production [26]. Compound JMV180 stimulates the release of [^{3}H]choline metabolites, predominantly phosphorylcholine, indicating that phosphatidylcholine hydrolysis might be involved in DAG production by rat pancreatic acini, as the result of stimulation by compound JMV180. Since compound JMV180 is believed to act as an agonist at the high-affinity CCK binding sites and as an antagonist at the low-affinity CCK binding sites, these results suggest that high-affinity CCK binding sites are correlated with phosphatidylcholine hydrolysis and subsequent DAG formation whereas low-affinity CCK binding sites are correlated with PIP_2 hydrolysis leading to both IP_3 formation and an early peak of DAG and a large transient in intracellular Ca^{2+} [26].

Effects on Adenylate Cyclase Activity

The second messenger system(s) by which CCK exerts its varied effects on pancreatic acini remain incompletely defined. CCK-8 is also known to induce in a dose-dependent manner cellular cyclic adenosine monophosphate (cAMP) accumulation. It has been proposed that CCK-8 activation of adenylate cyclase is mediated through low-affinity CCK receptors [32]. This assumption has been confirmed by the findings that neither compound JMV180 nor its N-terminal extended analogue was able to promote cellular cAMP accumulation, and they further antagonize the effects of CCK-8 [24,33].

Other Biological Effects

Effects on Pancreatitis

Recently, compound JMV180 has enabled studies that may identify the cell biology and pathological events mediated by high- and low-affinity CCK receptors. Saluja and colleagues reported that cerulein but not compound JMV180 can induce edematous pancreatitis in rats, and that it prevents cerulein-induced pancreatitis. These authors concluded that cerulein-induced pancreatitis is dependent on the inhibition of secretion that results from low-affinity receptor occupancy and that other methods of inhibiting secretion (e.g., somatostatin) may not be sufficient to induce pancreatitis [34]. These authors also demonstrated that compound JMV180 fails to protect against pancreatitis induced by methods that do not involve CCK.

These findings are of great interest for those interested in the search for CCK analogues selective for the peripheral CCK receptor (CCK-A type). CCK analogues, selective agonists for the CCK-A receptor, should be useful as satieting agents, but their ability to induce pancreatitis has to be taken into account. In this respect, compounds acting at the peripheral CCK receptor as antagonists at the low-affinity CCK binding site might be of great value in determining which CCK binding site(s) (high-affinity, low-affinity or both) is(are) involved in the control of food intake, and should direct thinking in this area.

In the mouse, high doses (10–50 mg/kg per hour, i.p.) of the compound JMV180 which acts as an agonist at the low-affinity CCK binding site, are able to induce acute pancreatitis [35]. These results strongly support the hypothesis that cerulein-induced pancreatitis results from occupation of the low-affinity CCK receptor by an agonist.

However, one should be concerned about the low potency of compound JMV180 in in vivo studies, probably due to the poor 2-phenylethyl ester stability. In in vivo studies on pancreatic secretion in the rat, the 2-phenylethylamide derivative [e.g., Boc-Tyr(SO_3H)-Nle-Gly-Trp-Nle-Asp-2-phenylethylamide, JMV170] was found more potent than compound JMV180 although it was less potent in in vitro studies [36–38].

Effects on Food Intake

It is known that CCK-8 is involved in the control of food intake, having a satieting effect. Compound JMV180 (10 μg/kg) was found about four times less potent in inhibiting food intake after intracerebioventricular injection in the rat than its 2-phenylethylamide analogue (compound JMV170). None of them affected food intake after i.p. administration, whatever the dose or time after injection [39,40]. The effects of JMV180 and analogues on food intake seem to be different from those of CCK-8 which has been found more active after i.p. injection. This contrast may also reflect differences in the CCK-8 and analogues degradation.

Effects on the Gastrin Receptor

Compound JMV180 and analogues lacking the C-terminal amide function have been shown to function as gastrin antagonists. They were able to inhibit binding of labeled gastrin to a rabbit (or rat) gastric mucosal cell preparation and to antagonize gastrin-stimulated acid secretion in the anesthetized rat [41, Martinez and Bali, unpublished results].

Effects on Smooth Muscle

Compound JMV180 and analogues were also found to inhibit the effects of gastrin and CCK on isolated smooth muscle cells from rabbit antrum [Martinez and Bali, unpublished results]. A 2-phenylethylamide analogue of CCK-7 (e.g., Suc-Tyr(SO_3H)-Met-Gly-Trp-Met-Asp-2-Phenylethylamide, 410) was shown to inhibit CCK-8 induced contractile responses of guinea pig gallbladder, ileum and muscle strips [42,43]. However, the N-terminal extended analogue of compound JMV180 was found as efficacious as CCK on gallbladder, although, as in pancreas, without expressing the supramaximal inhibition of activity typical of CCK [14].

Conclusions

These studies showed the importance of the C-terminal amide function for the expression of the entire biological activity of CCK, although this functional group appeared not to be crucial for binding to CCK receptors. However, if suppression of the C-terminal amide function led to CCK analogues that act as agonists at the high-affinity CCK binding sites and as antagonists at the low-affinity binding sites, the remaining biological activity can be modulated by modifications affecting the tryptophan residue or the peptide bonds surrounding the tryptophan. In JMV180 or analogues, replacing the tryptophan by a D-tryptophan produced full and potent CCK antagonists [e.g., Boc-Tyr(SO_3H)-Nle-Gly-DTrp-Nle-Asp-2-phenylethyl ester JMV179] [44], while modifying the peptide bonds surrounding the tryptophan residue produced partial CCK agonists [45].

Compound JMV180 is unique in that it can discriminate between high-affinity CCK receptors and low-affinity CCK receptors in pancreatic acini, in terms of biological activity. This compound acts as an agonist at the high-affinity CCK binding site and as an antagonist at the low-affinity CCK binding sites. This particular property has been of great help in more precisely defining the intracellular events and biological activities associated with both CCK binding sites.

The present results further support the concept that occupancy of specific affinity states of the CCK receptors are correlated with different biological actions. Although it seems more likely that high- and low-affinity CCK receptors are a unique protein that can be converted between states showing a high- or a low-affinity for CCK under different conditions, further work is clearly needed to determine the biochemical differences in the CCK receptor in the high- versus low-affinity state.

References

1. Spanarkel M, Martinez J, Briet C, Jensen RT, Gardner JD (1983) Cholecystokinin-27-32-amide a member of a new class of cholecystokinin receptor antagonists. J Biol Chem 258:6746–6749
2. Worms P, Martinez J, Briet J, Castro B, Biziere K (1986) Evidence for dopaminomimetic effect of intrastriatally injected cholecystokinin octapeptide in mice. Eur J Pharmacol 121:395–401
3. MacVicar B, Kerrin JP, Davidson JS (1987) Inhibition of synaptic transmission in the hippocampus by cholecystokinin (CCK) and its antagonism by a CCK analog (CCK_{27-33}) Brain Res 406:130–135
4. Sankaran H, Goldfine ID, Bailey A, Licko V, Williams JA (1982) Relationship of cholecystokinin receptor binding to regulation of biological functions in pancreatic acini. Am J Physiol 242:G250–G257
5. Williams JA, Bailey AC, Roach E (1988) Temperature dependence of high-affinity CCK receptor binding and CCK internalization in rat pancreatic acini. Am J Physiol 254:G513–G521
6. Sankaran H, Goldfine ID, Deveney CW, Wong EY, Williams JA (1980) Binding of cholecystokinin to high affinity receptors on isolated rat pancreatic acini. J Biol Chem 255:1849–1853
7. Younes M, Jensen RT, Gardner JD (1987) Cholecystokinin-induced residual stimulation of enzyme secretion from mouse pancreatic acini. Biochim Biophys Acta 930:410–418
8. Fulcrand P, Rodriguez M, Galas MC, Lignon MF, Laur J, Aumelas A, Martinez J (1988) 2-Phenylethylester and 2-phenylethylamide derivatives analogues of the C-terminal hepta- and octa-peptide of cholecystokinin. Int J Pept Protein Res 32:384–395
9. Galas MC, Lignon MF, Rodriguez M, Mendre C, Fulcrand P, Laur J, Aumelas A, Martinez J (1988) Structure activity relationship studies on cholecystokinin: analogues with partial agonist activity. Am J Physiol 254:G176–G182
10. Rodriguez M, Lignon MF, Mendre C, Galas MC, Martinez J (1987) Synthesis of pseudopeptide analogues of the C-terminal heptapeptide of cholecystokinin and preliminary results on their in vitro activity on stimulation of amylase release from rat pancreatic acini. In: Theodoropoulos D (ed) Peptides 1986. 19th European peptide symposium. de Gruyter, Berlin, pp 455–458
11. Stark HA, Sharp CM, Stuliff VE, Martinez J, Jensen RT, Gardner JD (1989) CCK-JMV-180: a peptide that distinguishes high-affinity cholecystokinin receptors from low-affinity cholecystokinin receptors. Biochim Biophys Acta 1010: 145–150
12. Matozaki T, Martinez J, Williams JA (1989) A new CCK analogue differentiates two functionally distinct CCK receptors in rat and mouse pancreatic acini. Am J Physiol 257:G594–G600

13. Gaisano HY, Klueppelberg UG, Pinon DI, Pfenning MA, Powers SP, Miller LJ (1989) Novel tool for the study of cholecystokinin-stimulated pancreatic enzyme secretion. J Clin Invest 83:321–325
14. Molero X, Hadac E, Miller LJ (1990) The type A cholecystokinin (CCK) receptor on gallbladder membranes exists in two-G-protein-regulated affinity. Gastroenterology 98:A511
15. Abdelmoumene S, Gardner JD (1980) Cholecystokinin-induced desensitization in dispersed acini from guinea pig pancreas. Am J Physiol 239:G272–G279
16. Menozzi D, Stark HA, Martinez J, Jensen RT, Gardner JD (1989) Cholecystokinin (CCK)-induced desensitization of pancreatic enzyme secretion is mediated by low affinity CCK receptors. Peptides 10:337–341
17. Streb H, Heslop JP, Irvine RF, Schulz I, Berridge MJ (1985) Relationship between secretagogue-induced Ca^{2+} release and inositol polyphosphate production in permeabilized pancreatic acinar cells. J Biol Chem 260:7309–7315
18. Merritt JE, Taylor CW, Rubin RP, Putney JW Jr (1986) Isomers of inositol triphosphate in exocrine pancreas. Biochem J 238:825–839
19. Berridge MJ (1984) Inositol triphosphate and diacylglycerol as second messengers. Biochem J 220:345–360
20. Noguchi M, Adachi H, Gardner JD, Jensen RT (1985) Calcium-activated, phospholipid-dependent protein kinase in pancreatic acinar cells. Am J Physiol 248:G692–G701
21. Pandol SJ, Schoeffield MS, Sachs G, Muallem S (1985) Role of free cytosolic calcium in secretagogue-stimulated amylase release from dispersed acini from guinea pig pancreas. J Biol Chem 260:10081–10086
22. Merritt JE, Rubin RP (1985) Pancreatic amylase secretion and cytoplasmic free calcium. Effects of ionomycin, phorbol dibutyrate and diacylglycerols alone and in combination. Biochem J 230:151–159
23. Burnham DP, Munowitz P, Hootman SR, Williams JA (1986) Regulation of protein phosphorylation in pancreatic acini. Distinct effects of calcium ionophore A23187 and 12-O-tetradecanoylphorbol 13-acetate. Biochem J 235:125–131
24. Lignon MF, Galas MC, Rodriguez M, Martinez J (1990) Correlation between phospholipid breakdown, intracellular calcium mobilization and enzyme secretion in rat pancreatic acini treated with Boc-[Nle^{28},Nle^{31}]-CCK-7 and JMV180, two cholecystokinin analogues. Cell Sign 2:339–346
25. Sato S, Stark HA, Martinez J, Beaven MA, Jensen RT, Gardner JD (1989) Receptor occupation, calcium mobilization, and amylase release in pancreatic acini: effects of CCK-JMV-180. Am J Physiol 257:G202–G209
26. Matozaki T, Göke B, Tsunoda Y, Rodriguez M, Martinez J, Williams JA (1990) Two functionally distinct cholecystokinin receptors show different modes of action on Ca^{2+} mobilization and phospholipid hydrolysis in isolated rat pancreatic acini. J Biol Chem 265:6247–6254
27. Tsunoda Y, Stuenkel E, Williams JA (1990) Oscillatory mode of calcium signaling in rat pancreatic acinar cells. Am J Physiol 258:C147–C155
28. Lignon MF, Galas MC, Rodriguez M, Guillon G, Jard S, Martinez J (1987) A CCK analogue that exhibits part of the CCK response on rat pancreatic acini: relationship among amylase release, receptor affinity and phosphoinositide breakdown. In: Bali JP, Martinez J (eds) Gastrin and cholecystokinin: chemistry, physiology and pharmacology. Elsevier, Amsterdam, pp 57–61
29. Martinez J, Rodriguez M, Lignon MF, Galas MC (1988) Selective cholecystokinin receptor antagonists. In: Wang R, Schoenfeld R (eds) Cholecystokinin antagonists, neurology and neurobiology, vol 47. Liss, New York, pp 29–51
30. Rowley WH, Sato S, Huang SC, Collado-Escobar DM, Beaven MA, Wang LH, Martinez J, Gardner JD, Jensen RT (1990) Cholecystokinin-induced formation of inositol phosphates in pancreatic acini. Am J Physiol 259:G655–G665
31. Matozaki T, Williams JA (1989) Multiple sources of 1,2-diacylglycerol in isolated rat pancreatic acini stimulated by cholecystokinin. J Biol Chem 264:14729–14734

32. Von Schrenk T, Jensen RT, Gardner JD (1987) Charateristics of the pancreatic acinar cell receptors with which cholecystokinin interacts to increase cyclic AMP. In: Bali JP, Martinez J (eds) Gastrin and cholecystokinin: chemistry, physiology and pharmacology. Elsevier, Amsterdam, pp 49–56
33. Leach SD, Marino CR, Miller LJ, Modlin IM, Gorelick FS (1990) Cholecystokinin activates adenylate cyclase via low-affinity CCK receptors. Gastroenterology 96:A224
34. Saluja AK, Saluja M, Printz H, Zavertnik A, Sengupta A, Steer ML (1989) Experimental pancreatitis is mediated by low-affinity cholecystokinin receptors that inhibit digestive enzyme secretion. Proc Natl Acad Sci USA 86:8968–8971
35. Powers RE, Grady T, Holt S, Steer ML, Saluja AK (1990) Supramaximal doses of a novel CCK analogue (JMV-180) induces acute pancreatitis in mice. Gastroenterology 98:A231
36. Nagain C, Rodriguez M, Martinez J, Roze C (1987) In vivo activities of peptide and pseudopeptide analogs of the C-terminal octapeptide of cholecystokinin on pancreatic secretion in the rat. Peptides 8:1023–1028
37. Nagain C, Rodriguez M, Martinez J, Roze C (1990) Deux peptides dérivés de la CCK8 ne désensibilisent pas la secrétion pancréatique externe et ont une action prolongée in vivo chez le rat. Gastroenterol Clin Biol 14:A35
38. Nagain C, Rodriguez M, Galas MC, Lignon MF, Martinez J, Roze C (1990) Synthetic CCK8 analogues with antagonist activity on pancreatic receptors: in vivo study in the rat, compared to non-peptidic antagonists. Pancreas 6:275–281
39. Orosco M, Gourch A, Rodriguez M, Martinez J, Jacquot C, Cohen Y (1990) Comparative activity of two cholecystokinin analogues with partial agonist activity: effects on food intake and brain monoamines. Peptides 11:873–877
40. Gourch A (1990) Monoamines cérébrales, comportement alimentaire et neuropeptide Y. Effects de la CCK8S et de nouveaux analogues peptidiques. Thesis, Université de Paris Sud, Centre d'Orsay, Orsay
41. Martinez J, Rodriguez M, Bali JP, Laur J (1986) Phenethyl ester derivatives analogues of the C-terminal tetrapeptide of gastrin as potent gastrin antagonists. J Med Chem 29:2201–2206
42. Rakovska A, Heinklein P, Milenov K, Nieber K, Oehme P (1987) Suc-Tyr(SE)-Met-Gly-Trp-Met-Asp-Phenethylamide (410): a competitive antagonist of cholecystokinin-induced contractions in smooth muscles in vitro. Methods Find Exp Clin Pharmacol 9:429–435
43. Nieber K, Milenov K, Rakovska A, Heinklein P, Oehme P (1988) Responses of guinea pig gastric, ileal and gall bladder smooth muscle to desamino-cholecystokinin-octapeptide (CCK-7). Methods Find Exp Clin Pharmacol 10: 513–520
44. Lignon MF, Galas MC, Rodriguez M, Laur J, Aumelas A, Martinez J (1987) A synthetic peptide that is a cholecystokinin receptor antagonist. J Biol Chem 262:7226–7231
45. Rolland M, Rodriguez M, Lignon MF, Galas MC, Laur J, Aumelas A, Martinez J (1991) Synthesis and biological activity of some 2-phenylethyl ester analogues of the C-terminal heptapeptide of cholecystokinin modified in the Trp 30 region. Int J Pept Protein Res (in press)

Part III: Physiological Application of CCK Antagonists

Cholecystokinin Receptor Antagonists In Vitro

R.T. JENSEN and J.D. GARDNER[1]

Introduction

Since the original observation in 1979 [48] that dibutyryl cyclic GMP (Bt_2cGMP) functions as a weak, but specific, cholecystokinin (CCK) receptor antagonist, five different classes of CCK receptor antagonists have been described in various in vitro studies (Tables 1, 2) [30,31]. Members of at least two of these classes [i.e., amino acid derivatives such as lorglumide (CR 1409) or loxiglumide (CR 1505) and substituted benzodiazepine analogues such as L-364 718 (MK-329), L-365 260 or A-65 186 have sufficient potency and specificity to be generally useful for in vivo studies that explore the importance of CCK-related peptides in various physiological processes. It is likely that additional useful CCK receptor antagonists which may further distinguish CCK receptor subtypes or have higher potency, will be developed, probably from one of the five different classes currently described. In this chapter the results of in vitro studies with each of the different classes of CCK receptor antagonists are reviewed.

General: CCK Receptor Subtypes

In the initial studies defining the action of various CCK receptor antagonists, the fact that more than one type of CCK receptor existed was not generally considered. It is now clear that there are at least two, and perhaps three, different types of CCK receptors [10,30,31,46]. Because the CCK receptor antagonists can have different affinities for the different types of receptors, it is important, when considering the in vitro results, to define first the type of CCK receptor being investigated. Numerous older functional studies demonstrated that the naturally occurring peptides, CCK and gastrin, had markedly different biologic actions [32] even though they were structurally similar in having an identical pentapeptide amide at the biologically active COOH-terminus of the molecule [32]. The presence of a

[1] Digestive Diseases Branch, National Institutes of Diabetes and Digestive and Kidney Diseases, National Institutes of Health, Bethesda, MD 20892, USA.

G. Adler and C. Beglinger (Eds.)
CCK Antagonists in Gastroenterology

Table 1. Classes of CCK receptor antagonists

	Antagonist class	Most potent members	Other potent members
I.	Cyclic nucleotide analogues	Bt_2cGMP (0.1 m*M*) [1,24,52]	$O^{2'}$ BtcGMP (1 m*M*) [1,24]
II.	Amino acid derivatives	CR 1409 (0.1–0.2 μ*M*)[a] [30,39,47,71]	CR 1505 (0.33 μ*M*) [53][a] Phenoxyacetyl proglumide (5 μ*M*) [27] Benzotript (0.3 m*M*) [17,25] CBZ-cystine (0.1 m*M*) [43]
III.	COOH-terminal CCK analogues	BOC-[D-Trp^{30}, Nle^{31}] CCK-27-32-Phenylethyl ester (0.05 μ*M*) [34]	CBZ-CCK-27-32-NH_2 (2.7 μ*M*) [62] BOC-CCK-31-33 (0.4 m*M*) [26]
IV.	D-Amino acid substituted substance P(SP)-4-11 analogues	[D-Pro^4,D-$Trp^{7,9,10}$]-SP-4-11 (5 μ*M*) [72]	
V.	Asperlicin and substituted benzodiazepines	L-364718 (0.08–2 n*M*)[b] [4,19,36,37,71]	Asperlicin (2.1 μ*M*)[b] [5,70] L-365260 (0.5 μ*M*)[b] [3,19,36] A-65186 (5 n*M*)[c] [33]

Numbers in parentheses refer to K_i for CCK_A receptors on pancreas.
[a] CR 1409 = D,L-4-(3,4-dichlorobenzoylamino)-5-(dipentylamino)-5-oxo-pentanoic acid is also called lorglumide, proglumide analogue 10, and compound B in various studies. CR 1505 = D,L-4-(3,4-dichlorobenzoylamino)-5-(N-3-methoxy-propylpentilamino)-5-oxo-pentanoic acid is also called loxiglumide [28,39–41,53].
[b] L-364718 = MK-329 = [3S(−)-*N*-(2,3-dihydro-1-methyl-2-oxo-5-phenyl-1 H-1, 4-benzodiazepin-3-yl)-1 H-indole-2-carboxide; L-365260 = 3*R*(+)-(*N*-2,3-dihydro-1-methyl-2-oxo-5-phenyl-1 H-1,4-benzodiazepin-3-yl)-*N*′-(3-methylphenyl) urea); Asperlicin = [2*S*-(2α,9β,9(R*),9αβ)]-6,7-dihydro-7-[[2,3,9,9α-tetrahydro-9-hydroxy-2-(2-methyl propyl)-3-oxo-1H-imidazo[1,2-α] indol-9-yl]methyl]guinazolino[3,2-α]1,4 benzodiazepine-5,13-dione [3,4,5].
[c] A-65186 = (*N*-[3′-quinolinoylcarbonyl]-D-Glu-N^{α},N^{α}-di-*n*-pentylamide) [33].

sulfate moiety in CCK in the 7th position from the COOH-terminus was essential in determining the ability of a CCK-related peptide to have high affinity for producing CCK-related actions [9,20,32,54]. Gastrin occurs naturally both with and without a sulfate moiety in the tyrosine in the 6th position from the COOH-terminus [32]. Gastrin's actions, such as stimulation of gastric acid secretion, were minimally affected by the presence of the sulfate and both forms had a very low potency for causing CCK-related actions such as stimulating pancreatic enzyme secretion or gallbladder contraction [9,18,32].

Both binding studies and studies of biological activity with agonists and antagonists demonstrate that there are CCK_A and CCK_B receptors [10,30,

Table 2. Proposed general classification of CCK receptors (modified from [30])

Type	Common name	Characteristic	Location (reference)
I.	CCK_A	1. CCK-8 = 500 × more potent $des(SO_3)CCK$-8 = 10 000 × CCK-4, gastrin[a] [24,30,56,67,71] 2. High affinity for antagonist L-364 718, A-65 186, CR 1409; low affinity for L-365 260 [4,19,33,36,37,71][b] 3. High affinity for selective agonist A-71 378; low affinity for A-72 962, cyclic cmpd II [7,35][c]	Pancreatic acini [24,37,71] Gallbladder muscle [54,58,63,67] Pancreatic islets [65] Rat anterior pituitary cells [51] Inhibitory neurons in LES [50] Area postrema and other CNS areas [10,46] Pyloric sphincter [60] AR4-2J tumor cells [57]
II.	CCK_B/gastrin	1. CCK-8 ≃ gastrin > CCK-4, $des(SO_3)CCK$-8 [6,22,40,55,70,71][a] 2. High affinity for antagonist L-365 260; low affinity for L-364 718 or CR 1409 [3,4,19,36,71][b] 3. High affinity for selective agonist A-72 962, cyclic cmpd II; low affinity for A-71 378 [7,35][c]	Cerebral cortex [18,22,55] GI smooth muscle [2,44] Parietal cells [61] Gastric chief cells [64] Gastric glands [6,49,61] Pancreatic acinar cells [12,70,71] AR4-2J tumor cells [57] Some human small cell lung cancer cell lines [69]

LES, lower esophageal sphincter
[a] *CCK-4* and *CCK-8* refer to the COOH-terminal tetra- and octapeptide of CCK.
[b] Structures for selective antagonists *L-364 718*, *A-65 186*, *CR 1409* and *L-365 260* are shown in Table 1.
[c] Structures for selective agonists *A-71 378*, *A-72 962* and *cyclic cmpd II* are shown in Table 3.

31,46] (Table 1). CCK_A receptors are characterized by having a high affinity only for CCK analogues that possess a sulfate in the 7th position from the COOH-terminus. In studies measuring both the ability of various CCK-related agonists to stimulate enzyme secretion from pancreatic acini or inhibit binding of radiolabeled CCK to pancreatic acinar cells or membranes [16,24,56], CCK-8 is 500 times more potent that desulfated CCK-8, and 10 000 times more potent than gastrin-17-I or CCK-4 (Table 2). Recently, selective agonists for CCK_A receptors, such as A-71 378 (Tables 2, 3), have been described that may be used increasingly to classify the type of CCK receptor mediating a particular response [35]. CCK_A receptors occur also on gallbladder muscle [54,58,63,67], rat anterior pituitary cells [51], inhibitory neurons of the lower esophageal sphincter (LES) [50], AR4-2J pancreatic tumor cells [57], islets of Langerhans [65], pyloric sphincter [60], myenteric

Table 3. Comparison of the affinities of various CCK receptor antagonists and agonists for CCK_A and CCK_B/gastrin receptors. Type of CCK receptors

	CCK_A K_i (μM)	CCK_B/gastrin K_i (μM)
Antagonist		
Bt_2cGMP	100 [1,24,67]	350–1700 [18,22,44,66,70,71]
CR 1409 (Lorglumide)[c]	0.15 [28,39,47,67,71]	30–300 [6,40,70]
CBZ-CCK-27-32-NH_2	2.7 [62,70]	3.3 [66,70,71]
BOC-[D-Trp^{30},Nle^{31}]-CCK-27-32-Phenylethyl ester	0.05 [34]	0.5 [34]
L-364718 (MK-329)[c]	0.0008–0.002 [4,19,37,67,71]	0.24–0.5 [4,71]
A-65186[c]	0.005 [33]	3.6 [33]
L-365260[c]	0.28 [3,19,36]	0.002 [3,19,36]
Agonist		
CCK-8[d]	0.001 [24,56,63,67]	0.4 [18,22,55]
Gastrin-17-I	2.5 [20,70,71]	0.0015 [20,70,71]
CCK-4[d]	29.1 [70,71]	0.1–0.65 [6,38,70,71] (pancrease, gastric cells) 0.05–0.1 [22,40] cerebral cortex
A-71378[a]	0.0004 [35]	0.3 [35]
A-72962[a]	0.11 [35]	0.0002 [35]
Cyclic cmpd II[b]	1.5 [7]	0.00092 [7]

[a] A-71318 = [des amino, $Nle^{28,31}$,*N*-Methyl-Asp^{32}]CCK-7 [35]; A-72962 = [des amino, Nle^{28},*N*-Methyl Leu^{31}]CCK-7[35].
[b] Cyclic cmpd II = BOC-8-D-Glu-Tyr(SO_3H)-Ahx-DLys-Trp-Ahx-Asp-Phe-NH_2, Ahx = 2-amino hexanoic acid [7].
[c] CR 1409, L-364718, A-65186, L-365260 (see Table 1 for structure).
[d] CCK-4 and CCK-8 refer to the COOH-terminal tetra- and octapeptide of CCK.

plexus [21], and the area postrema and other areas of the brain [10,46] (Table 1). CCK_B receptors have approximately equal affinities for CCK, gastrin-17-I (nonsulfated), and gastrin-17-II (sulfated), and, compared to CCK_A receptors, relatively high affinities for des(SO_3)CCK-8 and CCK-4 (Table 2). Recently, highly selective agonists for CCK_B receptors such as A-72962 [35] or cyclic cmpd II [7] (Tables 2, 3) have been described that may be increasingly used to classify the CCK_B receptors. Previously [31] we proposed that there are three functionally distinct classes of CCK receptors: CCK_A receptors, CCK_B receptors and gastrin receptors [30]. Because the functional characteristics of gastrin receptors are only marginally different from those of CCK_B receptors, it seems to us to be appropriate to group these receptors, for the purposes of this review, into a single type referred to as "CCK_B/gastrin receptors." It should be realized that development of selective agonists or antagonists for CCK_B receptors, or gastrin receptors, or determination of the receptor amino acid sequences, will be necessary to confirm or deny the existence of three classes of CCK receptors. CCK_B/gastrin receptors are widely distributed in the CNS and are present on parietal cells, gastric chief cells, gastric glands, gastrointestinal smooth muscle, pancreatic acinar cells, AR4-2J pancreatic tumor cells, and some human small cell lung cancer cell lines [2,6,8,19,38,44,57,61,69,70] (Table 2).

In the initial in vitro characterization of the ability of various substances to function as CCK_A receptor antagonists, the functional and binding studies were usually done using pancreatic acini or membranes. In vitro characterization of the abilities of various substances to function as CCK_B receptor antagonists has been complicated by the fact that the biologic function of the CCK_B/gastrin receptors in the CNS is in general unknown. Therefore, in vitro affinity for CCK_B/gastrin receptors was usually assessed by binding studies to cerebral cortical membranes, gastric glands or gastric mucosal membranes, and functional studies on the ability of the substances to inhibit gastrin-stimulated acid secretion in vitro or in vivo.

CCK-Receptor Antagonists In Vitro: General Features

The five different classes of inhibitors (Table 1) of the action of CCK in vitro show several common features. Each class functions as a full antagonist and there is no partial agonist activity in most species. Each class inhibits CCK-stimulated amylase secretion, CCK-stimulated mobilization of cellular calcium, and the binding of ^{125}I-BH-CCK to pancreatic CCK receptors (Fig. 1). For each class the inhibition is reversible and occurs whether the antagonist is added prior to, or after, the addition of the agonist. The inhibitory action of each class, except the D-amino acid substituted substance P-4-11 analogues, is specific for the CCK receptor. In particular, for each class of CCK receptor antagonist in pancreatic acinar cells, the antagonist inhibits the stimulation by CCK-related peptides [28], but has no effect on stimulation by carbachol, bombesin, substance P, or VIP, which interact with distinct receptors, or the calcium ionophore A23 187, which has a postreceptor mechanism of action [15,23,28,37,62]. For each class of antagonist the inhibition is competitive in nature, similar to that shown in Fig. 2 for CR 1409 [28]. Increasing concentrations of the antagonist causes a parallel rightward shift of the dose-response curve for the ability of CCK-8 to stimulate amylase release with no change in the maximal release (Fig. 2, left), and a Schild plot of the data demonstrated a slope not significantly different from unity for CR 1409 (Fig. 2, right). Furthermore, for each class of antagonist there was a very close correlation for the dose-response curves for the ability of the antagonist to inhibit the binding of ^{125}I-BH-CCK to the pancreatic CCK_A receptors and to inhibit CCK-stimulated amylase release

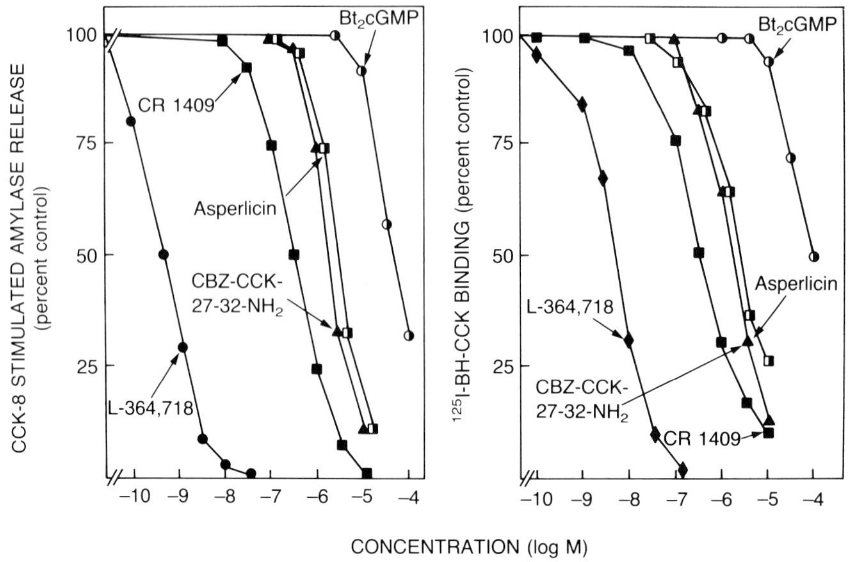

Fig. 1. Comparison of the abilities of various classes of CCK receptor antagonists to inhibit CCK-8-stimulated amylase release (*left panel*) and binding of ^{125}I-BH-CCK-8 (*right panel*) to CCK_A receptors on guinea pig pancreatic acini. (Data from [70,71])

(Fig. 1) or calcium mobilization [15,16,37,67,71]. Each CCK receptor antagonist also interacts with both CCK_A and CCK_B/gastrin receptors; however, some have more selectivity for one type than the others (Table 3).

CCK-Receptor Antagonists In Vitro: Results with Specific Classes

Cyclic Nucleotide Derivatives

Dibutyryl guanosine 3′, 5′-cyclic monophosphate (Bt_2cGMP) is the most potent member of this class and was the first CCK receptor antagonist described [48]. Since this report Bt_2cGMP was found to be a specific inhibitor of the action of CCK in a number of tissues including gallbladder muscle, gastric smooth muscle, gastric chief and parietal cells and the myenteric plexus [15]. Subsequent studies in pancreatic acinar cells examining the interaction of CCK with CCK_A receptors demonstrated that the unsubstituted cyclic nucleotide had no inhibitory action; however, other substituted cyclic nucleotides of cAMP, cIMP or cGMP also functioned as CCK_A receptor antagonists [1,52]. The dibutyryl moiety was not essential for antagonism as 8-bromo-derivatives also caused inhibition; however, of 15 different cyclic analogues tested, Bt_2cGMP was the most potent [1,52]. Even though Bt_2cGMP was specific in action and useful in certain in vitro

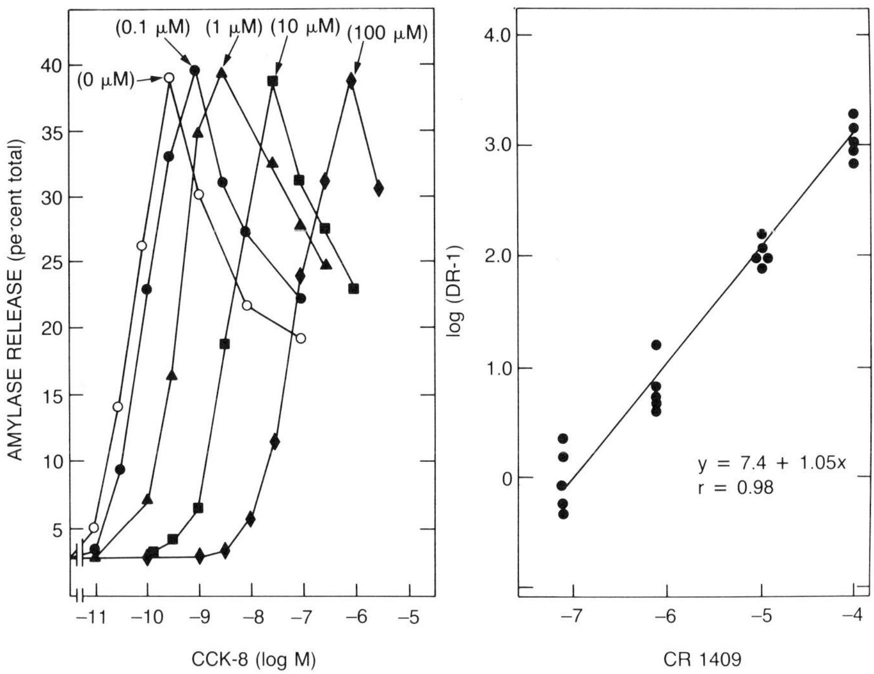

Fig. 2. Effect of increasing concentrations of the CCK receptor antagonist, CR 1409 (lorglumide), on CCK-8-stimulated amylase release (*left panel*), and a Schild plot (*right panel*) of the results. (Data from [28].) *Numbers* in parenthesis in the *left panel* are the concentration of CR 1409 (lorglumide) present. In the *right panel*, results from five experiments are shown and the best fit line determined by linear regression

studies, because of its low potency ($K_i = 0.1\,mM$, Tables 1, 3) the cyclic nucleotides were not useful generally for in vivo experiments.

Subsequent studies have demonstrated that Bt_2cGMP also interacts with CCK_B receptors (Fig. 3, Table 3). Bt_2cGMP was reported to have a 10- to 100-fold lower affinity for the CNS CCK_B/gastrin receptor and to be 10-fold less potent for CCK_B/gastrin receptors in the GI tract than for CCK_A receptors on pancreatic acini [4,6,66,70]. Although the mechanism of the ability of Bt_2cGMP to function as a CCK receptor antagonist has been debated [14,15], at least two studies demonstrated inhibition of binding of ^{125}I-BH-CCK or ^{125}I-gastrin to antibodies that recognized the C-terminal of CCK, suggesting that the Bt_2cGMP might have a similar structural configuration to CCK [1,52].

Amino Acid Derivatives

In 1981, Hahne et al. [17] reported that proglumide (DL-4-benzamido-*N*, *N*-di-*n*-propylglutaramic acid) as well as benzotript (*N*-*p*-chlorobenzoyl-L-

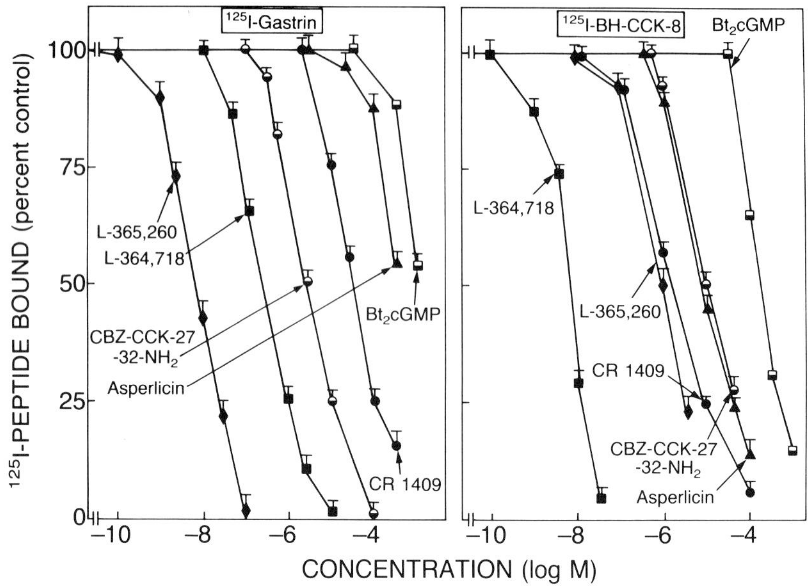

Fig. 3. Comparison of the abilities of various classes of CCK receptor antagonists to inhibit binding of ^{125}I-labeled gastrin-17-I to CCK_B/gastrin receptors (*left panel*) or ^{125}I-BH-labeled-CCK-8 to pancreatic CCK_A receptors (*right panel*). Guinea pig pancreatic acini were incubated with 150 p*M* ^{125}I-gastrin-17-I or 50 p*M* ^{125}I-BH-CCK-8 plus 0.1 μ*M* gastrin, conditions under which ^{125}I-gastrin-17-I only binds to CCK_B/gastrin receptors and ^{125}I-BH-CCK-8 to CCK_A receptors. (Data from [70,71])

tryptophan) functioned as CCK_A receptor antagonists. Benzotript was 1.5 times more potent than proglumide and proglumide was fivefold (K_i = 0.4 m*M*) less potent than Bt_2cGMP (Table 1). Proglumide in vitro has subsequently been shown to antagonize the action of CCK on gastric muscle, ileal muscle, gallbladder muscle, satiety, and in the CNS [15]. Structure-function studies of benzotript-related peptides demonstrated that the inhibitory activity was not limited to the benzoyl derivative of tryptophan, with numerous other acyl derivatives of L-tryptophan able to function as CCK receptor antagonists [25]. The inhibitory ability was not restricted to tryptophan analogues and most CBZ-substituted amino acids function as CCK antagonists with CBZ-cystine (K_i = 0.1 m*M*) being the most potent and approximately equally potent to Bt_2cGMP (K_i = 0.1 m*M*) (Table 1) [43]. The sterospecificity of the amino acid moiety was not important [25] but the hydrophobicity of the amino acid side chain was important in determining potency [43].

Whereas derivatives of tryptophan or other CBZ-amino acids were not more potent than Bt_2cGMP, relatively minor modifications of either the dialkyl amide or the benzoyl moieties of proglumide gave rise to several compounds that were more potent at inhibiting the action of CCK on

CCK_A receptors on pancreatic acini or gallbladder muscle [13,27,28,39–41]. Replacement of the benzoyl moiety with either a phenoxyacetyl group or *p*-chloro-phenoxyacetyl group [27] resulted in a 75-fold increase in potency (Tables 1, 4). A large number of proglumide analogues have been tested for their abilities to interact with CCK_A receptors on gallbladder muscle or pancreatic acinar cells. CR 1409 (lorglumide), the di-*n*-pentyl 3,4-dichloro analogue of proglumide, was one of the most potent proglumide derivatives, having a K_i of 0.1–0.3 μ*M* in guinea pig, rat and mouse pancreas, and in each species was 1500–4000 times more potent than proglumide [28, 39–41,47] (Tables 1, 4). Structure-function studies demonstrated that for both the pancreatic and gallbladder CCK_A receptors, alterations in both the di-*n*-alkyl group and substitutions on the benzoyl moiety of proglumide are equally important determinants of affinity for the CCK receptor (Table 4). Specifically, for the di-*n*-alkyl groups there was an optimum chain length with relative potencies of di-*n*-pentyl > di-*n*-hexyl > di-*n*-butyl > di-*n*-propyl. For the benzoyl moiety, adding two electron withdrawing groups increased potency more than adding a single electron withdrawing group or adding electron donating groups [28,39–41].

Studies have reported that proglumide and its derivatives also interact with CCK_B/gastrin receptors, with the relative affinities compared to those for CCK_A receptors differing for the different proglumide derivatives. For the CNS CCK_B/gastrin receptor, proglumide had a similar affinity to that for pancreatic CCK_A receptors [66], CR 1409 (lorglumide) (Table 3) had a 400-fold higher affinity for CCK_A receptors on pancreatic acini than for the CCK_B/gastrin receptors in the CNS, whereas CR 1392 had a 1660-fold higher, and CR 1372 a 39-fold higher, affinity for the CCK_A receptor [40]. For CCK_B/gastrin receptors in the GI tract, proglumide varied from being equivalent to ten-fold less potent than for that of CCK_A receptors [4,6,38, 61,70]. In contrast, CR 1409 was greater than 10000 times more potent at inhibiting the ability of CCK to cause gallbladder contraction (CCK_A receptors) than inhibiting pentagastrin-stimulated acid output (CCK_B/gastrin receptors), whereas the proglumide analogues CR 1392 and CR 1372 were 333- and 95-times, respectively, less potent for inhibiting acid secretion than gallbladder contraction [39–41]. In contrast to proglumide, which interacts with approximately equally low affinity with each class of CCK receptors, CR 1409 and analogue CR 1392 are much more selective for CCK_A receptors, each having a greater than 300-fold higher affinity for CCK_A than either CCK_B/gastrin receptors in the CNS or the GI tract (Table 3).

COOH-terminal Analogues of CCK: In Vitro Studies

This class of CCK receptor antagonists was first described in studies on pancreatic acini in 1983 when it was reported that both CCK fragments containing the last one, two or three amino acids of the COOH-terminus (phenylalanine amide, CCK-32-33, CCK-31-33) [26], as well as an analogue containing a partial sequence of the COOH-terminus of CCK (CBZ-CCK-27-32-NH_2) [62], functioned as specific CCK receptor antagonists. Structure-function studies of the COOH-terminal fragments of CCK demonstrated that the addition of a butyloxycarbonyl (BOC) moiety increased the affinity as much as 75-fold for the CCK_A receptor; however, the most potent CCK fragment described, BOC-CCK-31-33, had an affinity that was approximately equal to proglumide (Table 1, $K_i - 0.4\,mM$) [26]. Structure-function studies were also carried out, determining the affinity of partial sequences of the COOH-terminal region of CCK for the CCK_A receptor. AC-CCK-26-30-NH_2 was the minimal partial sequence with inhibitory activity. Adding acyl groups to the amino terminus did not increase potency. Removing the COOH-terminal amide decreased potency tenfold. The importance of the sulfate ester depended on the length of the partial CCK sequence [15,16]. Specifically, for the CCK_A receptor, for longer partial sequences such as AC-CCK-26-32-NH_2, removing the sulfate ester caused a tenfold decrease in potency, whereas for shorter sequences such as AC-CCK-26-30-NH_2, removing the sulfate ester had no effect on potency [15]. Recently, it has been demonstrated that BOC-Tyr(SO_3)-Met-Gly-D-Trp-Nle-Asp-2-phenylethyl ester (BOC-[D-Trp^{30},Nle^{31}]-CCK-27-32-phenylethy ester) (Table 1) functions as a specific CCK_A receptor antagonist in rat and guinea pig pancreas [34]. At present, this analogue is one of the most potent members of the COOH-terminal CCK analogue class of antagonists (Table 1).

COOH-terminal CCK analogues have been shown also to interact with CCK_B/gastrin receptors. Some members of this class of antagonists appear to have very little selectivity for one type of CCK receptor with the affinity of a given analogue for the various receptors generally not varying by more than tenfold. Specifically, CBZ-CCK-27-32-NH_2 has been shown to have equal affinity for CCK_A receptors and CCK_B/gastrin receptors in the CNS or GI tract ($K_i = 3\,\mu M$) [4,6,66,70]. One analogue, [D-Trp^{30},Nle^{31}]-CCK-27-32- phenylethyl ester, has been shown to have a 50-fold higher affinity for CCK_A receptors ($K_i = 0.05\,\mu M$, Table 1) than CCK_B/gastrin receptors in the CNS [34]. Gastrin and CCK have the same COOH-terminal pentapeptide, and the COOH-terminal tetrapeptide of CCK (CCK-4) possesses the full range of biological activity of gastrin at CCK_B/gastrin receptors, whereas it has a greater than 10000-fold lower affinity and is only a partial agonist at CCK_A receptors [16,24,32,70,71]. A number of des Met analogues of CCK-4 have been shown to be potent antagonists of the action of gastrin at CCK_B/gastrin receptors [42].

D-Amino Acid Substituted Substance P-4-11 Analogues

Various D-amino acid substituted substance P (SP)-4-11 analogues that function as substance P receptor antagonist and bombesin receptor antagonists also inhibit the action of CCK on CCK_A receptors [29,72]. [D-Pro^4,D-Trp^{7,9,10}]SP-4-11 and [D-Pro^4,D-Trp^{7,9}]SP-4-11, but not the SP receptor antagonists [D-Arg^1,D-Trp^{7,9},Leu^{11}]SP (spantide), each inhibit the action of CCK-8 by functioning as CCK receptor antagonists [29,72]. Each SP-4-11 analogue inhibited binding of ^{125}I-BH-CCK-8 to CCK$_A$ receptors on pancreatic acini over the same range as that in which it inhibited biologic activity; the inhibition was competitive in nature and the Schild plot had a slope not different from unity, also suggesting inhibition was mediated by occupying the CCK$_A$ receptor [72]. These analogues also inhibit SP and bombesin-stimulated amylase release by occupying SP and bombesin receptors [29,72]; however, their action was specific for these three receptors (CCK$_A$, bombesin and SP), because they did not inhibit the action of other secretagogues [29,72]. The basis for the broad inhibitory action of these peptides is not known, nor whether they also function as CCK$_B$/gastrin receptor antagonists. The low affinity of this group of CCK receptor antagonists and their relative lack of specificity make it unlikely that this class of antagonists will be useful for in vivo studies.

Substituted Benzodiazepines and Related Compounds

Asperlicin, originally isolated from the fungus, *Aspergillus alliaceus*, was described in 1985 as functioning as a specific CCK$_A$ receptor antagonist inhibiting the action of CCK on pancreas, gallbladder and ileum [5]. Subsequent structure-function studies of asperlicin, as well as studies which involved combining the 1,4-benzodiazepine ring found in asperlicin with L-tryptophan, an important amino acid in the COOH-terminal of CCK, led to a number of substituted 1,4-benzodiazepine derivatives with high affinities for CCK$_A$ receptors [11]. L-364 718, a 3-(acylamino) benzodiazepine analogue (Table 1), was one of the most potent analogues found [11]. L-364 718 (MK-329) is currently the most potent antagonist generally used to characterize CCK$_A$ receptors, and is reported to cause half-maximal inhibition of ^{125}I-BH-CCK-8 binding to rat pancreas at 0.08–0.5 nM, bovine gallbladder at 0.05 nM, and guinea pig pancreatic acini at 3 nM (Table 1) [4,37,71]. L-364 718, A-65 186 and asperlicin are highly selective for CCK$_A$ receptors [3,4,5,19] having at least a 500-fold greater affinity for CCK$_A$ receptors than CCK$_B$/gastrin receptors.

Recently, a new series of benzodiazepine analogues has been described, one of which (the 3-(benzoylamino) benzodiazepine analogue, L-365 260), has high selectivity for CCK$_B$/gastrin receptors in the CNS or GI tract [3]. L-365 260 has a 140- to 280-fold higher affinity for CCK$_B$/gastrin receptors than CCK$_A$ receptors, and functions in the nanomolar range [3,19,30,36].

Selectivity of CCK Receptor Antagonists

All five classes of CCK receptor antagonists will interact with each class of CCK receptor antagonist if sufficiently high concentrations are used. Table 3 summarizes the ability of the most potent members of the various classes of receptor antagonists to interact with CCK_A and CCK_B/gastrin receptors. L-364 718 has the greatest affinity for CCK_A receptors on various tissues – an affinity approximately 5-fold higher than that of A-65 186, 50-fold higher than BOC-[D-Trp^{30},Nle^{31}]CCK-27-32-phenylethyl ester, 150-fold higher than CR 1409, 100–280–fold higher than L-365 260, 2700-fold higher than CBZ-CCK-27-32-NH_2, and 100 000-fold greater than Bt_2cGMP (Tables 1, 3; Fig. 3) [4,19,31,34,37,71]. Of the various antagonists, L-365 260 has the highest affinity (K_i = 1–7 nM) for CCK_B/gastrin receptors in the CNS or GI tract (Table 3) [3,19,36]. Comparison of the abilities of the various antagonists to interact with CCK_A receptors or CCK_B/gastrin receptors on guinea pig pancreatic acini are shown in Fig. 3. L-365 260 has an approximately 100-fold higher affinity for both CCK_B/gastrin receptors in the CNS or GI tract than L-364 718 or BOC-[D-Trp^{30},Nle^{31}]CCK-27-32-phenylethyl ester, a 700-fold higher affinity than carbobenzoxy-CCK-27-32-NH_2, an 1800-fold higher affinity than A-65 186, a 6000-fold higher affinity than CR 1409, and a 160 000-fold greater affinity than Bt_2cGMP (Table 3) [3,19,30,34,36,70,71].

In comparing the relative affinities of the different types of CCK receptor antagonists for the two different classes of CCK receptors, a number of points can be made. L-364 718, A-65 186 and CR 1409 (lorglumide) have a high selectivity for CCK_A receptors (Table 3). L-364 718 has a 120- to 3300-fold, A-65 186 a 720-fold, and CR 1409 (lorglumide) a 120- to 2307-fold higher affinity for CCK_A receptors than for CCK_B/gastrin receptors [5,6, 36,40,71]. In contrast, Bt_2cGMP and BOC-[D-Trp^{30}, Nle^{31}]-CCK-27-32-phenylethyl ester have only an eight- to tenfold higher affinity for CCK_A receptors (Table 3). The affinities of these potent and selective antagonists, L-364 718, A-65 186, and L-365 260, for CCK_A receptors and CCK_B/gastrin receptors, respectively, were comparable to that of the naturally occurring agonists, gastrin or CCK-8, respectively. Specifically, the K_d of L-364 718 for the pancreatic CCK_A receptor was in the nanomolar range and varied from equipotent to sevenfold less potent than CCK-8 [4,6,19,36,37,71]. Similarly, the K_d of L-365 260 for the CCK_B/gastrin receptors was in the nanomolar range, and was two- to fourfold less than gastrin in different studies [3,19, 31,36]. Because of their selectivity and high affinity relative to the presumed endogenous agonist, it is likely that L-365 260, A-65 186, and L-364 718 will prove useful in distinguishing different types of CCK receptors even when present on the same cell. Recently, a number of cells have been shown to possess both CCK_B/gastrin and CCK_A receptors, including pancreatic acini, guinea pig chief cells and the pancreatic AR4-2J tumor cell line [7,8,57,71]. Because the various peptides of the gastrin/CCK family can interact with both types of CCK receptors, in tissues possessing both types of receptors it may be difficult to determine which effect of a given peptide in this family is due to occupation of which receptor. It is likely that similar situations exist in vivo, with both CCK_A and CCK_B/gastrin receptors existing on neuronal elements or on the effector, such as muscle tissue.

Some results suggest that there may be different subtypes of CCK_A receptors. Various CCK analogues, such as Suc-[Trp^{29}]-CCK-7, have different potencies for stimulating gallbladder contraction and pancreatic enzyme release [68]. Similarly, a recent study reported that the ability of some analogues of proglumide to inhibit CCK-stimulated pancreatic amylase release differed from those reported previously by another group for the ability of the same proglumide analogues to inhibit gallbladder contraction mediated by CCK_A receptors [30]. Furthermore, recent studies characterizing CCK_A receptors by chemical cross-linking techniques demonstrate that the size of the bovine gallbladder CCK receptor was M_r-70 000–85 000 which differed from that in rat pancreas which was M_r-85 000–95 000 [59]. In addition, CCK_A receptors on pancreatic acini differ from CCK_A receptors on gallbladder muscle in that in all species examined [16,56,71] more than one binding site are found, whereas in the gallbladder muscle only a single binding site is described [63,67]. Each of these results raised the possibility that the CCK_A receptors on gallbladder or pancreas might represent different subtypes of the CCK_A receptor. These comparisons, however, are limited because data from different species were compared under different experimental conditions. However, the results suggesting differences in subtypes of CCK_A receptors on pancreatic and gallbladder are supported by studies comparing results characterizing CCK_A receptors on rat anterior pituitary cells and rat pancreatic acini [51]. For stimulation of pancreatic secretion, desulfated CCK-8 was 1000-fold, and gastrin 3000-fold, less potent than CCK-8, whereas for adrenocorticotropic hormone (ACTH) release from anterior pituitary cells, des(SO_3)CCK-8 was 10 000-fold and gastrin-17-I 30 000-fold, less potent than CCK-8 [51].

Recently, the abilities of various agonists and antagonists to interact with CCK_A receptors on guinea pig pancreas and gallbladder were investigated using identical binding conditions [67]. The ability of various CCK receptor agonists and antagonists to inhibit binding of ^{125}I-BH-CCK-8 to pancreatic tissue sections using this method was shown not to be significantly different from that for inhibition of binding to pancreatic acini [67]. The abilities of some of the compounds to inhibit ^{125}I-BH-CCK-8 binding to gallbladder and pancreas tissue sections are shown in Fig. 4 (for antagonists) and Table 4 (for antagonists and agonists). As is evident, the abilities of agonists or antagonists to inhibit binding to each tissue agree closely. For both gallbladder and pancreas, L-364 718 was the most potent, being 150 times more potent than CR 1409, 400 times more potent than asperlicin, 700 times more potent than CBZ-CCK-27-32-NH_2 and 65 100 times more potent than Bt_2cGMP (Table 4). Comparison of the ability of 11 different proglumide analogues to inhibit binding of radiolabeled CCK-8 to gallbladder and pancreas tissue sections also demonstrated no significant differences between the potencies for inhibiting binding to either tissue [67] (Table 4). For the agonists, the potencies of each for inhibiting binding of ^{125}I-BH-CCK-8 to gallbladder and pancreas tissue sections were also nearly

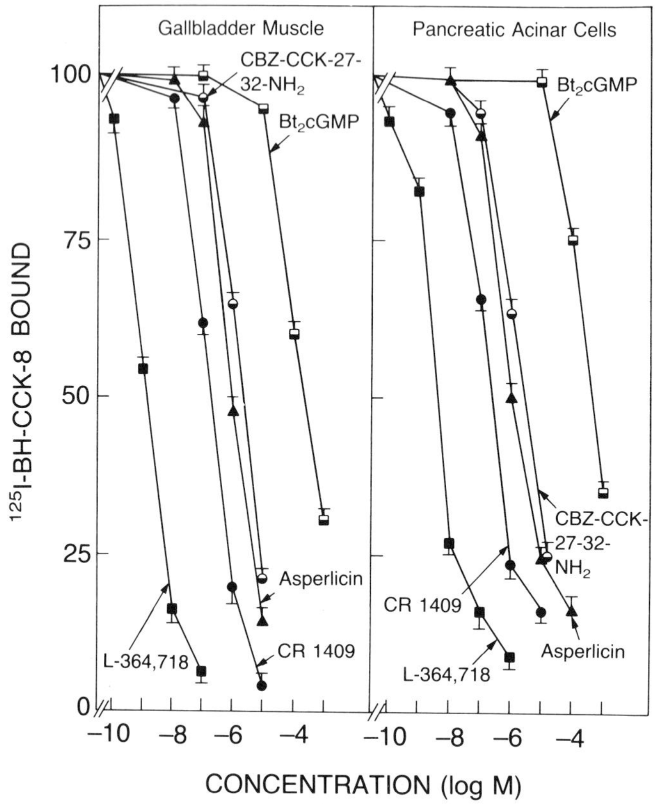

Fig. 4. Comparison of the abilities of various classes of CCK receptor antagonists to inhibit binding of ^{125}I-BH-CCK-8 to CCK_A receptors on guinea pig gallbladder (*left panel*) or pancreas (*right panel*) tissue sections. (Data from [67])

identical (Table 4). CCK-8 was the most potent for inhibiting binding to both gallbladder and pancreas tissue sections, with des(SO_3)CCK-8 being 300-fold less potent and gastrin 2500-fold less potent than CCK-8 (Table 4). These results demonstrate that CCK_A receptors on pancreatic receptors cannot be distinguished pharmacologically by currently available agonists or antagonists, and provide no functional evidence that they represent different subtypes of CCK_A receptors.

Finally, pancreatic acini studies of binding of ^{125}I-BH-CCK-8 as well as CCK-8-stimulated enzyme secretion (for review see [16]) indicate that there are high and low affinity CCK_A receptors on pancreatic acini. All CCK receptor antagonists described to date have the same apparent affinity for the high affinity as for the low affinity binding sites of the pancreatic CCK_A receptors [19,71].

Table 4. Comparison of the ability of various CCK receptor antagonists and agonists to interact with CCK_A receptors on gallbladder and pancreas

	K_i (μ*M*)			IC_{50} (μ*M*)	EC_{50} (μ*M*)
	Ability to inhibit binding of ^{125}I-BH-CCK-8 to tissue sections		Ability to inhibit binding of ^{125}I-BH-CCK-8 to pancreatic acini	Ability to inhibit 0.1 n*M* CCK-8-stimulated amylase release	Ability to inhibit 0.1 n*M* CCK-8-stimulated amylase release (EC_{50})
	Gallbladder	Pancreas			
Antagonist					
Bt_2cGMP	120 ± 28	130 ± 17	91 ± 17	120 ± 10	
CBZ-CCK-27-32-NH_2	1.8 ± 0.3	1.4 ± 0.3	2.7 ± 0.2	3 ± 1	
Proglumide analogues[c]					
di-*n*-propyl (CR 1287)	3.7 ± 0.3	4.6 ± 0.8	3.6 ± 1.2	2.7 ± 1.0	
di-*n*-butyl (CR 1404)	0.7 ± 0.3	0.8 ± 0.2	0.5 ± 0.1	0.61 ± 0.3	
di-*n*-pentyl (CR 1409)	0.2 ± 0.1	0.3 ± 0.1	0.2 ± 0.1	0.2 ± 0.1	
di-*n*-hexyl (CR 1413)	0.2 ± 0.1	1.0 ± 0.4	0.4 ± 0.1	0.4 ± 0.1	
L-364 718[a]	0.0015 ± 0.0002	0.002 ± 0.001	0.006 ± 0.001	0.003 ± 0.001	
Asperlicin[a]	0.8 ± 0.2	0.8 ± 0.1	1.3 ± 0.6	2.5 ± 1	
Agonist					
CCK-8[b]	0.0004 ± 0.0001	0.001 ± 0.0001	0.001 ± 0.0002	—	0.0001 ± 0.0000
des(SO_3)CCK-8	0.70 ± 0.02	0.300 ± 0.03	0.49 ± 0.2	—	0.49 ± 0.2
Gastrin-17-I	1.7 ± 0.3	2.5 ± 0.5	1.0 ± 0.3	—	1.0 ± 0.2

Data from [67,70,71].
[a] L-364 718, asperlicin – see Table 1 for structures.
[b] CCK-8 = COOH-terminal octapeptide of CCK.
[c] Proglumide – DL-4-benzamide-*N*,*N*-dipropylglutaramic acid; CR 1287 – 3,4-dichloro-di-*n*-propyl-derivative of proglumide; CR. 1404 – 3,4-dichloro-di-*n*-butyl derivative of proglumide; CR 1409 – 3,4-dichloro-di-*n*-pentyl derivative of proglumide; CR 1413 – 3,4-dichloro-di-*n*-hexyl derivative of proglumide [40,41].

References

1. Barlas N, Jensen RT, Beinfeld MC, Gardner JD (1982) Cyclic nucleotide antagonists of cholecystokinin: structural requirements for interaction with the cholecystokinin receptor. Am J Physiol 242:G161–G167
2. Bitar KN, Makhlouf GM (1982) Receptors on smooth muscle cells: characterization by contraction and specific antagonists. Am J Physiol 242:G400–G407
3. Bock MG, DiGardo RM, Evans BE, Rittle KE, Whitter WE, Veber DF, Anderson PS, Freidingger RM (1989) Benzodiazepine gastrin and cholecystokinin receptor ligands: L-365 260. J Med Chem 32:13–16
4. Chang RSL, Lotti VJ (1986) Biochemical and pharmacological characterization of an extremely potent and selective nonpeptide cholecystokinin antagonist. Proc Natl Acad Sci USA 83:4923–4926
5. Chang RSL, Lotti VJ, Monaghan RL, Birnbaum J, Stapley EO, Goetz MA, Albers-Schonberg G, Patchett AA, Liesch JM, Hensens OD, Springer JP (1985) A potent nonpeptide cholecystokinin antagonist selective for peripheral tissues isolated from Aspergillus Allicaceus. Science 230:177–179
6. Chang RSL, Lotti VJ, Keenan ME, Kristie KA (1986) Characterization of (^{3}H) pentagastrin binding in guinea pig gastric glands. Biochem Biophys Res Commun 134:895–899
7. Charpentier B, Pelaprat D, Durieux C, Dor A, Reibaud M, Blanchard J-C, Rogues BP (1988) Cyclic cholecystokinin analogues with high selectivity for central receptors. Proc Natl Acad Sci USA 85:1968–1972
8. Cherner JA, Sutliff VE, Grybowski DA, Jensen RT, Gardner JD (1988) Functionally distinct receptors for cholecystokinin and gastrin on dispersed chief cells from guinea pig stomach. Am J Physiol 254:G151–G155
9. De Castiglione R (1977) Structure-activity relationships in ceruletide-like peptides. In: Bonfils S, Fromageot P, Rosselin G (eds) 1st International symposium on hormonal receptors in digestive tract physiology. Elsevier/North-Holland, New York, pp 33–42
10. Durieux C, Coppey M, Zajac JM, Roques B (1986) Occurrence of two cholecystokinin binding sites in guinea pig brain cortex. Biochem Biophys Res Commun 137:1167–1173
11. Evans BE, Brock MG, Rittle KE, DiPardo RM, Whittier WL, Veber DF, Anderson PS, Freidinger RM (1986) Design of potent, orally effective, nonpeptidal antagonists of the peptide hormone cholecystokinin. Proc Natl Acad Sci USA 83:4918–4922
12. Fourmy D, Zahid A, Fabre R, Pradayrol L, Ribet A (1987) Receptors for cholecystokinin and gastrin peptides display specific binding properties and are structurally different in guinea pig and dog pancreas. Eur J Biochem 165: 683–692
13. Freidinger RM, Whitter WK, Gould NP, Holloway MK, Chang RSL, Lotti VJ (1990) Novel glutamic acid derived cholecystokinin receptor ligands. J Med Chem 33:591–595
14. Gardner JD (1983) Mechanism by which dibutyryl cyclic guanosine monophosphate antagonizes the action of cholecystokinin. Gastroenterology 85:1619–1621
15. Gardner JD, Jensen RT (1984) Cholecystokinin receptor antagonists. Am J Physiol 246:G471–G476
16. Gardner JD, Jensen RT (1987) Secretagogue receptors on pancreatic acinar cells. In: Johnson LR (ed) Physiology of the gastrointestinal tract, 2nd edn. Raven, New York, pp 1109–1127
17. Hahne WF, Jensen RT, Lemp GF, Gardner JD (1981) Proglumide and benzotript: members of a different class of cholecystokinin receptor antagonists. Proc Natl Acad Sci USA 78:6304–6308

18. Hays SE, Beinfeld MC, Jensen RT, Goodwin FIC, Paul SM (1980) Demonstration of a putative receptor site for cholecystokinin in rat brain. Neuropeptides 1:53–62
19. Huang SC, Zhang L, Chiang HCV, Wank SA, Maton PN, Gardner JD, Jensen RT (1989) Comparison of the ability of the 3-substituted 1,4 benzodiazapine analogues L-365260 and L-364718 to function as gastrin and pancreatic CCK receptor antagonists. Am J Physiol 257:G169–G174
20. Huang SC, Yu D-H, Wank SA, Mantey S, Gardner JD, Jensen RT (1989) Importance of sulfation of gastrin or cholecystokinin (CCK) on affinity or gastrin and CCK receptors. Peptides 10:785–789
21. Hutchinson JB, Dockray GB (1980) The inhibition of action of cholecystokinin octapeptide on the guinea pig myenteric plexus by dibutyryl cyclic guanosine monophosphate. Brain Res 20:501–505
22. Innes RB, Synder S (1980) Cholecystokinin receptors in brain and pancreas. Proc Natl Acad Sci USA 77:6917–6921
23. Jensen RT, Gardner JD (1981) Identification and characterization of receptors for secretagogues on pancreatic acinar cells. Fed Proc 40:2486–2496
24. Jensen RT, Lemp GF, Gardner JD (1980) Interaction of cholecystokinin with specific membrane receptors on pancreatic acinar cells. Proc Natl Acad Sci USA 77:2079–2083
25. Jensen RT, Jones SW, Gardner JD (1983) Structure-function studies of N-acyl derivatives of tryptophan that function as specific cholecystokinin receptor antagonists. Biochim Biophys Acta 761:269–277
26. Jensen RT, Jones SW, Gardner JD (1983) COOH-terminal fragments of cholecystokinin receptor antagonists. Biochim Biophys Acta 757:250–258
27. Jensen RT, Murphy RB, Trampota M, Schneider LH, Jones SW, Howard JM, Gardner JD (1985) Proglumide analogues: potent cholecystokinin receptor antagonists. Am J Physiol 249:G214–G220
28. Jensen RT, Zhou Z-C, Murphy RB, Jones SW, Setnikar I, Rovati LA, Gardner JD (1986) Structural features of various proglumide-related cholecystokinin receptor antagonists. Am J Physiol 251:G839–G846
29. Jensen RT, Heinz-Erian P, Jones SW, Mantey S, Gardner JD (1988) Mechanism of the ability of various substance P antagonists to inhibit the action of bombesin. Am J Physiol 254:G883–G890
30. Jensen RT, Wank SA, Rowley WH, Sato S, Gardner JD (1989) Interaction of CCK with pancreatic acinar cells. Trends Pharmacol Sci 10:418–423
31. Jensen RT. Huang SC, von Schrenck T, Wank SA, Gardner JD (1990) Cholecystokinin receptor antagonists: ability to distinguish various classes of cholecystokin receptors. In: Thompson JC (ed) Gastrointestinal endocrinology: receptors and post-receptor mechanisms. Academic, New York, pp 95–133
32. Jorpes JE, Mutt V (1973) Secretin and cholecystokinin (CCK). In: Jorpes JE, Mutt V (eds) Secretin, cholecystokinin, pancreozymin and gastrin. Springer Berlin Heidelberg, New York, pp 1–179
33. Kerwin JF, Nadzan AM, Kopecka H, Lin CW, Miller T, Witte D, Burt S (1989) Cholecystokinin (CCK) antagonists: new implications in the design and modification of CCK antagonists. J Med Chem 32:730–742
34. Lignon M-F, Galas M-C, Rodriquez M, Laur J, Aumelas A, Martinez J (1987) A synthetic peptide derivative that is a cholecystokinin receptor antagonist. J Biol Chem 262:7226–7231
35. Lin CW, Holladay, Witte DG, Miller TR, Wolfram CAW, Bianchi BR, Bennett MJ, Nadzan AM (1990) A71378: a CCK agonist with high potency and selectivity for CCK-A receptors. Am J Physiol 258:G648–G651
36. Lotti VJ, Chang RSL (1989) A new potent and selective non-peptide gastrin antagonist and brain cholecystokinin receptor (CCK-B) ligand: L-365260. Eur J Pharmacol 162:273–280

37. Louie DS, Liang J-P, Owyang C (1988) Characterization of a new antagonist, L-364718 in vitro and in vivo studies. Am J Physiol 255:G261–G266
38. Magous R, Bali J-P (1981) High affinity sites for gastrin on isolated rabbit gastric mucosal cells. Eur J Pharmacol 82:47–54
39. Makovec F, Christe R, Bani M, Pacini MA, Setnikar I, Rovati LA (1985) New glutaramic acid derivatives with potent competitive and specific cholecystokinin-antagonistic activity. Arzneimittelforschung 35:1048–1051
40. Makovec F, Bani M, Christe R, Revel L, Rovati LC, Rovati LA (1986) Differentiation of central and peripheral cholecystokinin receptors by new glutaramic acid derivatives with cholecystokinin-antagonistic activity. Arzneimittelforschung 36:98–101
41. Makovec F, Christe R, Bani M, Revel L, Setnikar I, Rovati AL (1986) New glutaramic and aspartic derivatives with potent CCK-antagonistic activity. Eur J Med Chem 21:9–20
42. Martinez J, Rodriquez M, Bali J-P, Laur J (1988) Phenylethyl ester derivatives analogues of the C-terminal tetrapeptide of gastrin as potent gastrin antagonists. J Med Chem 29:2201–2206
43. Maton PN, Sutliff VE, Jensen RT, Gardner JD (1985) Carbobenzoxy amino acids: structural requirements for cholecystokinin receptor antagonist activity. Am J Physiol 248:G479–G484
44. Menozzi D, Gardner JD, Jensen RT, Maton PN (1989) Properties of receptors for gastrin and CCK on gastrin smooth muscle cells. Am J Physiol 257:G73–G79
45. Miller LJ, Reilly WM, Rozenweig SA, Jamieson JD, Go VLW (1983) A soluble interaction between dibutyryl cyclic guanosine 3′:5′-monophosphate and cholecystokinin: a possible mechanism for the inhibition of cholecystokinin activity. Gastroenterology 84:1505–1511
46. Moran T, Robinson P, Goldrich M, McHugh PR (1986) Two brain cholecystokinin receptors: implication for behavioral actions. Brain Res 362:175–179
47. Niederau C, Niederau M, Williams JA, Grendell JH (1986) New proglumide-analogue CCK receptor antagonists: very potent and selective for peripheral tissues. Am J Physiol 251:G856–G860
48. Peikin SR, Costenbader CL, Gardner JD (1979) Actions of derivatives of cyclic nucleotides on dispersed acini from guinea pig pancreas: discovery of competitive antagonists of the action of cholecystokinin. J Biol Chem 254:5321–5327
49. Praissman M, Walen M (1984) The binding characteristics of ^{125}I-gastrin and ^{125}I-CCK-8 to guinea pig gastric glands differ. Biochem Biophys Res Commun 123:641–647
50. Rattan S, Goyal RK (1986) Structure-activity relationship of subtypes of cholecystokinin receptors in the cat lower esophageal sphincter. Gastroenterology 90:94–102
51. Reisine T, Jensen RT (1986) Cholecystokinin-8 stimulates adrenocorticotropin release from anterior pituitary cells. J Pharmacol Exp Ther 236:621–626
52. Robberecht P, Deschodt-Lanckman M, Woussen-Colle M-C, DeNeef P, Camus JC, Christophe J (1980) Butyryl derivatives of cyclic GMP interfere with the biological and immunological properties of the pancreozymin-gastrin family of peptides. Mol Pharmacol 17:268–274
53. Rovati LC, Makovec F (1988) New pentanoic acid derivatives with potent CCK antagonistic properties: different activity on the periphery vs central nervous system. Neurol Neurobiol 47:1–11
54. Rubin B, Engel SL (1972) Some biological characteristics of cholecystokinin (CCK-PZ) and synthetic analogs. Nobel Symp 16:41–56
55. Saito A, Sankaran H, Goldfine ID, Williams JA (1980) Cholecystokinin receptors in brain: characterization and distribution. Science 208:1155–1156
56. Sankaran H, Goldfine ID, Deveney CW, Wong K-Y, Williams JA (1980) Binding of cholecystokinin to high affinity receptors on isolated rat pancreatic acini. J Biol Chem 255:1849–1853

57. Scemama JL, de Vries L, Pradayrol K, Seva C, Trochere H, Vaysse N (1989) Cholecystokininin and gastrin peptides stimulate ODC activity in a rat pancreatic cell line. Am J Physiol 256:G846–G850
58. Schjoldager B, Shaw MJ, Powers SP, Schmalz P, Szurszewski J, Miller LJ (1988) Bovine gallbladder muscularis: source of a myogenic receptor for cholecytokinin. Am J Physiol 254:G294–G299
59. Shaw MJ, Hadac EM, Miller LJ (1987) Preparation of enriched plasma membranes from bovine gallbladder muscularis for characterization of cholecystokinin receptors. J Biol Chem 14:313–318
60. Smith GJ, Moran TH, Coyle JT, O'Donahue TL, McHugh RP (1984) Anatomic localization of cholecystokinin receptors to the pyloric sphincter. Am J Physiol 246:R127–R130
61. Soll AH, Amiran DA, Thomas LP, Reedy TJ, Elashoff JD (1984) Gastrin receptors on isolated canine parietal cells. J Clin Invest 73:1434–1447
62. Spanarkel M, Martinez J, Briet C, Jensen RT, Gardner JD (1983) Cholecystokinin-27-32-amide. A member of a new class of cholecystokinin receptor antagonists. J Biol Chem 258:6746–6749
63. Steigerwalt RW, Goldfine ID, Williams JA (1984) Characterization of cholecystokinin receptors on bovine gallbladder membranes. Am J Physiol 247:G709–G714
64. Sutliff A, Cherner JA, Jensen RT, Gardner JD (1990) Binding of ^{125}I-CCK-8 and ^{125}I-gastrin-I to dispersed chief cells from guinea pig stomach. Biochem Biophys Acta 1052:9–16
65. Verspohl EJ, Ammon HPT, Williams JA, Goldine ID (1986) Evidence that cholecystokinin interacts with specific receptors and regulates insulin release in rat islet of langerhans. Diabetes 35:38–43
66. Vigna SR, Szecowska J, Willians JA (1985) Do antagonists of pancreatic cholecystokinin receptors interact with central nervous system cholecystokinin receptors? Brain Res 343:394–397
67. Von Schrenck T, Moran TH, Heinz-Erian P, Gardner JD, Jensen RT (1988) Cholecystokinin receptors on gallbladder muscle and on pancreatic acinar cells. Am J Physiol 255:G512–G521
68. Yanaihara C, Sugiura N, Kashimoto K, Kondo M, Kawamura M, Naruse S, Yausi A, Yanaihara N (1985) Dissociation of pancreoszymin (PZ) activity from cholecystokinin (CCK) activity by N^a-carboxyacyl CCK-7 and CCK-8 analogues with a substituted glycine. Biomed Res 6:111–115
69. Yoder DG, Moody TW (1987) High affinity binding of cholecystokinin to small cell lung cancer cells. Peptides 8:103–107
70. Yu D-H, Noguchi M, Zhou Z-C, Villanueva ML, Gardner JD, Jensen RT (1987) Characterization of gastrin receptors on guinea pig pancreatic acini. Am J Physiol 253:G793–G801
71. Yu D-H, Huang SC, Wank SA, Mantey S, Gardner JD, Jensen RT (1990) Pancreatic receptors for cholecystokinin: evidence for interaction with 3 receptor classes. Am J Physiol 258:G86–G95
72. Zhang L, Mantey S, Jensen RT, Gardner JD (1988) An analogue of substance P with broad receptor antagonist activity. Biochem Biophys Acta 972:37–44

Effects of Cholecystokinin Receptor Antagonists in Animal Models*

C. Niederau, M. Niederau, R. Lüthen, G. Strohmeyer[1], and J.H. Grendell[2]

Effects of CCK Receptor Antagonists on Rat Pancreatic Secretion

Several peptide and nonpeptide compounds which have recently been described as CCK receptor antagonists in vitro [4–6,17,46] also act as specific antagonists of CCK's action on exocrine pancreatic secretion of protein and enzymes in vivo. The antagonists display the same rank order of potency in antagonizing CCK's action on the pancreas in vivo as that which they show in antagonizing CCK's action and binding in vitro [4–6,17,46] (Fig. 1). However, in particular, the most potent antagonists CR 1409 and L-364718 were 10–33 times less potent in vivo than in vitro. The effects of antagonists on the pancreatic CCK receptor are similar to those recently reported for antagonism of CCK's action on gastric emptying [17] where a similar difference between in vitro and in vivo potencies had been reported for CR 1409 and L-364718. The reason for the lower in vivo potencies of both peptide and nonpeptide antagonists in relation to their in vitro potencies is unknown. It has been speculated that proglumide (and probably other substances with low in vitro potencies) may be metabolized in vivo to more potent entities [17]. However, very potent antagonists such as CR 1409 or L-364718 may just as well be metabolized in vivo to less active entities. Although CCK antagonists possess different potencies in antagonizing binding of CCK to peripheral and central CCK receptors, suggesting that the peripheral and central CCK receptors appear to be different [5,6,46], the similarity of their effects on pancreatic versus gastric functions suggests that the peripheral type of CCK receptor is similar at different organs.

Experiments studying effects of the antagonists on secretin-stimulated secretion suggest that the CCK antagonists also show specificity for the CCK

* Dr. Claus Niederau was supported by grants from the Deutsche Forschungsgemeinschaft (Ni 224/1-1, 224/2-1 and 224/2-2) and from the Minister für Wissenschaft und Forschung des Landes Nordrhein-Westfalen. Dr. James H. Grendell was supported by a grant from the National Institute of Health (DK 38939).

[1]Medizinische Klinik und Poliklinik, Abteilung für Gastroenterologie, Heinrich-Heine-Universität, 4000 Düsseldorf, FRG; and [2]Depts. of Medicine, Physiology, and Pathology, University of California, San Francisco, CA 94143, USA.

G. Adler and C. Beglinger (Eds.)
CCK Antagonists in Gastroenterology

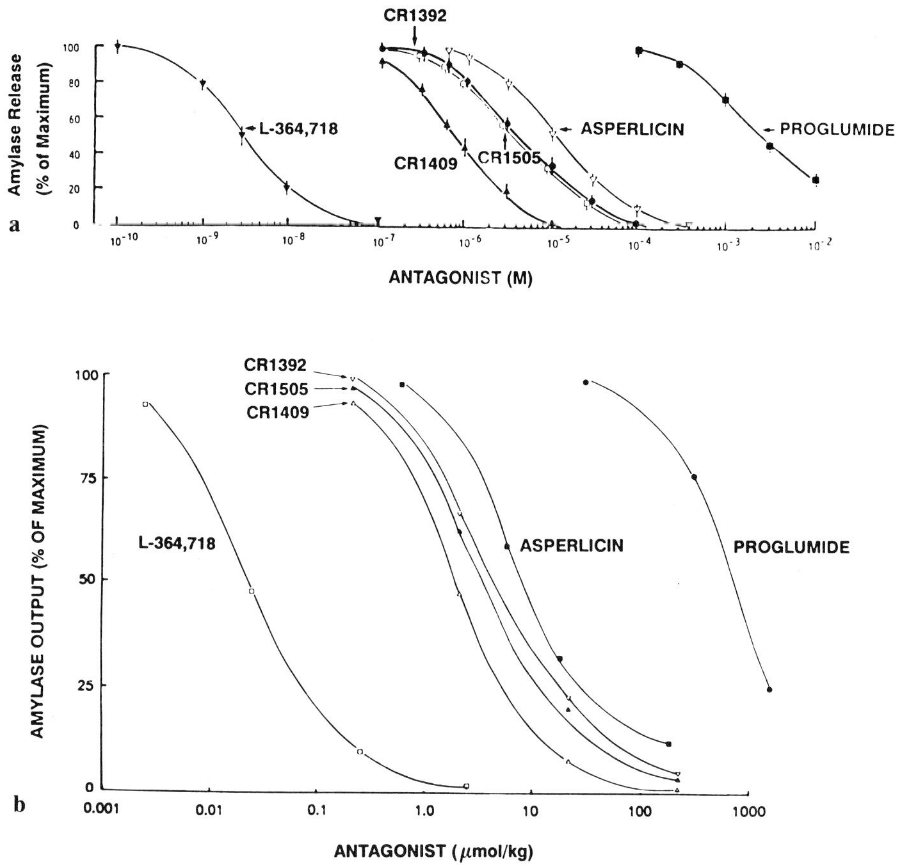

Fig. 1. **a** In vitro experiments. Effects of various antagonists on amylase release from isolated rat pancreatic acini stimulated by 60 p*M* CCK-8. In each experiment, basal release was subtracted and stimulated release was calculated as a percentage of maximal release in that experiment ($n = 6$). **b** In vivo experiments. Effects of various antagonists on mean integrated 1-h response of pancreatic amylase secretion to 0.25 μg/kg cerulein in the anesthetized rat. Data are calculated as a percentage of the response to this cerulein dose in the absence of antagonists and are shown as mean values for 4–8 experiments. For CR 1409, CR 1505, and CR 1392 doses of 2 μmol/kg or more significantly inhibited the response to 0.25 μg/kg cerulein ($p < 0.05$, analysis of variance) [3,15]; for proglumide only the dose of 1.5 mmol/kg significantly inhibited the response ($p < 0.05$). For L-364 718 the dose of 0.025 μmol/kg already significantly inhibited the response ($p < 0.05$); for asperlicin 5.5 μmol/kg, or higher doses, significantly inhibited the response ($p < 0.05$). [From 46,48]

receptor in vivo. The CCK antagonists CR 1409 and L-364 718 did not alter secretin-stimulated secretion of volume or bicarbonate. The antagonists did not significantly alter basal (nonstimulated) secretion of protein and enzymes, indicating a lack of partial agonist activity. In vitro experiments had shown that the antagonists studied here act as competitive antagonists at the CCK receptor [4–6,17,29,46,69]. In vivo, increasing doses of antagonists also caused a rightward shift of the dose-response curve to cerulein, indicating competitive-like kinetics although the actual form of the kinetics did not exactly mimic true competitive inhibition [48]. In particular, the upward part of the dose-response curve for cerulein became less steep with increasing doses of the antagonist than would be expected for the rightward shift of competitive kinetics. Thus, the dose of antagonist needed to reverse inhibition by supramaximal doses of caerulein was smaller than expected for a pure rightward shift of the dose-response curve. However, competitive kinetics can only be clearly established in a situation where the concentrations of agonists and antagonists at the receptor level are exactly known. This is not the case for the present in vivo experiments. Thus, the results in vivo appear to be compatible with in vitro competitive kinetics data. The experiments on the action of the antagonists on CCK-stimulated pancreatic secretion offer data on the doses of antagonists needed to inhibit the action of various CCK doses in vivo [48]. Both the new potent peptidal and nonpeptidal antagonists are powerful tools for further investigating the physiologic actions of CCK in vivo and, potentially, may also prove useful therapeutically [44,45].

Effects of CCK Antagonists on Pancreatic and Intestinal Growth, Morphology, and Function

Short-Term Studies

It is well established that exogenous CCK and CCK analogues, like cerulein, stimulate pancreatic growth in the experimental animal [12,21]. Feeding of trypsin inhibitors [7,20] and pancreaticobiliary diversion [27,37] also stimulate pancreatic growth, in each case by decreasing intraduodenal activity of proteases. The inhibition of intraduodenal proteolytic enzymes by protease inhibitors, such as camostate [72], or their diversion from the duodenum [37] increase plasma CCK which may mediate pancreatic growth under these conditions [27,37,72]. It has, however, been speculated that other hormones like enteroglucagon may contribute to pancreatic growth after pancreaticobiliary diversion [14]. Recent studies have tried to establish the hormone responsible for pancreatic growth after pancreaticobiliary diversion or feeding of a protease inhibitor by administration of proglumide, a specific CCK-inhibitor [14,25,37,72]. Proglumide significantly inhibited pancreatic growth after pancreaticobiliary diversion and camostate feeding [25,37] as well as after exogenous administration of CCK [71]. However, proglumide only partly blocked pancreatic growth due to these stimuli. Furthermore, large doses of proglumide itself exerted trophic effects which were interpreted as a partial agonist activity [25,71]. To further evaluate the physiologic impact of CCK's trophic effects, pancreatic growth was monitored after exogenous CCK-8 and after chronic feeding of camostate (FOY 305, Schwarz; Monheim, FRG) which is a potent inhibitor of serine proteases [72]. The same conditions were also studied with administration of the CCK receptor antagonist CR 1409 which is at least 1000 times more potent than proglumide in vitro [46]. Further experiments studied pancreatic growth following the combination of exogenous CCK and feeding of camostate, and with administration of the CCK antagonist alone. In addition, plasma CCK concentrations were monitored under these experimental conditions.

Feeding of the protease inhibitor camostate for 10 days exerted a marked stimulatory effect on the growth of the mouse pancreas [47] (Fig. 2). These results also indicate that an increase in plasma CCK is responsible for the stimulatory effect of camostate [47]. Not only was it found that chronic camostate feeding increased plasma CCK to eight times that of control values of chow-fed mice, but simultaneous administration of a CCK inhibitor greatly reduced the stimulatory effect of camostate. It is also remarkable that plasma CCK in fasted mice increased fourfold 30 min after a single dose of camostate given by an orogastric tube. This shows that the feedback effect causing a CCK release in response to inhibition of intraduodenal proteases, previously described in the rat [27,37,72], exists in the mouse, too. Exogenous CCK-8 had qualitatively similar but quantitatively smaller stimulatory effects on pancreatic growth than camostate feeding. The relatively small effect of CCK-8 compared to camostate feeding is, however, to be expected in view of the CCK plasma concentrations measured under these conditions. Although plasma CCK after s.c. injection of 2 μg/kg CCK-8 increased to a range similar to that observed in camostate-fed mice [47], this increase peaks after 30 min and then rapidly decreases toward previous control values [47]. Thus, the plasma CCK in camostate-fed mice, integrated over the entire study period of 10 days, was substantially higher than in chow-fed mice which received s.c. injections of CCK-8. Injections of the CCK antagonist before each injection of CCK-8 completely blocked CCK's stimulatory effect on pancreatic growth. In view of the rapid, long-lasting and marked stimulatory effects of camostate on plasma CCK concentrations, it is not surprising that three daily s.c. injections of the CCK antagonist were not sufficient to completely block camostate's, and thus probably CCK's, stimulatory actions on pancreatic growth. In two recent reports about proglumide's inhibitory action on CCK-stimulated pancreatic growth, proglumide was reported to have a partial agonist activity [25,71]. The antagonist CR 1409, however, did not show any partial agonist activity [47]. Instead, the CCK antagonist given without exogenous CCK or camostate exerted a small antitrophic effect. Thus, the short-term studies suggested that physiologic increases of CCK in response to feeding may have trophic effects on the exocrine pancreas. In most previous rat studies CCK increased both the absolute DNA content of the pancreas and the ratio of protein/

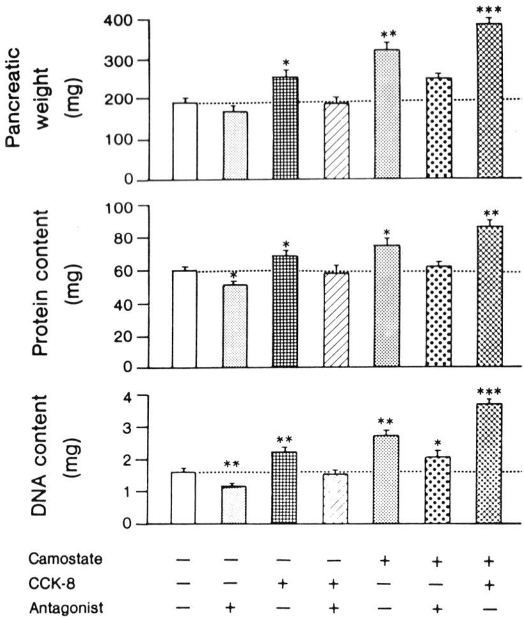

Fig. 2. Mean ± SE of mouse pancreatic weight ($n = 24$), protein content ($n = 12$), and DNA content ($n = 12$). The experimental conditions are as indicated: Camostate was mixed with regular chow and fed to achieve a daily dose of 400 mg/kg for 10 days; no camostate (-) indicates that regular chow was fed ad libitum; CCK-8 (1 µg/kg) was injected s.c. every 8 h for 10 days; the CCK-receptor antagonist (10 mg/kg) was given s.c. every 8 h. In mice, which received CCK-8 injections, the antagonist was given 15 min prior to the injection of CCK-8. Mean data for the various conditions were statistically compared to the corresponding group of mice which received no camostate, CCK-8, or antagonist by analysis of variance using Duncan's methods [3,15]. $^{*}p \leq 0.05$, $^{**}p \leq 0.01$, $^{***}p \leq 0.001$. No *asterisk* means NS, $p \geq 0.05$. [From 47]

DNA, and thus exerted both hypertrophic and hyperplastic effects [14,21]. In the mouse, camostate feeding and exogenous CCK appeared to induce almost exclusively hyperplasia [47] (Fig. 2). The lack of hypertrophy may, however, be due to the fact that mice were kept on the diets ad lib. Thus, particularly in camostate-fed mice, there was still an ongoing stimulation of exocrine secretion resulting in depletion of cellular protein at the time of sacrifice. It might be that fasting of mice prior to sacrifice would result in a greater increase in protein content and show hypertrophy. As in previous reports in the rat [25,59], both exogenous CCK and to an even greater degree feeding of the protease inhibitor, markedly increased the content of the proteolytic enzyme chymotrypsinogen, but left that of the starch-splitting enzyme amylase unaffected [47].

Long-Term Studies

Further studies were designed to examine the hypothesis that CCK plays a physiologic role in long-term maintenance of pancreatic growth. Pancreatic growth was monitored during a 9-month period of feeding of the protease inhibitor camostate [72] with or without simultaneous feeding of the CCK antagonist CR 1409 [46]. Further experiments studied pancreatic growth following feeding of the CCK antagonist alone, i.e., without camostate. It has been reported that chronic increases of circulating CCK, either by oral administration of a protease inhibitor or by pancreaticobiliary diversion, induce formation of hyperplastic or adenomatous nodules in the rat pancreas [33,37,64]. Therefore, the long-term experiments also evaluated whether feeding of camostate leads to formation of pancreatic nodules and whether this nodule formation can be inhibited by simultaneous feeding of a CCK receptor antagonist. Since feeding of a protease inhibitor like camostate is thought to act by release of CCK from the intestinal mucosa, one might speculate whether a long-term stimulation induces not only pancreatic hypertrophy but also hypertrophy of the intestinal mucosa. Thus, the present studies also evaluated morphology and composition of small intestinal mucosa. Finally, body weight and food intake were also monitored throughout long-term feeding of the protease inhibitor and of the CCK antagonist because it had been speculated that CCK is involved in regulation of satiety. Several previous experiments had shown that administration of exogenous CCK reduces food intake [35,41]. It is, however, unknown whether this mechanism is of physiologic importance and whether it is mediated by central or peripheral CCK receptors.

Acute and chronic feeding of the protease inhibitor camostate releases CCK from the small intestine and increases its circulating concentrations [24,47]. Although, the present experiments did not monitor plasma CCK during the 9 months of camostate feeding, the results suggest that camostate continuously released CCK throughout this period. Such long-term release of endogenous CCK greatly increased pancreatic weight by induction of marked pancreatic hypertrophy (increase of protein content) and of moderate hyperplasia (increase in DNA content; Fig. 3) [50]. Increase in chymotrypsinogen content was more pronounced than increase in amylase content. Feeding of camostate also increased maximal secretory capacity [50]. The CCK antagonist markedly inhibited the effects of camostate which are therefore mainly mediated by CCK [50]. The feedback-regulation induced by inhibition of intraduodenal proteases still functions after 9 months of continuous feeding of the protease inhibitor. The target-organ of this mechanism, the exocrine pancreas, does not adapt to such long-term stimulation. Compared with previous studies, in which camostate was fed for 10 days [47], long-term feeding induced a more pronounced increase in pancreatic growth [50]. Fed animals under all experimental conditions

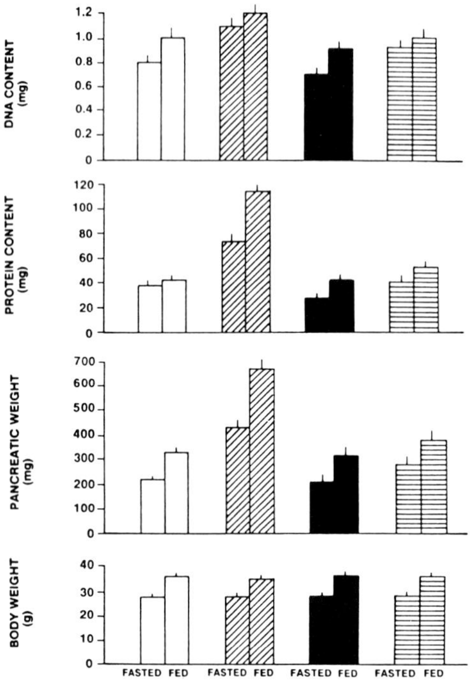

Fig. 3. Mean ± SE of body weight, pancreatic weight and content of DNA and protein of Naval Medical Research Institute (NMRI) mice ($n \pm 12-24$) which had been fed different diets for 9 months: Control diet mice (*open bars*) which received regular chow. In a second group of mice (*diagonally lined bars*) camostate was mixed with chow at a daily dose of 100 mg/kg to induce release of endogenous CCK. In a third group (*solid bars*) CR 1409 was mixed with chow to achieve a daily dose of 50 mg/kg. A fourth group received chow with camostate + CR 1409 (*horizontally lined bars*) to achieve a daily dose of 100 mg/kg camostate and 50 mg/kg CR 1409. *Fed* indicates mice which received the corresponding diets until they were killed (12 mice per group). *Fasted* indicates mice which were fasted for 24 h prior to killing (24 mice per group). Body weight and pancreatic weight were significantly increased in fed mice compared to fasted mice ($p < 0.01$; analysis of variance) [3,15]. Body weights were identical between the four experimental groups ($p > 0.2$). Pancreatic weights and contents of protein and DNA were increased in camostate-fed mice when compared to the control group both under fed and fasted conditions ($p < 0.01$). Under fasted conditions pancreatic weight was slightly but significantly increased in mice which received both camostate and CR 1409 when compared to the control group ($p < 0.05$); under fed conditions pancreatic weight in mice which received camostate and CR 1409 did not differ from control ($p > 0.1$). Simultaneous feeding of CR 1409 and camostate reduced contents of DNA and protein to levels which were not different from control ($p > 0.1$). Pancreatic weight and content of protein and DNA did not differ between mice which received only CR 1409 and the control group both in fasted and fed mice ($p > 0.1$). [From 50]

showed an increase in pancreatic content of protein and DNA compared to animals which had been fasted for 24 h. This increase also occurred in mice which received the CCK antagonist without camostate. Thus, feeding exerts short-term trophic effects on the pancreas which are not mediated by CCK.

Despite the long-term and marked hypertrophy and hyperplasia, formation of hyperplastic or neoplastic nodules could be observed in none of the mice [50]. In previous rat studies the long-term feeding of protease inhibitors and diversion of pancreaticobiliary juice induced formation of hyperplastic and adenomatous nodules [33,37,64], the discrepancy may be due to a species difference. Long-term effective blockade of the CCK receptor only slightly inhibited pancreatic growth and secretory capacity [50] (Fig. 3). This inhibition was less pronounced than that seen after short-term administration of CR 1409 [47]. CCK is, therefore, not an essential growth factor for the pancreas although increases of endogenous and exogenous CCK markedly stimulate pancreatic growth. Neither long-term CCK-stimulation nor CCK-blockade altered morphology or composition of the duodenal mucosa. Thus, despite continuous release of CCK from the small intestine, there was no indication of intestinal hypertrophy [50]. Neither long-term, effective, and continuous blockade of the peripheral CCK receptor nor long-term and continuous release of endogenous CCK altered food intake or body weight [50]. These observations suggest that the peripheral CCK receptor is not involved in physiologic modulation of food intake and satiety and support other recent studies which also suggested that the satiety effect induced by exogenous CCK is not of physiologic importance [35,41]. Administration of an antiemetic substance could greatly reduce the satiety effect induced by peripheral administration of exogenous CCK [41]. The present results, however, do not exclude the possibility that the central CCK receptor may be involved in regulation of food intake because the CCK antagonist used in the present experiments shows a 100-fold weaker affinity to central CCK receptors than to peripheral CCK receptors.

Effects of CCK Antagonists on Plasma Concentrations of Glucose and Insulin After Oral Administration of Glucose and Camostate

Insulin release after ingestion of nutrients is thought to be facilitated by the release of various gut factors which have been termed insulinotropic factors or incretins [9,10,67]. Since the first report of the insulinotropic effect of extracts of intestinal mucosa [36], several investigators have shown that CCK is one of several gastrointestinal hormones capable of stimulating insulin secretion in vitro and in vivo [26,67,68]. Since CCK is released from the small intestine into the circulation in response to a meal [32], it might act as a physiologic incretin. Gastric inhibitory polypeptide (GIP) has been suggested as another major factor involved in the enteroinsular axis [9,10, 16,54], and further studies support the involvement of yet other factors [17,18]. Pure preparations of natural CCK [53], synthetic COOH-terminal octapeptide of CCK (CCK-OP) [57,70], and synthetic cerulein, which contains a COOH-terminal pentapeptide identical to CCK [51–53,57], have also been shown to stimulate insulin secretion in vivo and in vitro. Nevertheless, it has been difficult to determine whether the insulinotropic action of these peptides administered exogenously is physiologic. In order to evaluate the *physiologic* influence of CCK on the plasma insulin response after ingestion of nutrients the studies employed the specific CCK receptor antagonist CR 1409.

CR 1409, at a dose which abolishes the actions of physiologic plasma concentrations of CCK and even the actions of pharmacologic doses of exogenous CCK [46–50,62], did not significantly alter the increase in circulating concentrations of glucose, insulin, and C-peptide after an oral glucose load with and without simultaneous oral administration of the protease inhibitor camostate (substances given by an orogastric tube; Fig. 4). The rise in plasma concentrations of glucose and CCK after feeding of glucose and camostate [47] did not potentiate the increase in insulin or C-peptide, i.e., no incretin effect was observed. Similar results were observed when a blenderized chow diet was fed by an orogastric tube instead of glucose and when mice were used instead of rats (data not shown). In the present animal studies we cannot exclude effects of the CCK antagonist on gastric emptying. Our present results are in contrast to previous animal work in which CCK receptor blockade antagonized the stimulatory effects of CCK on glucose-mediated insulin secretion in vitro [67,68] and on meal-induced insulin secretion in vivo [56]. Although the present study does not

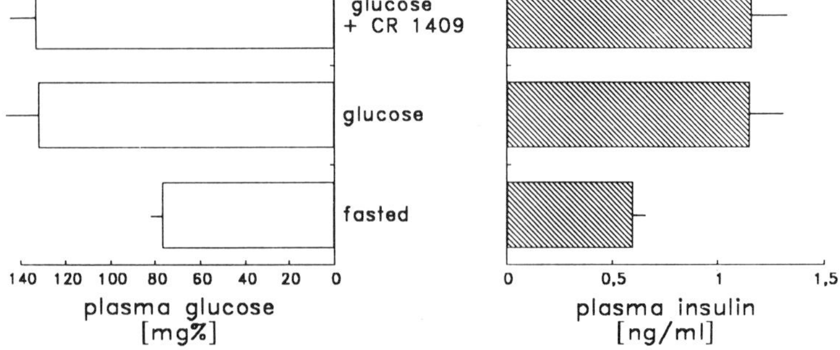

Fig. 4. Maximal plasma concentrations of insulin and glucose after tube feeding of 1 mg/kg glucose, 1 mg/kg glucose + 50 mg/kg CR 1409, 1 mg/kg glucose + 100 mg/kg camostate, and 1 mg/kg glucose + 50 mg/kg CR 1409 + 100 mg/kg camostate. Plasma insulin and glucose significantly increased after glucose administration by orogastric tube ($p < 0.01$ by analysis of variance) [3,15]. However, simultaneous administration of CR 1409 or camostate, or both, did not alter the increase in plasma insulin and glucose ($p < 0.2$). Values are given as mean ± SD for 10 rats

exclude the possibility that at some physiologic condition CCK may increase insulin secretion in man and in the experimental animal, the results make it unlikely that CCK acts as a major physiologic incretin after ingestion of regular meals in healthy humans as well as in rats and mice.

The Effect of CCK Antagonists on Feedback Regulation of Rat Pancreatic Secretion

The diversion of pancreaticobiliary secretions from the small intestine produces a marked increase in pancreatic secretion in the rat [27,28,38,39]. A similar increase in secretion is seen if rats are fed trypsin inhibitors [19], or after the infusion of trypsin inhibitors into the duodenum [31,59]. This stimulation of secretion is thought to be due to feedback inhibition of pancreatic secretion which is suppressed when the protease activity in the duodenum is lowered. On the other hand, intraduodenal administration of proteases abolishes the increase in pancreatic secretion seen after diversion of pancreaticobiliary juice. Feedback-regulation has been demonstrated in the rat [27,28,31,38,39], chicken [1,7], pig [8,30], hamster [2], mouse [47], and calf [11], but appears to be absent in the dog [13,58]. Several studies indicate that the increase in pancreatic secretion induced by diversion of pancreaticobiliary juice or administration of protease inhibitors is associated with an increase in endogenous CCK [22,63]. Our own experiments show that, in the anesthetized rat amylase output in pancreaticobiliary secretion only slightly increased after diversion of pancreaticobiliary juice [43,48]. This increase was completely inhibited by both the CCK antagonists CR 1409 and L-364 718. The potent CCK antagonists CR 1409 or L-364 718 did not alter basal enzyme secretion prior to diversion of pancreaticobiliary juice [43].

In conscious rats equipped with pancreatic and biliary cannulas pancreatic protein output markedly increased after diversion of pancreaticobiliary juice (Fig. 5) [43]. The CCK antagonists CR 1409 and L-364 718 significantly inhibited this increase in pancreatic protein secretion after diversion of pancreaticobiliary juice. However, after diversion there was still some increase in protein output compared to prior basal values despite complete blockade of CCK receptors (Fig. 5). Pancreatic protein secretion during recirculation of pancreaticobiliary juice tended to be lower in the presence of CCK antagonists although the differences compared to the infusion of 0.9% NaCl did not reach statistical significance (Fig. 5). Atropine, however, markedly decreased basal pancreatic protein secretion during recirculation of pancreaticobiliary juice when compared to control studies with NaCl infusion (Fig. 5). Atropine only partly inhibited the increase in pancreatic protein secretion after diversion of pancreaticobiliary juice, similar to what was reported previously [38]. Only the simultaneous administration of atropine and CR 1409 completely inhibited the increase in pancreatic secretion after diversion of pancreaticobiliary juice in conscious rats. The simul-

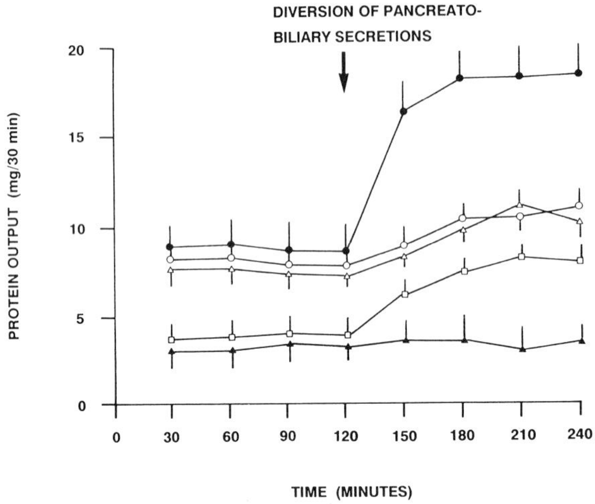

Fig. 5. Effects of the CCK antagonists CR 1409 and L-364718 and of atropine on ductal amylase output in pancreatic secretion in the conscious rat equipped with pancreatic and biliary cannulas. Data are mean ± SD of 4–6 independent experiments. Amylase output increased 30 min after diversion of pancreatobiliary secretion ($p < 0.01$ by analysis of variance) [3,15]. This increase was markedly reduced but not completely abolished by CR 1409 and L-364178. Neither CCK antagonist altered amylase secretion under recirculation of pancreatobiliary secretion ($p > 0.05$). Atropine, however, markedly reduced secretion under recirculation ($p < 0.01$) and partly reduced the increase in amylase secretion after diversion. Only the simultaneous administration of both atropine and CR 1409 completely abolished the increase in amylase secretion after diversion. [From 43]. The i.v. infusions were 0.9% NaCl (*solid circles*), 10 mg/kg per hour CR 1409 (*open circles*), 1 mg/kg per hour L-364718 (*open triangles*), 0.1 mg/kg per hour atropine (*squares*), and 0.1 mg/kg per hour atropine + 10 mg/kg per hour CR 1409 (*solid triangles*)

taneous administration of atropine and CR 1409 also caused a marked inhibition of basal pancreatic secretion (pancreatic juice recirculated). Thus, the basal tone of rat pancreatic secretion under the physiologic conditions of drainage of pancreatic and biliary juice into the proximal small intestine appears to be mainly regulated by cholinergic mechanisms. In the rat, atropine had no effect on pancreatic enzyme output during intraduodenal infusion of a protease inhibitor [23]. The stimulation of pancreatic secretion after diversion of pancreaticobiliary juice appears to be regulated mainly by CCK and to a lesser degree also by cholinergic factors. In addition, other factors such as secretin might be involved in the mediation of feedback stimulation after diversion of pancreaticobiliary juice [65]. As in results obtained with CCK receptor antagonists, immunoneutralization of circulating free CCK with an anti-CCK serum also inhibited the increase in secretion induced by diversion in the rat [63]. Thus, several recent studies using specific CCK antagonists and anti-CCK serum support the original proposal of Green and Lyman [27,28] that CCK plays the central role in the mechanism of exocrine pancreatic feedback inhibition in the rat.

References

1. Alumot E, Nitsan Z (1961) The influence of soybean antitrypsin on the intestinal proteolysis of the chicken. J Nutr 73:71–77
2. Andrén-Sandberg A, Ihse I (1983) Regulatory effect on the pancreas of intraduodenal pancreatic juice and trypsin in the Syrian golden hamster. Scand J Gastroenterol 18:697–706
3. Byrkit SJ (1980) Elements of statistics, 3rd edn. van Nostrand, New York, pp 305–358
4. Chang RSL, Lotti VJ (1986) Biochemical and pharmacological characterization of an extremely potent and selective nonpeptide cholecystokinin receptor antagonist. Proc Natl Acad Sci USA 83:4923–4926
5. Chang RSL, Monaghan RL, Birnbaum J, Stapley AA, Goetz MA, Albers-Schonberg G, Patchett AA, Liesch JM, Hensens OD, Springer JP (1985) A potent nonpeptide cholecystokinin antagonist selective for peripheral tissues isolated from *Aspergillus alliaceus*. Science 230:177–179
6. Chang RSL, Lotti VJ, Chen TB, Kunkel KA (1986) Characterization of the binding of (^{2}H)-(±)-L364 218: a new potent, nonpeptide cholecystokinin antagonist radioligand selective for peripheral receptors. Mol Pharmacol 30: 212–217
7. Chernick SS, Lepkovsky S, Chaikoff IL (1948) A dietary factor regulating the enzyme content of the pancreas: changes induced in size and proteolytic activity of the chick pancreas by ingestion of raw soybean meal. Am J Physiol 115:33–41
8. Corring T (1973) Mechanisme de la secrétion pancréatique exocrine chez le porc: régulation par rétro inhibition. Ann Biol Anim Biochim Biophys 13:755–6
9. Creutzfeldt W (1979) The incretin concept today. Diabetologia 16:75–85
10. Creutzfeldt W, Ebert R (1985) New development in the incretin concept. Diabetologia 28:565–573
11. Davicco MJ, Lefaivre J, Thivend P, Bartlet JP (1979) Feedback regulation of pancreatic secretion in the young milk-fed calf. Ann Biol Anim Biochim Biophys 19:1147–1152
12. Dembinski AR, Johnson LR (1978) Stimulation of pancreatic growth by secretin, cerulein, and pentagastrin. Endocrinology 106:232–238
13. Diaz GR, Devaux MA, Johnson CD (1981) Physiological condition for the study of basal and meal stimulated exocrine pancreatic secretion in the dog. Absence of feedback inhibition of basal secretion. Can J Physiol Pharmacol 60:1287–1295
14. Dowling RH (1982) Small bowel adaption and its regulation. Scand J Gastroenterol 74:53–74
15. Duncan DB (1957) Multiple range tests for correlated and heteroscedastic means. Biometrics 13:164–176
16. Dupre J, Ross SA, Watson D, Brown JD (1973) Stimulation of insulin secretion by gastric inhibitory polypeptide in man. J Clin Endocrinol Metab 37:826–828
17. Evans BE, Block MG, Rittle KE, DiPardo RM, Whitter WL, Veber DF, Anderson PS, Freidinger RM (1986) Design of potent, orally effective, nonpeptidal antagonists of the peptide hormone cholecystokinin. Proc Natl Acad Sci USA 83:4918–4922
18. Ebert R, Unger H, Creutzfeldt W (1983) Preservation of incretin activity after removal of gastric inhibitory polypeptide (GIP) from rat gut extracts by immunoabsorption. Diabetologia 24:449–454
19. Fölsch UR, Creutzfelt W (1985) Adaptation of the pancreas during treatment with enzyme inhibitors in rats and man. Scand J Gastroenterol 20:54–63
20. Fölsch UR, Winckler K, Wormsley KG (1974) Effect of soybean diet on enzyme content and ultrastructure of the rat exocrine pancreas. Digestion 11:161–171
21. Fölsch UR, Winckler K, Wormsley KG (1978) Influence of repeated administration of cholecystokinin and secretin on the pancreas of the rat. Scand J Gastroenterol 13:663–671

22. Fölsch UR, Cantor P, Wilms HM, Schafmayer A, Becker HD, Creutzfeldt W (1987) Role of cholecystokinin in the negative feedback control of pancreatic enzyme secretion in conscious rats. Gastroenterology 92:449–458
23. Fushiki T, Fukuoka S, Kajiura H, Iwai K (1978) Atropine-non-sensitive feedback regulatory mechanism of rat pancreatic enzyme secretion in response to food protein intake. J Nutr 117:948–954
24. Göke B, Printz H, Koop I (1986) Endogenous CCK release and pancreatic growth in rats after feeding a proteinase inhibitor (camostate). Pancreas 1: 509–515
25. Göke B, Printz, H, Richter G, Adler G, Arnold R (1986) Beeinflussung der Pankreashypertrophie infolge Camostategabe durch Injektion des CCK-Antagonisten Proglumid. Klin Wochenschr 64:A54
26. Goldfine ID, Williams JA (1983) Receptors for insulin and CCK in the acinar pancreas: relationship to hormone action. Int Rev Cytol 85:1–38
27. Green GM, Lyman RL (1972) Feedback regulation of pancreatic enzymes secretion as a mechanism for trypsin inhibitor-induced hypersecretion in rats. Proc Soc Exp Biol Med 140:6–12
28. Green GM, Olds BA, Matthews G, Louis DS (1973) Protein, as a regulator of pancreatic enzyme secretion in the rat. Proc Soc Exp Biol Med 142:1162–1167
29. Hahne WF, Jensen RT, Lemp GF, Gardener JD (1981) Proglumide and benzotript: members of a different class of cholecystokinin receptor antagonists. Proc Natl Acad Sci USA 78:6304–6308
30. Ihse I, Lilja P (1979) Effect of intestinal amylase and trypsin on pancreatic secretion in the pig. Scand J Gastroenterol 14:1009–1013
31. Ihse I, Lilja P, Lundquist I (1974) Trypsin as a regulator of pancreatic secretion in the rat. Scand J Gastroenterol 14:875–880
32. Jansen JBMJ, Lamers BHHW (1983) Radioimmunoassay of cholecystokinin in human tissue and plasma. Clin Chim Acta 33:2197–2205
33. Longnecker LS (1987) Interface between adaptive and neoplastic growth in the pancreas. Gut 28:253–258
34. Louie DS, May D, Miller P, Owyang C (1986) Cholecystokinin mediates feedback regulation of pancreatic enzyme secretion in rats. Am J Physiol G252–G259
35. Makovec F, Bani M, Chistè R, Revel L, Rovati LC, Setnikar I (1986) Different peripheral and central antagonistic activity of new glutaramic acid derivatives on satiety induced by cholecystokinin in rats. Regul Pept 16:281–290
36. Meade RC, Kneubuhler HA, Schulte WJ, Barboiak JJ (1967) Stimulation of insulin secretion by pancreozymin. Diabetes 16:141–147
37. Miazza BM, Turberg Y, Guillaume P, Hahnen W, Chayvialle JA, Loizeau E (1985) Mechanism of pancreatic growth induced by pancreatico-biliary diversion in the rat. Digestion 20:75–83
38. Miyasaka K, Green GM (1983) Effect of atropine on rat basal pancreatic secretion during return or diversion of bile-pancreatic juice. Proc Soc Exp Biol Med 174:187–192
39. Miyasaka K, Green GM (1984) Effect of partial exclusion of pancreatic juice of rat basal pancreatic secretion. Gastroenterology 86:114–119
40. Miyasaka K, Kurosawa H, Kitani K (1987) Proglumide stimulates basal pancreatic secretion in the conscious rat. Digestion 37:135–143
41. Moore BO, Deutsch JA (1985) An antiemetic is antidotal to the satiety effects of cholecystokinin. Nature 315:321–322
42. Niederau C, Karaus M (1990) Effects of cholecystokinin antagonists on myoelectric and motor activities of ideal colonic muscle in vitro. Gastrointest Motil 2:169–175
43. Niederau C, Niederau M (1990) Effects of CCK-receptor antagonist on pancreatic feedback regulation. In: Beger HG, Büchler M, Ditschuneit H, Malfertheiner P (eds) Chronic pancreatitis. Springer, Berlin Heidelberg New York, pp 186–197

44. Niederau C, Ferrell LD, Grendell JH (1985) Caerulein-induced acute necrotizing pancreatitis in mice: protective effects of proglumide, benzotript, and secretin. Gastroenterology 88:1192–1204
45. Niederau C, Ferrell LD, Liddle RA, Grendell JH (1986) Beneficial effects of cholecystokinin receptor blockade and inhibition of proteolytic enzyme activity in experimental acute hemorrhagic pancreatitis in mice. J Clin Invest 78: 1056–1063
46. Niederau C, Niederau M, Williams JA, Grendell JH (1986) New proglumide analogue CCK receptor antagonists: very potent and selective for peripheral tissues. Am J Physiol 251:G856–G860
47. Niederau C, Liddle RA, Williams JA, Grendell JH (1987) Pancreatic growth: interaction of exogenous cholecystokinin, a protease inhibitor and a cholecystokinin receptor antagonist in mice. Gut 28:63–69
48. Niederau M, Niederau C, Strohmeyer G, Grendell JH (1989) Comparative effects of CCK receptor antagonists on rat pancreatic secretion in vivo. Am J Physiol 256:G1–G8
49. Niederau C, Heindges T, Rovati L, Strohmeyer G (1989) Effects of loxiglumide in gall bladder emptying in healthy volunteers. Gastroenterology 97:1331–1336
50. Niederau C, Lüthen R, Niederau M, Strohmeyer G, Ferrell LD, Grendell JH (1990) Long-term effects of stimulation and inhibition at the CCK-receptor on morphology, function and growth of pancreas and intestine. Digestion 46:217–225
51. Ohneda A, Horigome K, Ishil S, Kai Y, Chiba M (1978) Effects of caerulein upon insulin and glucagon secretion in dogs. Horm Metab Res 10:7–14
52. Otsuki M, Sakamoto C, Maeda M, Yuu H, Morita S, Baba S (1979) Effect of caerulein on exocrine and endocrine pancreas in the rat. Endocrinology 105: 1396–1402
53. Otsuki M, Sakamoto C, Maeda M, Morita S, Ohki A, Kobayashi N, Terashi K, Okano K, Baba S (1979) Discrepancies between the doses of cholecystokinin- or caerulein stimulating exocrine and endocrine responses in perfused isolated rat pancreas. J Clin Invest 63:478–484
54. Pederson RA, Brown JC (1976) The insulinotropic action of gastric inhibitory polypeptide in the perfused isolated rat pancreas. Endocrinology 99:780–785
55. Petersen H, Grossman MI (1977) Pancreatic exocrine secretion in anesthetized and conscious rats. Am J Physiol 233:E530–E536
56. Rosetti L, Shulman GI, Zawalich WS (1987) Physiologic role of cholecystokinin in meal-induced insulin secretion in conscious rats. Studies with L-364718, a specific inhibitor of CCK-receptor binding. Diabetes 36:1212–1215
57. Sakamoto C, Otsuki M, Ohki A, Mitsuo M, Yamasaki T, Baba S (1985) Glucose-dependent insulinotropic action of cholecystokinin and caerulein in the isolated perfused rat pancreas. Endocrinology 110:398–402
58. Sale JK, Goldberg DM, Fawcett N, Wormsley KG (1977) Chronic and acute studies indicating absence of exocrine pancreatic feedback inhibition in dogs. Digestion 15:540–555
59. Schick J, Kern H, Scheele G (1984) Hormonal stimulation of the exocrine pancreas results in coordinate and anticoordinate regulation of protein synthesis. J Cell Biol 99:1569–1574
60. Schneemann BO, Lyman RL (1975) Factors involved in the intestinal feedback regulation of pancreatic enzyme secretion in the rat. Proc Soc Exp Biol Med 148:897–903
61. Schwarzendrube J, Lüthen R, Niederau M, Niederau C (1990) Ist CCK beim Menschen ein physiologisches Inkretin? Aktuel Endokrinol Stoffwechsel 11: A130
62. Setnikar I, Bani M, Cereda R, Chiste R, Makovec F, Pacini MA, Revel L, Rovati LC, Rovati LA (1987) Pharmacological characterization of a new potent and specific nonpolypeptide antagonist. Arzneimittelforschung 6:703–707

63. Shiratori K, Chen YF, Chey WY, Lee KY, Chang TM (1986) Mechanism of increased exocrine pancreatic secretion in pancreatic juice-diverted rats. Gastroenterology 91:1171–1178
64. Stace NH, Palmer TJ, Vaja S, Dowling RH (1987) Longterm pancreaticobiliary diversion stimulates hyperplastic and adenomatous nodules in the rat pancreas: a new model for spontaneous tumor formation. Gut 28:253–258
65. Sun G, Lee KY, Chang TM, Chey WY (1989) Effect of pancreatic juice diversion on secretin release in rats. Gastroenterology 96:1173–1179
66. Unger RH, Eisentraud AH (1969) Entero-insular axis. Arch Intern Med 123: 261–266
67. Verspohl EJ, Wunderle G, Ammon HPT, Williams JA, Goldfine ID (1986) Proglumide (gastrin and cholecystokinin receptor antagonist) inhibits insulin secretion in vitro. Naunyn-Schmiedebergs's Arch Pharmacol 332:284–287
68. Verspohl EJ, Ammon HPT, Williams JA, Goldfine ID (1986) Evidence that cholecystokinin interacts with specific receptors and regulates insulin release in isolated rat islets of Langerhans. Diabetes 35:38–43
69. Williams JA, Bailey A, Steigerwalt RW (1983) Effects of proglumide on pancreatic acinar cell function. Digestion 27:227–233
70. Williams RH, Champagne J (1979) Effects of cholecystokinin, secretin, and pancreatic polypeptide on secretion of gastric inhibitory polypeptide, insulin, and glucagon. Life Sci 22:947–953
71. Yamaguchi T, Tabat K, Johnson LR (1985) Effect of proglumide on rat pancreatic growth. Am J Physiol 249:G294–G298
72. Yonezawa H (1984) Discrepancy between the potency of various trypsin inhibitors to inhibit trypsin activity and the potency to release biologically active cholecystokinin-pancreozymin. Jpn J Physiol 34:849–856

Role of Cholecystokinin in Regulating Gallbladder Contraction and Pancreatic Secretion in Man: Studies with Loxiglumide*

C. BEGLINGER[1] and G. ADLER[2]

Introduction

The gallbladder and the exocrine pancreas are two principal sites of action of cholecystokinin (CCK) in the gastrointestinal tract [1]. However, it has been difficult to demonstrate that these actions are truly physiologic events.

The elaboration of specific peptide hormone antagonists with CCK as a model has been a keystone in biomedical research [2]. CCK antagonists should open the way for the investigation of physiological roles of this important gastrointestinal regulatory peptide.

Loxiglumide is one of the potent and highly specific antagonists of CCK that has become available for use in man [3–5]. It is specific for peripheral (A-type) CCK receptors and antagonizes the effects of CCK by competitive binding. This chapter summarizes some of our results obtained in human subjects. The objectives of these studies were (a) to evaluate the role of CCK in regulating postprandial gallbladder contraction and exocrine pancreatic secretion and (b) to determine whether CCK interacts with the cholinergic system to regulate gallbladder contraction and exocrine pancreatic secretion.

Effect of Loxiglumide on Gallbladder Contraction and Exocrine Pancreatic Secretion

To determine whether loxiglumide is an effective antagonist of CCK, subjects received i.v. infusions of loxiglumide or, as control, saline prior to stimulation with CCK-8 in a randomized, controlled fashion [6]. Dose-response curves were constructed in six healthy subjects with CCK-8 (1–27 pmol/kg per hour) with and without loxiglumide treatment. Gallbladder

* Supported by a grant from the Swiss National Science Foundation (grant 3.890–0.88).

[1] Division of Gastroenterology, University Hospital, 4031 Basel, Switzerland.
[2] Department of Internal Medicine, University of Marburg, Baldingerstr. 1, 3550 Marburg, FRG.

G. Adler and C. Beglinger (Eds.)
CCK Antagonists in Gastroenterology

contraction was measured by abdominal sonography, pancreatic enzyme secretion was measured by a multilumen intestinal tube and marker perfusion technique, and plasma CCK by a specific RIA [7]. Gallbladder and pancreatic responses are given in Figs. 1 and 2. Baseline gallbladder volumes ranged from 12.5 to 17.6 ml and pancreatic amylase and lipase

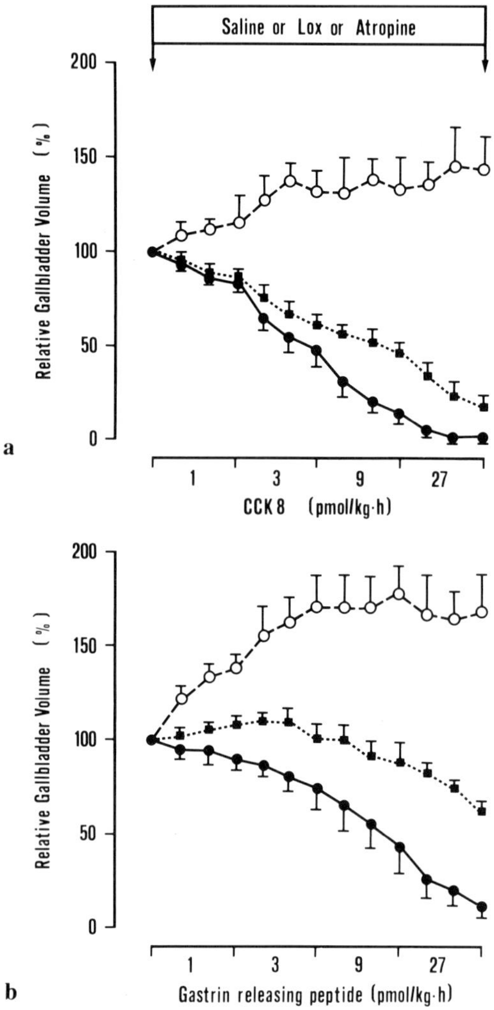

Fig. 1a,b. Effect of loxiglumide (10 mg/kg per hour; *open circles*) or atropine (5 µg/kg per hour; *squares*) on gallbladder volumes during infusion of graded doses of CCK-8 (**a**) or gastrin-releasing peptide (**b**). Gallbladder volumes were measured sonographically in six healthy subjects. Gallbladder volumes are expressed as a percentage of initial volume, and results are mean ± SEM. Both loxiglumide ($p < 0.01$) and atropine ($p < 0.05$) induced a significant inhibition of gallbladder contraction to both stimuli compared to placebo (saline; *closed circles*)

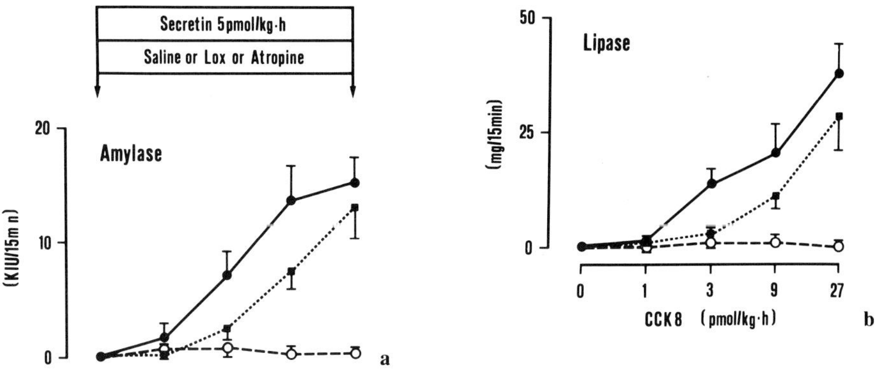

Fig. 2a,b. Effect of loxiglumide (10 mg/kg per hour; *open circles*) or atropine (5 μg/kg per hour; *squares*) on incremental CCK-8-stimulated pancreatic amylase (**a**) and lipase (**b**) outputs in six healthy subjects. Loxiglumide abolished the pancreatic response ($p < 0.01$). Atropine induced a significant inhibition of pancreatic response at the lower two dose of CCK-8 ($p < 0.05$, respectively). Results are expressed as mean ± SEM. *Closed circles*, control experiment (saline)

outputs from 1.62 to 4.3 kilo international units (KIU)/15 min and from 4.2 to 20.0 mg/15 min, respectively. An i.v. dose of 10 mg/kg per hour loxiglumide completely abolished CCK-8-stimulated gallbladder contraction and pancreatic enzyme responses (Figs. 1,2). Other studies support these findings by demonstrating a dose-dependent inhibition of gallbladder contraction and pancreatic secretion [5,8]. These studies demonstrate two important points. Firstly, CCK-stimulated gallbladder contraction and pancreatic enzyme secretion can be completely inhibited by loxiglumide administration. Secondly, the degree of inhibition is dose dependent, thus suggesting competitive kinetics. The results suggest, furthermore, that loxiglumide is a specific tool to study the physiology of CCK in man.

Effect of Loxiglumide on Postprandial Gallbladder Contraction and Pancreatic Enzyme Secretion

In order to evaluate the effects of blocking CCK receptors with loxiglumide on postprandial gallbladder contraction and pancreatic enzyme secretion, subjects received the same dose of loxiglumide (10 mg/kg per hour i.v.) or saline as a control together with a standard liquid meal (500 ml Ensure). There was no significant difference between fasting gallbladder volume after placebo and after loxiglumide treatment (19.1 ± 2.1 vs 16.7 ± 3.5 ml). Oral intake of the liquid meal was followed by a significant time-dependent contraction of the gallbladder (Fig. 3). However, when the CCK antagonist loxiglumide was given before the test meal, gallbladder contraction was

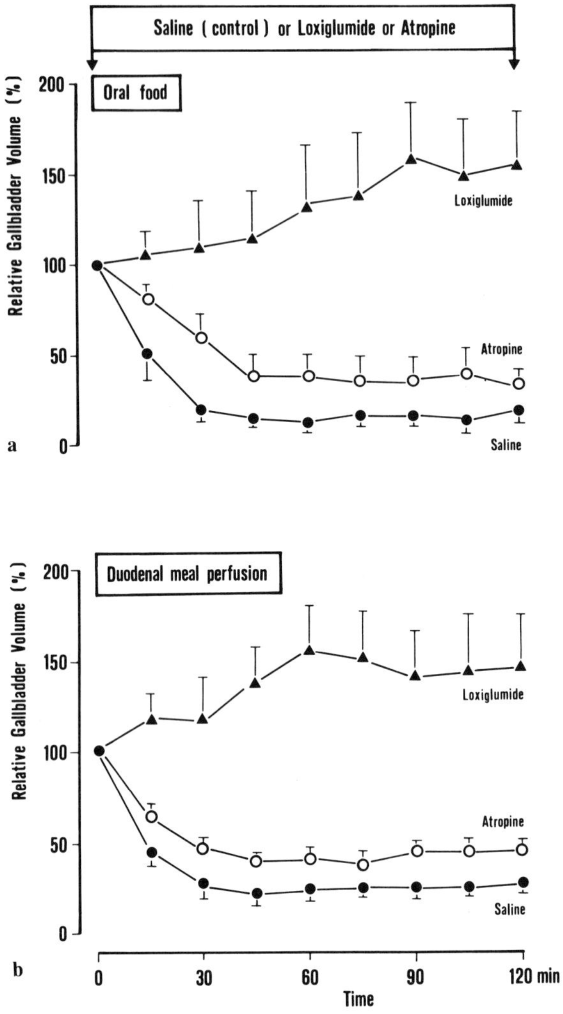

Fig. 3a,b. Effect of loxiglumide (*triangles*) or atropine (*open circles*) on gallbladder volumes after oral ingestion (**a**) or duodenal perfusion (**b**) of a liquid testmeal. Results are expressed as a percentage of initial (premeal) gallbladder volume. Values given are mean ± SEM. Loxiglumide abolished ($p < 0.01$) and atropine induced ($p < 0.05$) a significant inhibition of gallbladder contraction compared to placebo (saline; *closed circles*)

completely abolished. The gallbladder even tended to increase during the observation period. Pancreatic amylase and lipase responses to oral food intake rose immediately after taking the meal (Fig. 4). Loxiglumide caused a significant reduction in pancreatic enzyme secretion which amounted to 26% for amylase and 31% for lipase output, respectively (Fig. 4).

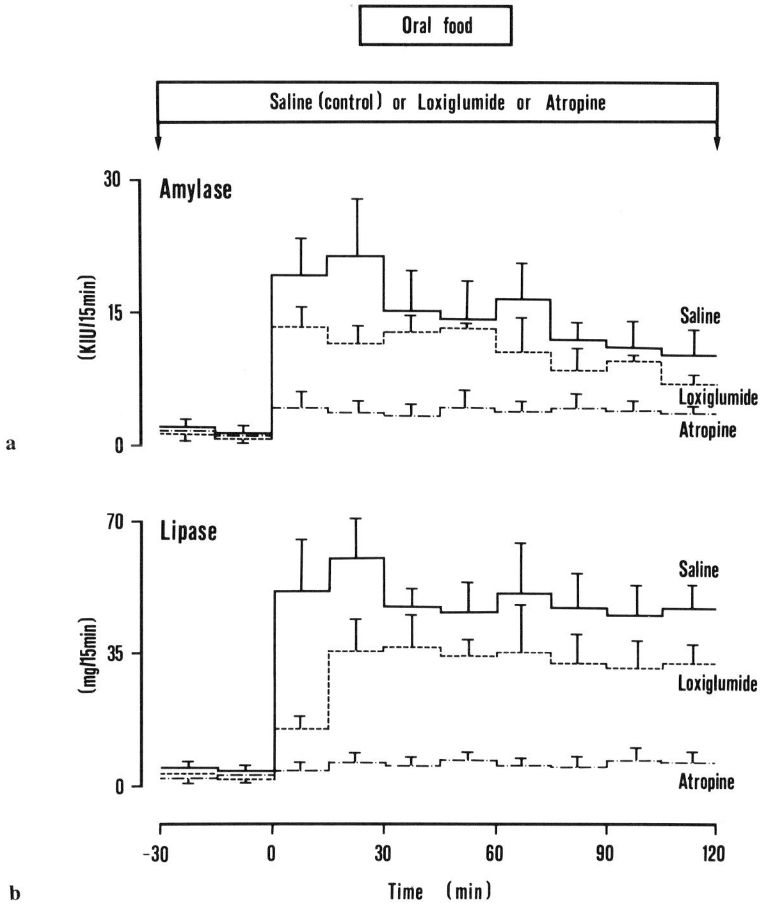

Fig. 4a,b. Effect of loxiglumide (*broken line*) or atropine (*dash-dot line*) on pancreatic amylase (**a**) and lipase (**b**) secretion after oral ingestion of a liquid meal. Loxiglumide caused a significant reduction in enzyme secretion ($p < 0.05$), whereas atropine virtually abolished pancreatic enzyme output ($p < 0.01$). Data are mean ± SEM in six healthy subjects. *Solid line*, control experiment (saline)

Conclusions Regarding the Effects of Loxiglumide

It has been known for many years that exogenously administered CCK can induce gallbladder contraction and pancreatic enzyme secretion [1]. The lack of hormone receptor antagonist has made it difficult to pursue this line of investigation. These studies demonstrate that loxiglumide is a potent and specific CCK antagonist. The complete inhibition of meal-stimulated gallbladder contraction demonstrates that endogenous CCK is a major regulator of the postprandial gallbladder response in man. The partial inhibition of pancreatic enzyme secretion observed after meal intake furthermore suggests that CCK participates in the physiologic control of enzyme secretion.

Effect of Atropine on Gallbladder Contraction and Pancreatic Enzyme Secretion

CCK has a central role in regulating postprandial gallbladder contraction and pancreatic enzyme secretion. On the other hand, it is well known that cholinergic control of gut functions is crucial for the coordination of normal digestion [9]. To determine the interactions of CCK with the cholinergic system, we performed the following studies: 1. dose-response curves to CCK-8 with and without concomitant i.v. infusion of atropine (5 μg/kg per hour) and 2. oral intake of a liquid test meal (500 ml Ensure) with and without atropine (5 μg/kg per hour). As expected, CCK-8 caused a dose-dependent contraction of the gallbladder and an increase in pancreatic enzyme secretion (Figs. 1, 2) Atropine caused a small, but significant inhibition of the dose response curve with a dose response relationship remaining apparent. Atropine caused a reduction of pancreatic enzyme secretion to each single dose of CCK-8, but this was most apparent and only significant at the lower two doses of CCK-8, where the inhibition amounted to 83% and 77%, respectively. These studies demonstrate an important point: both the gallbladder and the exocrine pancreas are dependent on a cholinergic background in order to react maximally to CCK stimulation. The meal studies revealed that atropine caused a small, but significant, decrease in gallbladder contraction (Fig. 3), but it virtually abolished the pancreatic enzyme response (inhibition 85%–99%).

Physiological Implications

The results of the studies summarized in this chapter clearly show that, while the gallbladder is less sensitive than the exocrine pancreas to cholinergic blockade, it is crucially dependent on CCK, whereas the exocrine pancreas is less dependent on CCK, but requires a cholinergic tone.

Several recent studies with different CCK-blockers have established the role for CCK in regulating gallbladder contraction in humans [4,5,10]. The present data extend these observations with the implication that any interference with CCK action will ultimately abolish gallbladder contraction. The cholinergic system participates in this control, but it is not a prime regulator of gallbladder contraction. Several mechanisms whereby atropine inhibits CCK-stimulated gallbladder contraction are possible. Firstly, cholinergic innervation may be necessary to maintain the gallbladder tone and/or CCK responsiveness. The cholinergic input would have a modulatory function on CCK's action. Secondly, CCK could stimulate the release of acetylcholine from cholinergic neurons within the wall of the gallbladder. Finally, CCK could activate inhibitory inputs whose actions only become evident when the cholinergic activity is blocked by atropine.

Recent work supports a role for CCK in regulating postprandial pancreatic secretion [6]. It has been known for a long time, however, that atropine inhibits pancreatic enzyme responses. The present observations extend these findings and suggest a predominant regulation of the exocrine pancreas by cholinergic pathways. The peptidergic (CCK) system participates in this control, but it is not a prime regulator of pancreatic exocrine secretion.

The physiological implications of these observations can be summarized as follows:

1. CCK appears to be the major regulator of postprandial gallbladder contraction in man, and interference with CCK abolishes the contraction. The findings furthermore show that cholecystokinin, previously also called cholecystokinin-pancreozymin for its enzyme-stimulating properties, is adequately named, as its prime action is on the gallbladder.
2. Pancreatic enzyme secretion is much more dependent on a cholinergic innervation, supporting the Pavlowian concept that the cholinergic system is the major regulator of pancreatic secretion.

References

1. Solomon TE (1987) Control of exocrine pancreatic secretion. In: Johnson LR (ed) Physiology of the gastrointestinal tract, 2nd edn. Raven, New York, pp 1173–1207
2. Snyder SH (1986) Virtuoso design of drugs. Nature 323:292–293
3. Meyer BM, Werth BA, Beglinger C, Hildebrand P, Jansen JBMJ, Zach D, Rovati LC, Stalder GA (1989) Role of cholecystokinin in regulation of gastrointestinal motor functions. Lancet 2:12–15
4. Adler G, Reinshagen M, Koop I, Göke B, Schafmayer A, Rovati LC, Arnold R (1989) Differential effects of atropine and a cholecystokinin receptor antagonist on pancreatic secretion. Gastroenterology 96:1158–1164
5. Hildebrand P, Beglinger C, Gyr K, Jansen JBMJ, Rovati LC, Zuercher M, Lamers CBHW, Setnikar I, Stalder GA (1990) Effects of a cholecystokinin receptor antagonist on intestinal phase of pancreatic and biliary responses in man. J Clin Invest 85:640–646
6. Beglinger C, Hildebrand P, Adler G, Werth B, Luo H, Delco F, Gyr K (1991) Control of gallbladder contraction and exocrine pancreatic secretion in humans: contrasting dependence on cholinergic system and cholecystokinin. Am J Physiol (submitted)
7. Meier R, Hildebrand P, Thumshirn M, Albrecht C, Studer B, Gyr K, Beglinger C (1990) Effect of loxiglumide, a cholecystokinin antagonist, on pancreatic polypeptide release in humans. Gastroenterology 99:1757–1762
8. Niederau C, Heintges T, Rovati L, Strohmeyer G (1989) Effects of loxiglumide on gallbladder emptying in healthy volunteers. Gastroenterology 97:1331–1336

9. Meyer JH (1987) Motility of the stomach and gastroduodenal junction. In: Johnson LR (ed) Physiology of the gastrointestinal tract, 2nd edn. Raven, New York, pp 613–629
10. Liddle RA, Gertz BJ, Kanayama S, Beccaria L, Coker LD, Turnbull TA, Morita ET (1989) Effects of a novel cholecystokinin (CCK) receptor antagonist, MK-329, on gallbladder contraction and gastric emptying in humans. Implications for the physiology of CCK. J Clin Invest 84:1220–1225

Effect of MK-329 on Pancreatic Secretion in Man

P. CANTOR[1]

Introduction

The relative importance of hormonal and neural factors in the regulation of pancreatic exocrine secretion in man has been much debated. Circulating cholecystokinin (CCK) is generally regarded as an important stimulant of the postprandial pancreatic enzyme output based on studies where the enzyme response to physiological doses of exogenous CCK have been compared to the food stimulated response [1,2]. Most of these studies have concluded that postprandial elevations in plasma CCK concentrations are sufficient to produce the pancreatic enzyme secretion normally occurring after a meal. However, such evidence does not prove conclusively that CCK is the sole, or major, physiologic regulator of pancreatic enzyme secretion compared to other hormonal or neural factors.

Specific blockade of the peripheral (type A) CCK receptors by MK-329 and loxiglumide has now enabled specific evaluation of the physiologic importance of CCK for the function of the pancreas and other organs. Several animal studies have shown that MK-329 effectively antagonizes the stimulatory actions of exogenous as well as endogenous CCK on pancreatic enzyme secretion and gallbladder contraction [3,4]. Following oral administration in man, this agent also antagonizes the effect of exogenous CCK on gallbladder emptying and blocks postprandial gallbladder contraction, indicating a major role of CCK in regulating gallbladder motility [5]. Recently, we completed the first human studies on MK-329 and pancreatic secretion [6,7], which will be summarized in the following sections.

Effect of MK-329 on CCK-Stimulated Pancreatic Secretion

At present, a preparation of MK-329 for parenteral administration in humans is not available. This renders studies of pancreatic exocrine secretion somewhat troublesome, since aspiration of duodenal contents for as-

[1]Department of Clinical Chemistry KK, Rigshospitalet, Blegdamsvej 9, 2100 Copenhagen O, Denmark.

G. Adler and C. Beglinger (Eds.)
CCK Antagonists in Gastroenterology

Table 1. Percentage difference in CCK-stimulated pancreaticobiliary output after MK-329 (10 mg orally) in relation to placebo in six normal subjects

	Basal (%)	CCK-8 dose 15 pmol $kg^{-1} h^{-1}$ (%)	40 pmol $kg^{-1} h^{-1}$ (%)
Trypsin	−39	−74**	−38
Bicarbonate	−26	−75*	−65*
Duodenal flow	+21	−72**	−39*
Bilirubin	−100	−98**	—

The data during CCK infusion were calculated from the integrated median increase *above* basal.
$^{*}p<0.05$; $^{**}p<0.01$.

sessment of pancreatic output may affect the absorption of the drug after oral intake. Preliminary pharmacokinetic studies in man have shown that peak plasma levels of MK-329 occur 2–4 h after oral intake, and that the half-life is in the order of 6–12 h (J. Lin, unpublished observation). Therefore, in order to obtain full absorption, the drug in our studies was given to the volunteers 2 h before starting duodenal aspiration. A previous study showed that an oral dose of 10 mg MK-329 is sufficient to block both CCK- and meal-stimulated gallbladder contraction in man [5].

The ability of 10 mg MK-329 orally to antagonize the effect of exogenous CCK on pancreaticobiliary secretion was tested in normal subjects using a duodenal marker perfusion technique and a background i.v. infusion of secretin in a physiologic dose (5 pmol/kg per hour) [6]. Compared to placebo, MK-329 was associated with non-significant reductions in the basal outputs of trypsin and bicarbonate of 39% and 26%, while the duodenal flow was slightly higher (Table 1; Fig. 1). Plasma CCK concentrations of 8–9 p*M*, similar to upper postprandial levels, were mimicked by an intravenous infusion of 15 pmol/kg per hour of CCK-8. During this infusion rate, MK-329 caused a marked inhibition (>70%) in the outputs of trypsin as well as bicarbonate and duodenal flow compared to placebo (Table 1; Fig. 1). This finding illustrates the synergistic effect of CCK and secretin in stimulating pancreatic bicarbonate and juice secretion. During a higher CCK-8 dose of 40 pmol/kg per hour, which produced supraphysiological plasma CCK levels of about 23 p*M*, the inhibitory action of MK-329 was still evident,

Fig. 1. Effect of MK-329 (10 mg orally) versus placebo on integrated trypsin output (**A**), bicarbonate output (**B**), and duodenal flow (**C**) in six normal subjects before and during CCK stimulation. Data are given as medians – 25th quartile, since strict normal distribution was not verified by statistical tests [6]. The results during CCK stimulation represent integrated response *above* basal. $^{*}p < 0.05$; $^{**}p < 0.01$

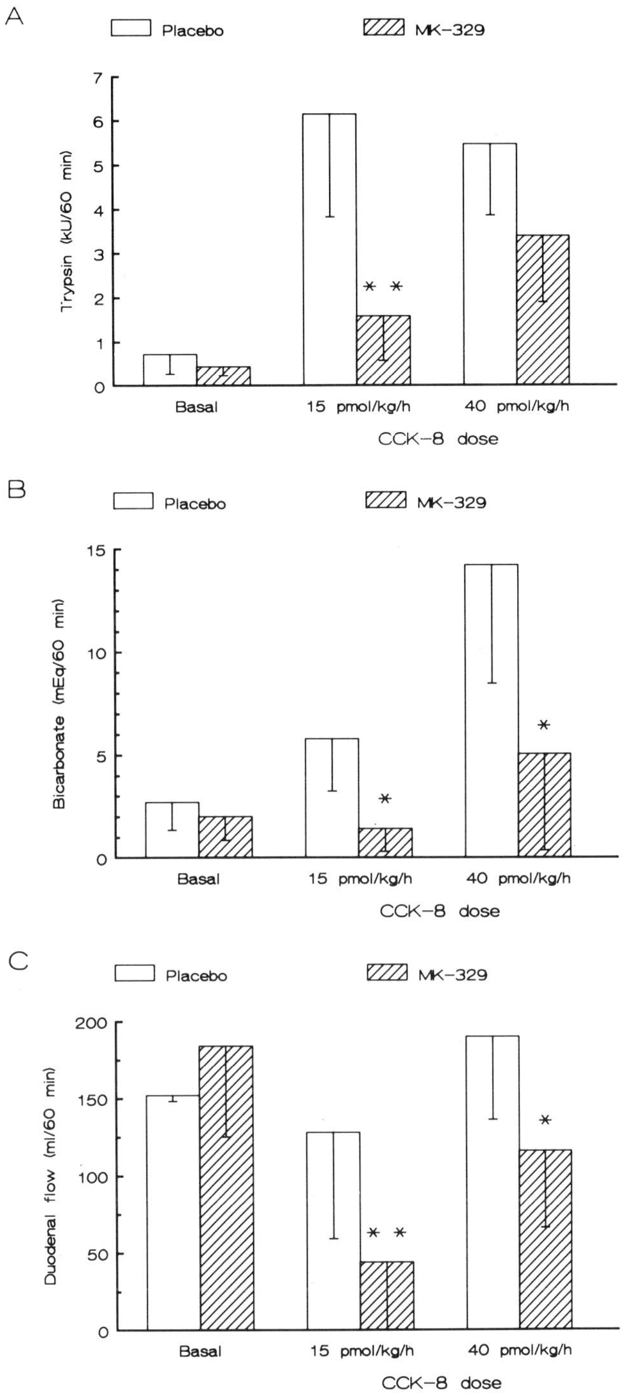
A
Placebo
MK-329
Trypsin (kU/60 min)
7
6
5
4
3
2
1
0
* *
Basal
15 pmol/kg/h
40 pmol/kg/h
CCK-8 dose
B
Placebo
MK-329
Bicarbonate (mEq/60 min)
15
10
5
0
*
*
Basal
15 pmol/kg/h
40 pmol/kg/h
CCK-8 dose
C
Placebo
MK-329
Duodenal flow (ml/60 min)
200
150
100
50
0
* *
*
Basal
15 pmol/kg/h
40 pmol/kg/h
CCK-8 dose

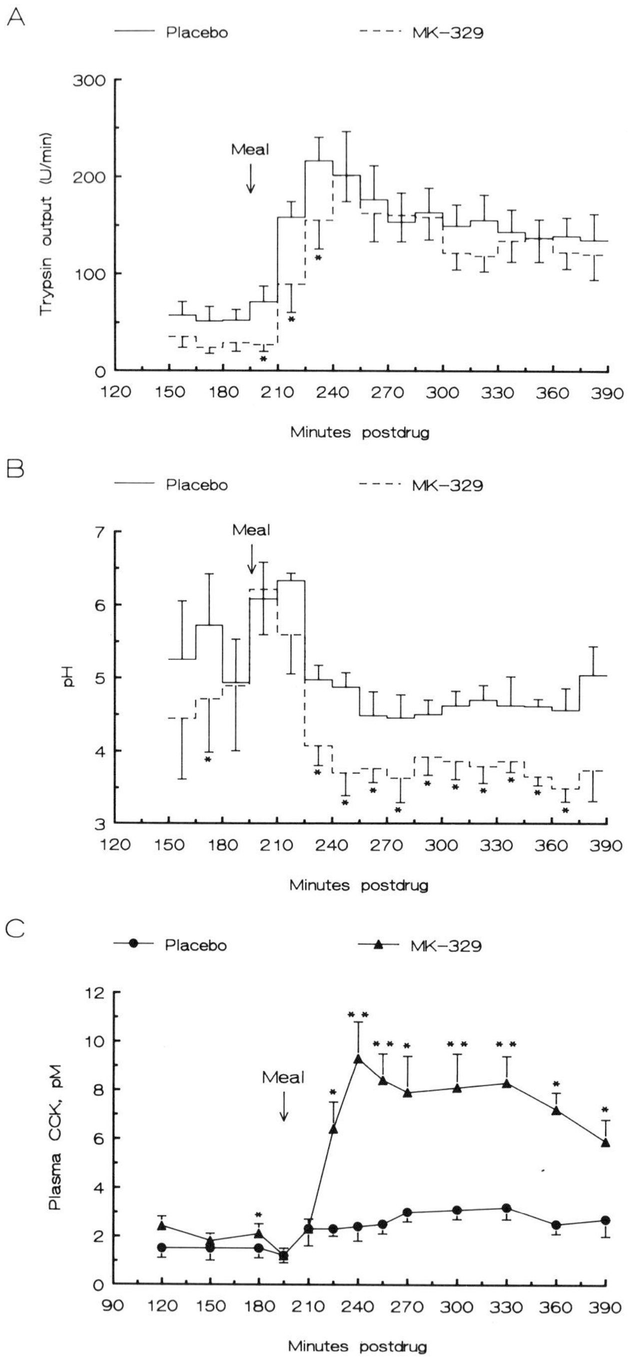

Fig. 2. Effect of MK-329 (10 mg orally) versus placebo on trypsin output (**A**), duodenal pH (**B**), and plasma CCK concentrations (**C**) after a mixed meal in six normal subjects. Data are given as mean ± SEM. $^{*}p < 0.05$; $^{**}p < 0.01$

although not significantly for trypsin (Table 1; Fig. 1). Bilirubin output was virtually abolished after MK-329 (Table 1), indicating almost complete inhibition of gallbladder contraction. The plasma CCK concentrations after MK-329 did not differ from those observed after placebo, neither basally nor during CCK infusions. Thus, MK-329 was found to be an orally effective antagonist of CCK-stimulated pancreaticobiliary output in man.

Effect of MK-329 on Meal-Stimulated Pancreatic Secretion

Assessment of pancreatic exocrine secretion after a meal using duodenal aspiration is complicated by the mixture of food components and pancreatic juice, which renders valid measurements of bicarbonate and volume output impossible. Sampling of pure pancreatic juice by endoscopic duct cannulation cannot guarantee complete recovery of pancreatic juice, which potentially may lead to inaccurate determinations.

In our study, the volunteers ingested a normal mixed meal 3 h, 15 min, after an oral dose of 10 mg MK-329 or placebo using a marker perfusion technique and aspirating at maximum 20 ml/15 min of the duodenal contents [7]. This set-up has previously been evaluated and found to yield reproducible intraindividual assessments of the pancreatic secretory capacity [8]. As in the first study (Table 1), the basal output of trypsin was nonsignificantly reduced, in this case by 43%, after MK-329 (Table 2). During the initial 45 min following the meal, trypsin secretion was inhibited by about 30%–60%, but thereafter the trypsin output was almost the same as after placebo (Fig. 2A). Thus, the integrated postprandial response was only reduced by 15% (NS) (Table 2). This finding strongly suggests that the action of circulating CCK is not essential for the pancreatic enzyme response after a normal meal in healthy subjects. In studies involving another type of CCK antagonist, loxiglumide (CR 1505), direct stimulation of CCK release by intraduodenal perfusion of nutrients reduced pancreatic enzyme secretion by 40%–75% compared to the response in controls [9,10], suggesting a major stimulatory role of CCK. However, these studies are not strictly physiological, since the cephalic and gastric phases of pancreatic secretion are bypassed, which may lead to insufficient activation of other stimulatory mechanisms, most importantly the cholinergic system. Our findings are in agreement with a recent study in normal subjects, where a 7-day treatment with loxiglumide only induced a 15% (NS) reduction in pancreatic enzyme secretion as determined by the para-aminobenzoic acid (PABA) test [11]. Although the PABA test only offers a rough, indirect extimate of pancreatic function, the study shows that, in man, even prolonged CCK antagonism does not cause a major reduction in pancreatic enzyme secretion. Taken together, these results indicate that the effect of neural regulation and/or other hormones is sufficient to maintain an almost normal postprandial enzyme response.

Table 2. Percentage difference in meal-stimulated trypsin secretion, bile acid output, and plasma CCK concentrations after MK-329 (10 mg orally) in relation to placebo in six normal subjects

	Basal (%)	Postprandial (%)
Trypsin	−43	−15**
Bile acid	−96*	−77**
Plasma CCK	+20	+175**

The data were calculated from the integrated mean values.
* $p < 0.05$; ** $p < 0.01$.

Since bicarbonate could not be precisely determined in the aspirates, due to the buffer capacity of the food components, the pH was used as an indirect estimate of the influence of MK-329 on bicarbonate secretion. The pH in the basal duodenal aspirates tended to be lower after MK-329, although the pH of 4.89 in the period immediately before the meal was almost identical to that of controls (Fig. 2B). After the meal, the pH increased to about 6 in both groups during the initial two periods, but thereafter MK-329 caused a sustained decrease in duodenal pH, with mean values ranging from 3.5–4.1 compared to 4.5–5.0 after placebo (Fig. 2B). Since no in vitro or animal studies suggest that MK-329 may stimulate gastric acid secretion, this pH difference is probably explained by a decreased output of pancreatic bicarbonate. Irrespective of the possibility that other sources of bicarbonate, most importantly bile and duodenal mucosal secretions, may play a significant role in neutralizing gastric acid entering the duodenum, the present results demonstrate that the action of CCK is important for the maintenance of a normal duodenal pH.

In contrast to the modest effect on enzyme secretion, MK-329 markedly inhibited the postprandial gallbladder contraction as determined by a 77% reduction in bile acid output (Table 2). Besides confirming the crucial role of CCK in regulating gallbladder motility, this also serves as an indirect proof of the presence of MK-329 in the circulation, at least in quantities sufficient to inhibit gallbladder emptying. The significance of this finding is further strengthened by in vitro studies showing that the relative binding affinities of MK-329 compared to CCK-8 are similar for the gallbladder and pancreatic receptors [12,13]. Valid data on the plasma concentrations of MK-329 await the development of a sensitive and specific assay.

The premeal plasma CCK concentrations tended to be slightly higher after MK-329 than after placebo (Fig. 2C; Table 2). However, the postprandial plasma CCK levels were markedly higher after MK-329 than after placebo (Fig. 2C), resulting in a 175% increase ($p < 0.01$) in the integrated meal-response (Table 2). The augmented plasma CCK concentrations after MK-329 were manifest 30 min after food ingestion and continued to be significantly elevated throughout the study (Fig. 2C) in spite of almost equal secretion of trypsin in the two groups (Fig. 1A). Thus, no inverse relationship was demonstrable between the trypsin activity in the duodenal lumen and the plasma CCK levels after MK-329. A detailed discussion on the mechanism(s) involved in the augmented postprandial CCK response during CCK receptor blockade is outside the topic of this chapter, but, at present, attractive explanations are (a) activation of a negative feedback mechanism due to low concentrations of bile constituents in the duodenal lume and, more speculatively (b) interference with autoregulating, inhibitory CCK receptors on the vascular side of the CCK cell leading to enhanced secretion of CCK to the bloodstream.

References

1. Beglinger C, Fried M, Whitehouse I, Jansen JB, Lamers CB, Gyr K (1985) Pancreatic enzyme response to a liquid meal and to hormonal stimulation. J Clin Invest 75:1471–1476
2. Cantor P (1989) Cholecystokinin in plasma. Digestion 42:181–201
3. Lotti VJ, Pendleton RG, Gould RJ, Hanson HM, Chang RSL, Clineschmidt BJ (1987) In vivo pharmacology of L-364718, a new potent nonpeptide peripheral cholecystokinin antagonist. J Pharmacol Exp Ther 241:103–109
4. Pendleton RG, Bendesky RJ, Schaffer L, Nolan TE, Gould RJ, Clineschmidt BJ (1987) Roles of endogenous cholecystokinin in biliary, pancreatic and gastric function: studies with L-364718, a specific cholecystokinin receptor antagonist. J Pharmacol Exp Ther 241:210–216
5. Liddle RA, Gertz BA, Kanyama S, Beccaria L, Coker LD, Turnbull TA, Morita ET (1989) Effects of a novel cholecystokinin receptor antagonist, MK-329, on gallbladder contraction and gastric emptying in humans: implications for the physiology of CCK. J Clin Invest 84:1220–1225
6. Cantor P, Olsen O, Gertz BJ, Gjorup I, Worning H (1991) Inhibition of cholecystokinin (CCK)-stimulated pancreaticobiliary output in man by the CCK-receptor antagonist MK-329. Scand J Gastroenterol 26:627–637
7. Cantor P, Mortensen PE, Myhre J, Gjorup I, Worning H, Stahl E, Survill TT (1990) The effect of the cholecystokinin receptor antagonist MK-329 on meal-stimulated pancreatico-biliary output and gastrointestinal motility in man. gastroenterology (submitted)
8. Myhre J, Mortensen PE, Astrup A, Worning H (1988) Normal human pancreatic secretion after ingestion of a solid meal. Digestion 40:103–104
9. Hildebrand P, Beglinger C, Gyr K, Jansen JBMJ, Rovati LC, Zuercher M, Lamers CBHW, Setnikar I, Stalder GA (1990) Effects of a cholecystokinin receptor antagonist on intestinal phase of pancreatic and biliary responses in man. J Clin Invest 85:640–646
10. Adler G, Reinshagen M, Koop I, Arnold R, Rovati L (1988) Inhibition of stimulated pancreatic secretion in man by a cholecystokinin antagonist (CR 1505). Digestion 40:67
11. Meyer BM, Beglinger C, Jansen JBMJ, Rovati LC, Werth BA, Hildebrand P, Zach D, Stalder GA (1989) Role of cholecystokinin in regulation of gastrointestinal motor functions. Lancet 2:12–15

12. Chang RSL, Lotti VJ (1986) Biochemical and pharmacologic characterization of a new extremely potent and selective nonpeptide cholecystokinin antagonist. Proc Natl Acad Sci USA 83:4923–4926
13. Von Schrenck T, Moran TH, Heinz-Erian P, Gardner JD, Jensen RT (1988) Cholecystokinin receptors on gallbladder muscle and pancreatic acinar cells: a comparative study. Am J Physiol 255:G512–G521

Regulation of Gallbladder Contraction and Gastric Emptying by the CCK Receptor Antagonist MK-329

R.A. LIDDLE[1]

Introduction

The gastrointestinal hormone cholecystokinin (CCK) has been proposed as having a number of physiologic actions. These include stimulation of gallbladder contraction and pancreatic protein secretion as well as regulation of gastric emptying, stimulation of intestinal motility, stimulation of insulin secretion, and induction of satiety [23]. However, it has been difficult to establish whether these are pharmacologic or true physiologic actions of CCK. Studies on the physiology of CCK have been hampered by difficulty in measuring plasma levels of the hormone, primarily because of the structural similarities between CCK and gastrin [25]. Both hormones share an identical pentapeptide sequence at the carboxyl terminus consisting of Gly-Trp-Met-Asp-Phe-NH_2. Since this portion of the molecule is the biologically active region of CCK, it is important that an assay for CCK be able to detect all molecular forms of the peptide without cross-reactivity with gastrin. Such a radioimmunoassay must be specific for the amino terminal region of CCK-8 which would confer the ability to recognize larger forms of CCK yet not cross-react with gastrin. Development of these radioimmunoassays has been difficult and an antibody is not yet universally available. An alternative method has been the development of a sensitive and specific bioassay based on the ability of CCK in plasma extracts to stimulate amylase release from isolated pancreatic acini [14,15].

The classical approach to determining whether a candidate transmitter acts as a hormone has been to measure plasma levels of the transmitter simultaneously, with its target tissue response. Then, by infusing exogenous hormone to reproduce the same plasma levels that occur endogenously, and measuring the same target tissue response, it is possible to determine if a transmitter functions in a physiologic manner, i.e., as a true hormone. This approach has been taken to determine the possible physiologic actions of CCK [1,13,15,17,18,26].

[1]Duke University Medical Center, Gastroenterology Section, Durham Veterans Administration Medical Center, Durham, NC 27710, USA.

G. Adler and C. Beglinger (Eds.)
CCK Antagonists in Gastroenterology

Another way of investigating, the role of candidate hormones is to selectively inhibit the hormone of interest by a specific antagonist. Recently, a nonpeptide CCK receptor antagonist has been developed, termed MK-329 (3*S*(-)-*N*-(2,3-dihydro-1-methyl-2-oxo-5-phenyl-1H-1,4 benzodiazepine-3-yl)-1H-indole-2-carboxamide, previously designated L-364718) [2,5]. MK-329 is specific for peripheral (type A) CCK receptors and has an approximately 1000-fold lower affinity for binding to cerebrocorticol CCK (type B) receptors [2,5]. *In vitro* studies have shown MK-329 to be an effective inhibitor of CCK binding to pancreatic membranes and gallbladder tissues with $IC_{50's}$ of 81 and 45 p*M*, respectively [2,5]. In animals, MK-329 has been shown to inhibit CCK-stimulated pancreatic exocrine secretion and colonic contraction as well as gallbladder contraction and CCK-induced inhibition of gastric emptying [20]. These data indicate that MK-329 is a specific CCK antagonist which may be used *in vivo*.

Our laboratory has recently had the opportunity of investigating MK-329 in humans [19]. The objectives of these studies were (a) to determine whether MK-329 was an effective CCK antagonist in humans, and (b) to establish whether CCK receptor antagonism could inhibit gallbladder contraction and modify gastric emptying after a meal.

Effect of MK-329 on CCK-Stimulated Gallbladder Contraction

To determine whether MK-329 was an effective antagonist of exogenous CCK, subjects were treated with MK-329 prior to infusion of CCK in a randomized, controlled trial [19]. Two hours before receiving an infusion of CCK-8 at a rate of 30 pmol $kg^{-1}h^{-1}$ subjects ingested placebo or 0.5, 2, or 10 mg of MK-329. Plasma CCK levels were measured by radioimmunoassay using an antibody directed against the amino terminus of CCK-8, thus allowing measurement of the multiple molecular forms of CCK [19]. Basal plasma levels of CCK averaged 0.8 p*M* and increased to between 7.7 and 10.4 p*M* within 15 min of starting the infusion. No significant differences in plasma CCK concentrations were achieved during CCK infusion with any of the drug or placebo treatments. Gallbladder volumes were measured by abdominal sonography (Fig. 1). Baseline gallbladder volumes were in the range 21.1–25.1 ml. In placebo-treated subjects, infusion of CCK caused a decrease in gallbladder volume of 26% within 20 min and a 57% decrease within 2 h of beginning the infusion. MK-329 inhibited CCK-induced gallbladder contraction in a dose-dependent manner. The 2 mg dose of MK-329 reduced the decrease in gallbladder volume to 36% at the end of 2 h, while 10 mg MK-329 completely inhibited CCK-stimulated gallbladder contraction. These studies demonstrated two important points. First, CCK infusion approximating postprandial CCK levels, stimulated gallbladder contraction, suggesting a hormonal role for CCK. Second, this degree of gallbladder contraction was completely inhibited by 10 mg of MK-329.

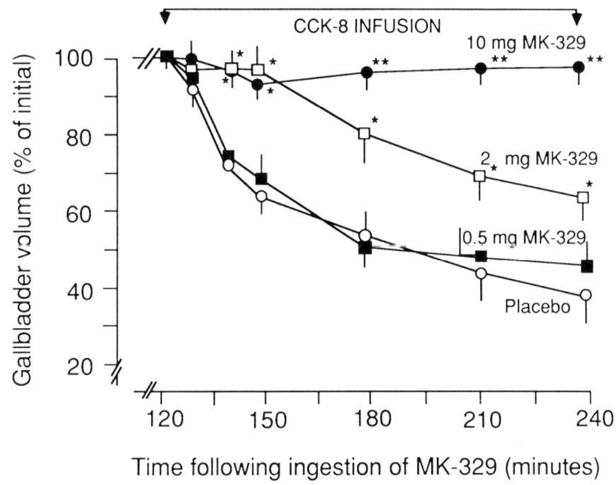

Fig. 1. Effect of MK-329 on gallbladder volumes during infusion of CCK. Gallbladder volumes are expressed as the percentage of initial volume. *Asterisks* indicate values statistically different from placebo [from 19]

Effect of MK-329 on Meal-Stimulated Gallbladder Contraction and Gastric Emptying

In order to determine the effect of MK-329 on meal-stimulated gallbladder contraction and gastric emptying rates, subjects received placebo or 10 mg MK-329 2 h before eating a mixed meal. The 10 mg dose was chosen because it was the maximally effective dose observed in the previous study. In patients treated with placebo, plasma CCK concentrations increased from basal levels of 0.6 p*M* to peak postprandial levels of 2.3 p*M* (Fig. 2). However, in subjects receiving MK-329, there was an accentuation of the postprandial increase in plasma CCK concentrations with median peak levels reaching 13.8 p*M*.

In placebo-treated subjects, gallbladder volume decreased by 68% 2 h after eating (Fig. 3). However, in subjects taking 10 mg MK-329, despite much higher circulating CCK concentrations, gallbladder contraction was completely inhibited after the meal.

Gastric emptying of both the solid and liquid components of a mixed meal were measured by gamma camera scintigraphy using ^{99m}Tc as a label of solid food and ^{111}In for liquids (Fig. 4). Gastric emptying of the solid component of the meal was based on the rate at which the ^{99m}Tc-labeled marker disappeared from the area of the stomach. With placebo treatment, the solid marker emptied slowly with a half-life of 128 min. Furthermore, there was no difference between placebo and MK-329 treatments. After placebo, liquids emptied more rapidly with a half-life of 58 min. The rate of emptying of liquids from the stomach was also unaffected by MK-329.

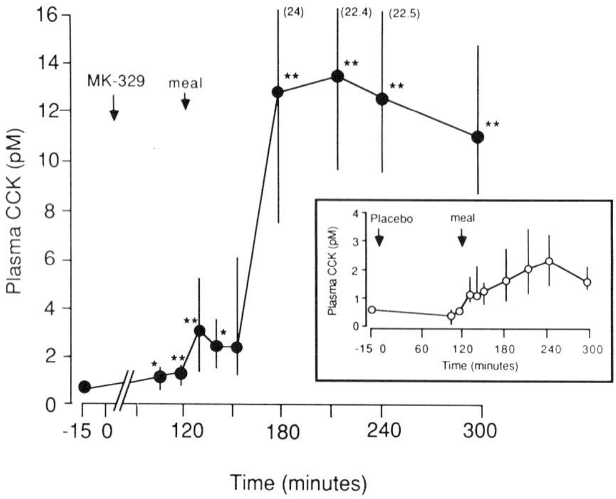

Fig. 2. Effect of MK-329 on plasma CCK concentration with ingestion of a mixed meal. Eight subjects received orally either placebo (*open circles*) or 10 mg MK-329 (*closed circles*) 2 h before ingestion of a 614 kcal mixed meal. Plasma CCK values are expressed as mean values and interquartile ranges. *Numbers in parentheses* indicate the 75th percentile. Placebo treatment is shown in the *insert* [from 19]

Adverse Effects

No serious adverse effects were observed after the administration of MK-329. Symptoms of diarrhea and abdominal cramping occurring in several patients may have been drug related but were self-limited and resolved within 24 h.

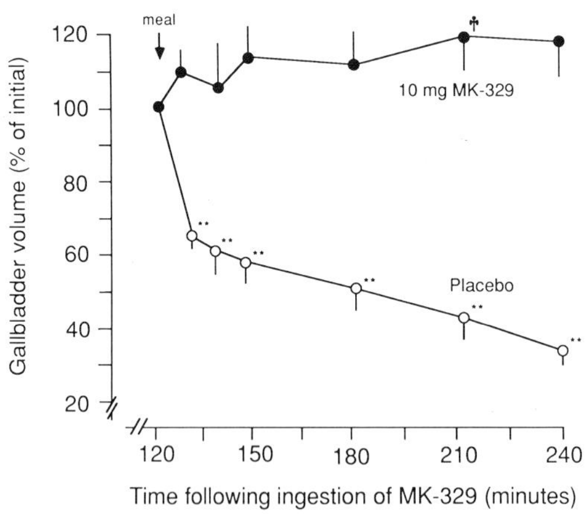

Fig. 3. Effect of MK-329 on gallbladder volumes after ingestion of a mixed meal. Values are the mean ±SEM [from 19]

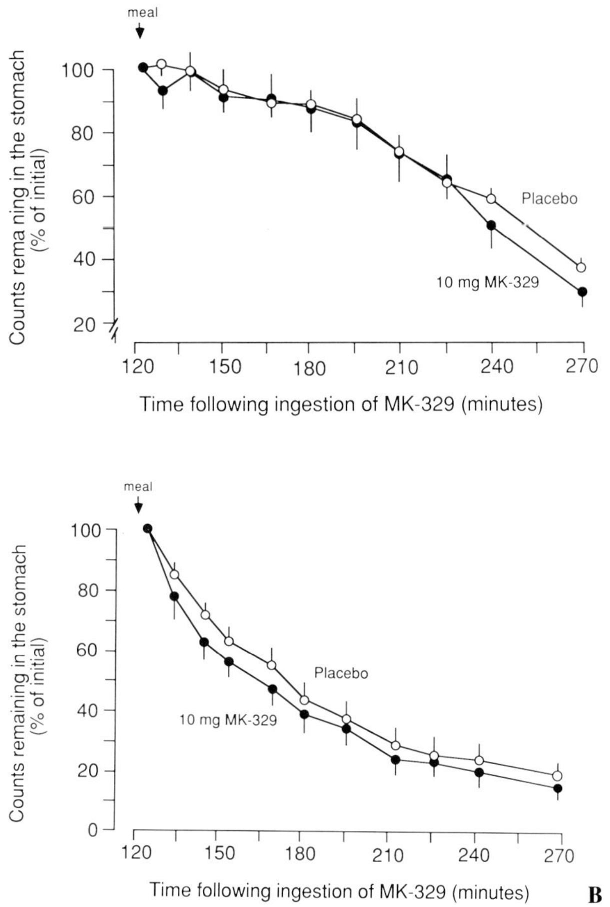

Fig. 4A.B. Effect of MK-329 on gastric emptying. Gastric emptying of solids (**A**) and liquids (**B**) were measured in subjects described in Figs. 2,3. The solid component of the meal as labeled with ^{99m}Tc sulfur colloid. The liquid component of the meal was labeled with ^{111}In-diethylene triamine penta-acetic acid [from 19]

Discussion

These studies demonstrate that MK-329 is a potent, orally active, CCK antagonist in humans. In a dose-dependent manner, MK-329 inhibited CCK-induced gallbladder contraction. To determine the effect of CCK receptor blockade on postprandial responses, 10 mg of the antagonist was shown to (a) completely inhibit meal-stimulated gallbladder contraction, (b) dramatically increase postprandial plasma CCK levels, and (c) have no effect on gastric emptying. The ability of MK-329 to completely inhibit meal-induced gallbladder contraction indicates that CCK is the major hormonal regulator of gallbladder contraction.

Similar effects of CCK receptor antagonism on gallbladder contraction have been supported by studies using another type of CCK receptor antagonist. Loxiglumide, a glutamic acid analogue has also recently been studied in humans. Several studies have confirmed that CCK receptor antagonism inhibits the decrease in gallbladder volume after a meal [4,9,10,22,24].

The observation that MK-329 markedly increased meal-stimulated plasma CCK concentrations could be explained by three possible mechanisms. First, the rate of CCK clearance could be reduced by MK-329, indicating that a receptor-mediated mechanism participates in removal of CCK from the circulation. However, with infusion of CCK, steady-state plasma CCK levels were achieved and there were no significant differences in CCK levels between any dose of MK-329 or placebo. These findings indicate that the receptor antagonist does not influence CCK clearance and, therefore, it is unlikely that a receptor-mediated mechanism is necessary for CCK metabolism.

A second possible reason CCK levels were higher after MK-329 treatment could be due to increased delivery of nutrients to the duodenum secondary to accelerated gastric emptying. However, gastric emptying rates were not increased after MK-329, thus excluding increased nutrient delivery to the small intestine. Therefore, this mechanism could not explain the increase in CCK responses after drug treatment.

The third and most likely possibility that could account for the higher postprandial CCK levels after MK-329, is a negative feedback mechanism regulating CCK secretion. It has been well demonstrated in the rat that diversion of pancreaticobiliary juice from the duodenum, or inhibition of duodenal pancreatic enzyme activity with trypsin inhibitors, causes a prompt increase in pancreatic exocrine secretion [8]. Furthermore, it has been confirmed that CCK is stimulated by both of these mechanisms [12,16]. Therefore, CCK appears to mediate negative feedback regulation of pancreatic secretion [21]. Recent evidence also suggests that bile acids participate in negative feedback regulation of CCK secretion [7,11]. In the present study, the observation that peak plasma CCK levels were much higher in subjects who received CCK receptor antagonist treatment suggests that MK-329 may have inhibited meal-induced pancreatic secretion and gallbladder contraction, thereby increasing the stimulus for CCK release. The absence or reduction of bile and pancreatic juice in the duodenum is a likely cause of the accentuated CCK response. These data support the concept of negative feedback regulation of CCK secretion in humans. Similarly, recent studies using loxiglumide have observed increased CCK levels after CCK receptor antagonist treatment [9,22].

At the dose studied, MK-329 had no effect on gastric emptying of solids or liquids. These findings suggest that CCK alone is not a major hormonal regulator of gastric emptying. However, these experiments must be interpreted with caution since other factors may compensate for, or obscure, the effects of CCK in the milieu of ingestion of a mixed meal. It is also possible that higher doses of MK-329 might have demonstrated an acceleration of gastric emptying. Since gastric emptying and CCK release are regulated by various properties of a meal, including nutrient composition, it is also possible that an alteration of gastric emptying with MK-329 would have been observed with a meal composed of different nutrients.

Conflicting reports have been published regarding the effects of loxiglumide on gastric emptying. One recent study indicated that CCK receptor antagonism with loxiglumide had no effect on gastric emptying of a meal [4]; however, another report demonstrated that gastric emptying of nondigestible markers was accelerated with loxiglumide treatment [22]. Therefore, the precise physiologic role of CCK in regulating gastric emptying may not yet be fully established.

In summary, these studies have demonstrated that CCK is an effective, orally active antagonist of CCK based on its ability to inhibit CCK-induced gallbladder contraction. We may also conclude that CCK has an important physiologic role in regulating postprandial gallbladder contraction. The significant effect of CCK antagonism on plasma CCK concentrations supports a mechanism of negative feedback regulation of CCK secretion. Finally, at present, it appears that CCK may have a limited role in regulating gastric emptying rates after a meal.

A number of postulated physiologic effects of CCK suggest several possible therapeutic applications for a CCK receptor antagonist drug [6]. Therefore, it will be important to examine the effects of such an agent on appetite, the treatment of eating disorders, and the modification of bowel motility. The selectivity of antagonists for peripheral (type A) CCK receptors such as MK-329, and central (type B) receptors such as L-365 260, should also make it possible to distinguish between the physiologic effects of CCK receptor subtypes [3]. Together these antagonists provide valuable tools for studying the physiologic actions of CCK.

References

1. Beglinger C, Fried M, Whitehouse I, Jansen JB, Lamers CB, Gyr K (1985) Pancreatic enzyme response to a liquid meal and to hormonal stimulation. J Clin Invest 75:1471–1476
2. Chang RSL, Lotti VJ (1986) Biochemical and pharmacological characterization of an extremely potent and selective nonpeptide cholecystokinin antagonist. Proc Natl Acad Sci USA 83:4923–4926
3. Chang RSL, Chen TB, Bock MG, Freidinger RM, Chen R, Rosegay A, Lotti VJ (1989) Characterization of the binding of [3H]L-365 260: a new potent and selective brain cholecystokinin (CCK-B) and gastrin receptor antagonist radioligand. Mol Pharmacol 35:803–808
4. Corazziari E, Ricci R, Biliotti D, Bontempo I, Demedici A, Pallotta N, Torsoli A (1990) Oral administration of loxiglumide CCK antagonist inhibits postprandial gallbladder contraction without affecting gastric emptying. Dig Dis Sci 35:50–54

5. Evans BE, Rittle KE, Bock MG, DiPardo RM, Freidinger RM, Whitter WL, Gould NP, Lundell GF, Homnick CF, Veber DF, Anderson PS, Chang RSL, Lotti VJ, Cerino DJ, Chen TB, King PJ, Kunkel KA, Springer JP, Hirshfield J (1987) Design of nonpeptidal ligands for a peptide receptor: cholecystokinin antagonists. J Med Chem 30:1229–1239
6. Gertz BJ (1988) Potential clinical applications of a CCK antagonist. In: Wang RY, Schoenfeld R (eds) Cholecystokinin antagonists. Liss, New York, pp 327–342
7. Gomez G, Upp JR Jr, Lluis F, Alexander RW, Poston GJ, Greeley GH Jr, Thompson JC (1988) Regulation of the release of cholecystokinin by bile salts in dogs and humans. Gastroenterology 94:1036–1046
8. Green GM, Lyman RL (1972) Feedback regulation of pancreatic enzyme secretion as a mechanism for trypsin inhibitor-induced hypersecretion in rats. Proc Soc Exp Biol Med 140:6–12
9. Hildebrand P, Beglinger C, Gyr K, Jansen JBMJ, Rovati LC, Zuercher M, Lamers CBHW, Setnikar I, Stadler GA (1990) Effects of a cholecystokinin receptor antagonist on intestinal phase of pancreatic and biliary responses in man. J Clin Invest 85:640–646
10. Konturek JW, Konturek SJ, Kurek A, Bogdal J, Oleksy J, Rovati L (1989) CCK receptor antagonism by loxiglumide and gall bladder contractions in response to cholecystokinin, sham feeding and ordinary feeding in man. Gut 30:1136–1142
11. Koop I, Koop H, Gerhardt C, Schafmayer A, Arnold R (1989) Do bile acids exert a negative feedback control of cholecystokinin release? Scand J Gastroenterol 29:315–320
12. Levan VH, Liddle RA, Green GM (1987) Jejunal bypass stimulation of pancreatic growth and cholecystokinin secretion in rats: importance of luminal nutrients. Gut 28 (S1):25–29
13. Liddle RA, Ensinck JW (1990) Cholecystokinin does not stimulate prosomatostatin-derived peptides in man. J Clin Endo Crinol Metab 70: 1403–1407
14. Liddle RA, Goldfine ID, Williams JA (1984) Bioassay of plasma cholecystokinin in rats: effects of food, trypsin inhibitor, and alcohol. Gastroenterology 87: 542–549
15. Liddle RA, Goldfine ID, Rosen MS, Taplitz RA, Williams JA (1985) Cholecystokinin bioactivity in human plasma: molecular forms, responses to feeding, and relationship to gallbladder contraction. J Clin Invest 75:1144–1152
16. Liddle RA, Green GM, Conrad CK, Williams JA (1986) Proteins but not amino acids, carbohydrates, or fats stimulate cholecystokinin secretion in the rat. Am J Physiol 251:G243–G248
17. Liddle RA, Morita ET, Conrad CK, Williams JA (1986) Regulation of gastric emptying in humans by cholecystokinin. J Clin Invest 77:992–996
18. Liddle RA, Rushakoff RJ, Morita ET, Beccaria L, Carter JD, Goldfine ID (1988) Physiological role for cholecystokinin in reducing postprandial hyperglycemia in humans. J Clin Invest 81:1675–1681
19. Liddle RA, Gertz BJ, Kanayama S, Beccaria L, Coker LD, Turnbull TA, Morita ET (1989) Effects of a novel cholecystokinin (CCK) receptor antagonist, MK-329, on gallbladder contraction and gastric emptying in humans: implications for the physiology of CCK. J Clin Invest 84:1220–1225
20. Lotti VJ, Pendleton RG, Gould RJ, Hanson HM, Chang RSL, Clineschmidt BV (1987) In vivo pharmacology of L-364718, a new potent nonpeptide peripheral cholecystokinin antagonist. J Pharmacol Exp Ther 241:103–109
21. Louie DS, May P, Miller P, Owyang C (1986) Cholecystokinin mediates feedback regulation of pancreatic enzyme secretion in rats. Am J Physiol 250: G252–G259
22. Meyer BM, Werth BA, Beglinger C, Hildebrand P, Jansen JBMJ, Zach D, Rovati LC, Stalder GA (1989) Role of cholecystokinin in regulation of gastrointestinal motor functions. Lancet 2:12–15

23. Mutt V (1988) Secretin and cholecystokinin. In: Mutt V (ed) Gastrointestinal hormones. Academic, San Diego, pp 251–320
24. Niederau C, Heintges T, Rovati L, Strohmeyer G (1989) Effects of loxiglumide on gallbladder emptying in healthy volunteers. Gastroenterology 97:1331–1336
25. Rehfeld JF (1984) How to measure cholecystokinin in plasma. Gastroenterology 87:434–438
26. Rushakoff RJ, Goldfine ID, Carter JD, Liddle RA (1987) Physiological concentrations of cholecystokinin stimulate amino acid-induced insulin release in humans. J Clin Endocrinol Metab 65:395–401

Regulation of CCK Release by Bile Acids

I. Koop[1]

Introduction

Cholecystokinin (CCK) is the most potent hormonal stimulus for contraction of the gallbladder [1–3] thereby markedly increasing the delivery of bile acids into the duodenum. Together with monoglycerides and phospholipids, bile acids form mixed micelles to facilitate fat absorption. Eventually, 95% of them are reabsorbed by the terminal ileum to finish the enterohepatic cycle [4]. Since bile acids presumably get in contact with intestinal CCK cells and are closely linked to the digestion and absorption of fat, a potent stimulus for CCK secretion, there is likely a relationship between bile acids and CCK release.

Acute Effects of Bile Acids and Bile Diversion on CCK Release

Duodenal perfusion of "bile excess" or chenodeoxycholic acid had marginal, if any, effects on basal plasma CCK concentrations in dogs and humans [5,6]. However, the influence on stimulated CCK release was far more pronounced. Bile acids decreased stimulated CCK release in humans, dogs and guinea pigs [5–9]. This inhibitory effect was independent of the chemical nature of the stimulus, such as amino acids [7], triglycerides [5] or a mixed liquid testmeal containing protein, long chain fatty acids and glucose [6,8] (Fig. 1). Furthermore, taurocholate, chenodeoxycholic acid and pooled bile exerted the inhibitory action in a similar way, irrespective of the site of administration (oral ingestion or intraduodenal infusion). Elevated plasma CCK concentrations due to diversion of pancreaticobiliary juice in rats were reduced by 70% following duodenal infusion of taurocholate [10].

Bile diversion can be achieved by either bile duct ligation or external or internal drainage of bile. In addition, the nonabsorbable bile salt binding resin cholestyramine [11] has been used as a tool to mimic intraluminal bile acid depletion. Almost unequivocal results have been obtained by the

[1] Department of Internal Medicine, Division of Gastroenterology and Metabolism, University of Marburg, Baldingerstr. 1, 3550 Marburg, FRG.

G. Adler and C. Beglinger (Eds.)
CCK Antagonists in Gastroenterology

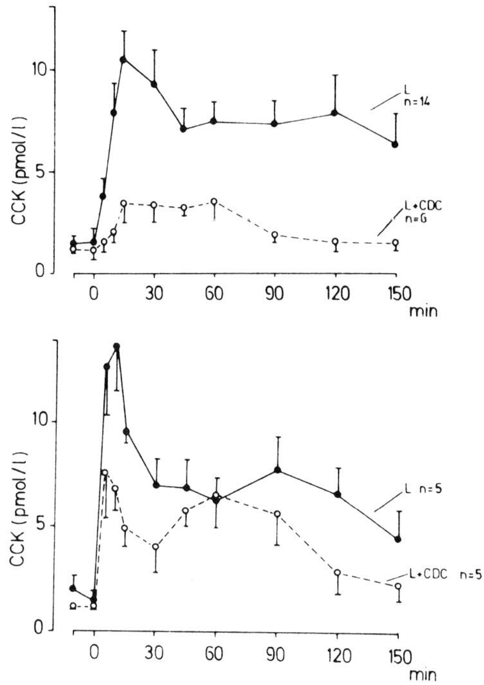

Fig. 1. Basal and stimulated plasma CCK concentrations in patients with bile duct obstruction (*upper panel*) and in healthy controls (*lower panel*). *L* liquid tastmeal; *L + CDC*, testmeal with 4 g chenodeoxycholic acid (from [8])

removal of functional bile acids from the intestine: augmentation of CCK release stimulated either by nutrients or pancreatic juice diversion [6,7, 10,12]. While amino acid- or meal-stimulated CCK levels were enhanced by bile diversion in dogs or by cholestyramine in humans, addition of bile acids reversed this effect [6,7] suggesting that bile acids are the key constituents of bile responsible for the modulation of CCK release. Basal CCK release was not at all or only weakly stimulated by bile diversion [5] or duodenal cholestyramine-infusion [6,7]. In contrast, oral ingestion of cholestyramine caused a significant rise of CCK [12].

It is unknown whether bile acids act directly on the CCK cell. Indirect modulation of CCK release may be due to increased trypsin activity in the upper intestine: bile acids enhance release of enterokinase from the duodenal mucosa to activate trypsinogen [13,14]. Furthermore, in vivo studies in rats suggested an important role for bile acids as a stabilizing factor for trypsin activity [15,16]. Recently, a trypsin-sensitive, CCK-releasing monitor peptide was discovered in pancreatic juice [17,18]. Thus, bile acids may affect CCK release by enhancing tryptic activity, thereby decreasing the activity of the monitor peptide and release of CCK.

Chronic Effects of Bile Acid Administration and Bile Depletion on CCK Release

After 1–5 weeks of either bile duct ligation or cholestyramine administration in animals [7,9,19,20] basal plasma CCK concentrations were unchanged. In humans, however, basal CCK levels were substantially elevated up to 21 days after initiation of cholestyramine treatment but had normalized after 28 days [12]. It was assumed that the CCK cell had changed its responsiveness to the chronic overstimulation by cholestyramine during the 4-week treatment, a phenomenon which has also been described in rats following long-term protein administration [21]. In parallel, patients with long-lasting bile duct obstruction due to a malignant tumor and marked hyperbilirubinemia showed normal CCK levels [8] (Fig. 1).

While basal CCK levels did not change at all, or returned to normal values after a certain period of time, CCK release in response to nutrients was reported to be enhanced both after 7 and 28 days of cholestyramine administration in dogs and humans [7,12]. Patients with chronic, advanced bile duct obstruction showed the same postprandial CCK response as healthy controls. However, inhibition of stimulated CCK release by concomitant administration of bile acids was more pronounced in patients with biliary obstruction than in healthy controls, suggesting again that the responsiveness of the CCK cell to bile acids had changed during long-term intraluminal bile depletion [8] (Fig. 1).

There is evidence that bile acids modulate the number of CCK receptors in guinea-pigs: cholestyramine feeding for 5 weeks resulted in an increase in CCK receptors on gallbladder muscle whereas taurocholate administration had the opposite effect [9].

Bile Acid-Induced Effects on the Exocrine Pancreas: Influence of CCK Receptor Antagonism

Changes in CCK release following intraduodenal bile salt infusion or depletion are paralleled by changes in gallbladder contraction/biliary output and exocrine pancreatic secretion and pancreatic growth. Proglumide, a CCK receptor antagonist of the first generation, almost entirely suppressed pancreatic protein output induced by intraduodenal infusion of amino acids and cholestyramine in dogs [7]. In humans, intravenous infusion of the highly specific CCK receptor antagonist loxiglumide inhibited pancreatic trypsin output by 60%. Inhibition of cholestyramine-enhanced enzyme secretion by loxiglumide amounted to 73%. Enzyme output did not differ in both groups during loxiglumide administration, suggesting that elevated plasma CCK levels were responsible for enhancement of pancreatic secretion by cholestyramine [22].

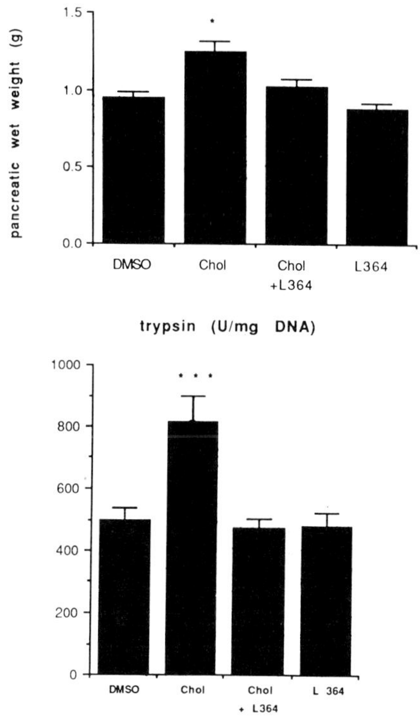

Fig. 2. Effect of 4-week administration of 6% cholestyramine and L-364718 (MK329) on pancreatic wet weight and trypsin content of the rat pancreas. *DMSO*, dimethylsulfoxide, vehicle for the antagonist; *Chol*, cholestyramine. $^{*}p < 0.05$, $^{***}p < 0.01$ vs. DMSO (from [6])

Long-term cholestyramine feeding has a trophic effect on the exocrine pancreas in rats and guinea-pigs [9,19,23]. The CCK receptor antagonist MK-329 (formerly L-364718) completely abolished this effect in rats [19], indicating that CCK was the mediator of the cholestyramine-induced trophic effect on the pancreas (Fig. 2). Furthermore, it antagonized the increase of trypsin and chymotrypsin content by cholestyramine.

Intraduodenal infusion of chenodeoxycholic acid reduced meal-stimulated CCK output but did not inhibit pancreatic enzyme secretion in humans [22]. In consequence, loxiglumide had no influence on enzyme release, suggesting that stimulation of pancreatic exocrine secretion by chenodeoxycholic acid involved a mediator other than CCK. However, in previous studies taurocholate has been shown to inhibit amino acid- and fat-stimulated enzyme release [24,25]. Thus, the effect of bile acids on exocrine pancreatic secretion may differ according to the type (and amount/concentration) of bile acid used whereas their inhibitory action on CCK release seems to be uniform (Fig. 3).

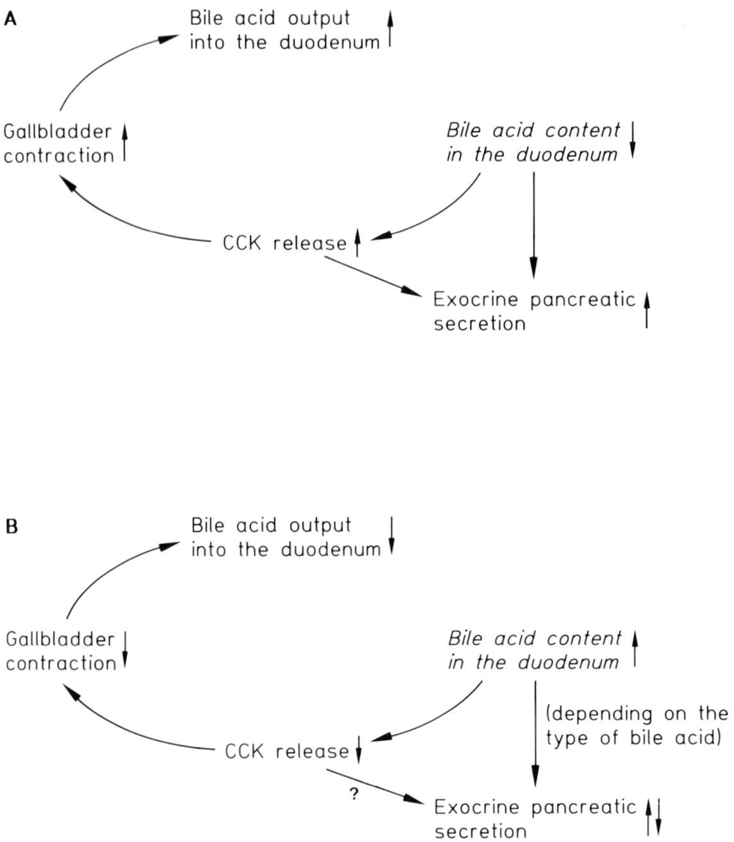

Fig. 3A,B. Proposed role of bile acids in the control of CCK release and biliary and pancreatic secretion. **A** Effect of bile acid depletion. **B** Effect of bile acid excess

Summary

Bile acids play a regulatory role in the control of CCK release, especially in the postprandial state. Though most studies have proven bile acids to inhibit and removal of bile acids to enhance stimulated release more investigations are needed to define the role of CCK in bile acid-induced changes of biliary and pancreatic secretion. Specific CCK receptor antagonists which are now available provide a useful tool to elucidate this interrelationship.

References

1. Maton PN, Selden AC, Fitzpatrick ML, Chadwick VS (1984) Infusion of cholecystokinin octapeptide in man: relation between plasma cholecystokinin concentrations and gallbladder emptying rates. Eur J Clin Invest 14:37–41
2. Anagnostides AA, Chadwick VS, Selden AC, Barr J, Maton PN (1985) Human pancreatic and biliary responses to physiological concentrations of cholecystokinin octapeptide. Clin Sci 69:259–263
3. Niederau C, Heintges T, Rovati L, Strohmeyer G (1989) Effects of loxiglumide in gallbladder emptying in healthy volunteers. Gastroenterology 97:1331–1336
4. Erlinger S (1987) Physiology of bile secretion and enterohepatic circulation. In: Johnson LR (ed) Physiology of the gastrointestinal tract. Raven, New York, pp 1557–1580
5. Gomez G, Lluis F, Guo YS, Greeley GH, Townsend CM, Thompson JC (1986) Bile inhibits release of cholecystokinin and neurotensin. Surgery 100:363–367
6. Koop I, Dorn S, Koop H, Witzleb S, Beglinger C, Schafmayer A, Arnold R (1990) Dissociation of cholecystokinin and pancreatico-biliary response to intraduodenal bile acids and cholestyramine in humans. Dig Dis Sci (in press)
7. Gomez G, Upp JR, Lluis F, Alexander RW, Poston GJ, Greeley GH, Thompson JC (1988) Regulation of the release of cholecystokinin by bile salts in dogs and humans. Gastroenterology 94:1036–1046
8. Koop I, Koop H, Gerhardt C, Schafmayer A, Arnold R (1989) Do bile acids exert a negative feedback control on cholecystokinin release? Scand J Gastroenterol 24:315–320
9. Gomez G, Townsend CM, Maani R, Singh P, Greeley G, Thompson JC (1989) Down-regulation of pancreatic growth and gallbladder contractility by bile salts. Am J Surg 157:20–26
10. Nakamura R, Miyasaka K, Kuyama Y, Kitani K (1990) Luminal bile regulates cholecystokinin release in conscious rats. Dig Dis Sci 35:55–60
11. Hagerman LM, Julow DA, Schneider DL (1973) In vitro binding of mixed micellar solutions of fatty acids and bile salts by cholestyramine. Proc Soc Exp Biol Med 143:89–92
12. Koop I, Fellgiebel A, Koop H, Schafmayer A, Arnold A (1988) Effect of cholestyramine on plasma cholecystokinin and pancreatic polypeptide levels and exocrine pancreatic secretion. Eur J Clin Invest 18:517–523
13. Nordstroem C (1972) Release of enteropeptidase and other brush-border enzymes from the small intestinal wall in the rat. Biochim Biophys Acta 289: 367–377
14. Götze H, Adelson JW, Hadorn HB, Portmann R, Troesch V (1972) Hormone-elicited enzyme release by the small intestinal wall. Gut 13:471–476
15. Green G, Nasset ES (1977) Effect of bile duct obstruction on pancreatic enzyme secretion and intestinal proteolytic enzyme activity in rats. Dig Dis Sci 22: 437–444
16. Green G, Nasset ES (1980) Importance of bile in regulation of intraluminal proteolytic enzyme activities in the rat. Gastroenterology 79:695–702
17. Miysaka K, Nakamura R, Funakoshi A, Kitani K (1989) Stimulatory effect of monitor peptide and human pancreatic secretory inhibitor on pancreatic secretion and cholecystokinin release in conscious rats. Pancreas 4:139–144
18. Iwai K, Fushiki T, Fukuoka S (1988) Pancreatic enzyme secretion mediated by novel peptide: monitor peptide hypothesis. Pancreas 3:720–728
19. Koop I, Lindenthal M, Schade T, Adler G, Arnold R (1991) Role of cholecystokinin in cholestyramine-induced changes of the exocrine pancreas. Pancreas (in press)
20. Baba N, Suzuki T, Tobe T, Inoue K, Chowdhury P, Change L, Rayford P (1986) Influence of obstructive jaundice on pancreatic growth and on basal plasma levels of cholecystokinin and gastrin in rats. Dig Dis Sci 31:1233–1241

21. Green G, Levan VH, Liddle RA (1986) Plasma cholecystokinin and pancreatic growth during adaptation to dietary protein. Am J Physiol 251:G70–G74
22. Koop I, Witzleb S, Adler G, Nustede R, Arnold R (1990) Effect of cholecystokinin (CCK) receptor blockade on bile acid-induced changes in CCK, neurotensin and pancreatic enzyme release. Gastroenterology 98:A222
23. Brand SJ, Morgan RGH (1982) Stimulation of pancreatic secretion and growth in the rat after feeding cholestyramine. Gastroenterology 83:851–859
24. Malagelada JR, Go VLW, DiMagno EP (1973) Interactions between intraluminal bile acids and digestive products on pancreatic and gallbladder function. J Clin Invest 52:2160–2165
25. Malagelada JR, DiMagno EP, Summerskill WHJ, Go VLW (1976) Regulation of pancreatic and gallbladder functions by intraluminal fatty acids and bile acids in man. J Clin Invest 58:493–499

Pyloric Cholecystokinin Receptors*

T.H. MORAN, L. SHNAYDER, G.J. SCHWARTZ, and P.R. MCHUGH[1]

Introduction

Central or peripheral administration of the brain gut peptide cholecystokinin (CCK) results in a range of biological actions. CCK binding sites at which these actions may be mediated have been identified in multiple brain regions and at various sites in the gastrointestinal tract. This chapter focuses on the anatomy, pharmacological characterization, and functional significance of a population of CCK receptors localized to the circular muscle layer of the pyloric sphincter.

Autoradiographic Demonstration of Pyloric CCK Receptors

Exogenous CCK exerts a potent inhibition on liquid gastric emptying in a variety of species at dose levels in the picomolar range [8]. Our efforts to identify the particular mechanisms and sites of actions through which CCK exerts this gastric inhibitory effect stimulated our search for specific CCK receptors in the gastrointestinal tract of the rat [20]. Utilizing autoradiographic techniques and computerized microdensitometry, an initial screening of the upper gastrointestinal tract demonstrated increases in specific binding in the areas of the proximal pyloric sphincter, the distal pyloric sphincter, and the proximal duodenum. As demonstrated in Fig. 1, the particular anatomical localization of CCK binding sites in this region corresponds to the area of a thickening of the gastric circular smooth muscle occurring in the most distal portion of the pyloric sphincter. Binding to this region was specific, reversible, and of high affinity. Some nonspecific binding was evident to the gastric mucosa and in the submucosal layer.

The discretely localized concentration of CCK receptor sites and their correspondence to the bands of circular muscle fibers suggested that these receptors are located directly on the muscle fibers. However, the gastric

---

* This work was supported by NIH grant DK 19302.
[1] Department of Psychiatry and Behavioral Sciences, Johns Hopkins University School of Medicine, 600 N, Wolfe Street, Baltimore, MD 21205, USA.

G. Adler and C. Beglinger (Eds.)
CCK Antagonists in Gastroenterology

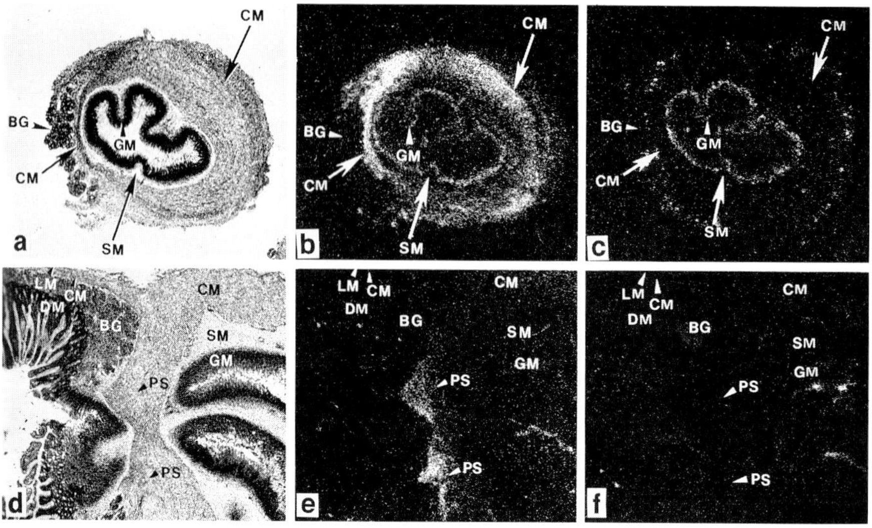

Fig. 1a-f. Photomicrographs of toluidine blue-stained tissue section of pyloric sphincter (*PS*) and corresponding autoradiographs, showing total and nonspecific CCK binding sites: **a** cross section of distal pyloric sphincter, **b** autoradiograph of section in **a** showing total CCK binding, **c** autoradiograph of adjacent tissue section showing non-specific CCK binding, **d** longitudinal section of pyloroduodenal junction, **e** and **f** autoradiographs showing total and nonspecific CCK binding respectively. *LM*, longitudinal smooth muscle; *CM*, circular smooth muscle; *SM*, submucosa; *BG*, Brunner's glands; *GM*, gastric mucosa; *DM*, duodenal mucosa [from 20]

branches of the vagus nerve also contain and transport CCK receptors [9], raising the possibility that the CCK receptors identified in the pylorus represent a terminus for the peripheral transport of vagal CCK receptors. In order to assess this possibility, we examined the effects of severing the vagus nerve on pyloric CCK receptors. Total subdiaphragmatic vagotomy did not significantly alter either the location or the density of pyloric CCK receptors [9]. This finding is consistent with the view that these receptors are located directly on the circular muscle fibers.

Pyloric CCK binding localized to the circular muscle layer has also been demonstrated in tissue samples from mouse [21], rhesus monkey [17], and man [17].

Pharmacological Characterization of Pyloric CCK Receptors

Pyloric CCK receptors fit the pharmacological profile of type A CCK receptors [10]. That is, while they demonstrate a high affinity for sulfated CCK, nonsulfated CCK and gastrin have only a low affinity for these receptors [9]. Figure 2 demonstrates a comparison of the relative ability of

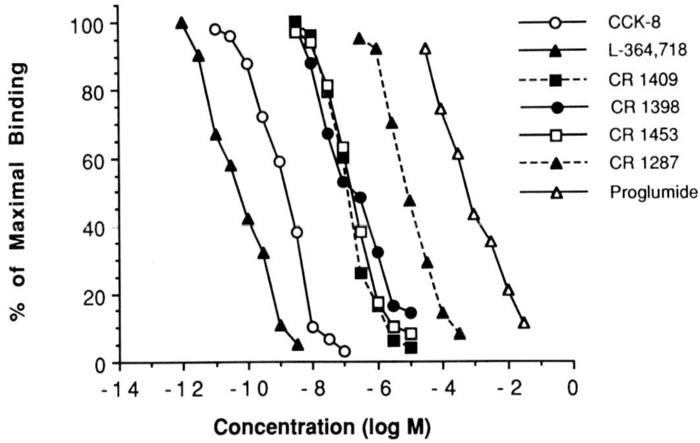

Fig. 2. Abilities of CCK and various CCK antagonists to inhibit the binding of 125I-CCK to pyloric CCK receptors. Values are expressed as a percentage of maximal binding and represent the means of three determinations. Values were generated by computerized microdensitometry from autoradiographs

CCK-8 and a series of CCK antagonists to inhibit the binding of ^{125}I-CCK to this population of pyloric CCK receptors. L-364 718 had the highest potency with an IC_{50} similar to that demonstrated for pancreatic CCK receptors. The relative affinities of proglumide and the proglumide analogues for pyloric CCK receptors are also similar to those that have been demonstrated for pancreatic CCK receptors [5]. Furthermore, the patterns of potencies of the antagonists in inhibiting CCK binding are consistent with those that would be expected for type A CCK receptors. That is, these receptors demonstrate a high affinity for the specific type A CCK antagonists L-364 718, CR 1409 (lorglumide), and other of the proglumide derivatives that have been demonstrated to differentiate between type A and type B CCK receptors [5].

Biological Actions Mediated by Pyloric CCK Receptors

CCK induces a variety of gastric events ranging from in vitro contraction of gastric muscle [1,2] to the inhibition of gastric emptying [7,8,15]. Only recently has a direct and separate role for pyloric CCK receptors in the mediation of these events been investigated. Work by Murphy et al. [13], Margolis et al. [6], and Schwartz et al. [18] demonstrated dose-related contractions of the isolated neonatal and adult rat pylorus in response to CCK. This contraction of the pylorus produced by CCK is different from the contractile effects of CCK on guinea pig fundus or gastric antrum in a number of ways. In contrast to CCK's actions on guinea pig antrum [1], CCK-induced contraction of the rat pylorus is resistant to either the addition of atropine or tetrodotoxin [13], indicating that CCK is probably acting through a CCK receptor population which does not lie upon vagal nerve endings or other neural elements but through a direct action on the circular muscle fibers.

CCK's action on the isolated pylorus is not mimicked by nonsulfated CCK or gastrin [13], while CCK's action on guinea pig smooth muscle is [2]. Furthermore, the type A CCK antagonists L-364 718 and CR 1409 block the pyloric contractile actions of CCK [14]. Together, these results indicate that CCK-induced pyloric contractions are mediated by type A CCK receptors while the antral and fundal contractile effects of CCK in guinea pig are probably mediated by type B or gastrin receptors.

The work of Murphy et al. [13], examining the in vivo actions of CCK on the pylorus, has suggested a physiological relevance of CCK-induced pyloric contractions observed during in vitro studies. They demonstrated that the intravenous administration of CCK resulted in fluctuations in pyloric perfusion pressure, again in a dose-related fashion. Thus, these CCK receptors appear to play a role in the regulation of pyloric sphincter function.

A direct role for pyloric CCK receptors in the mediation of the inhibition of gastric emptying by the exogenous administration of CCK has recently been demonstrated. In the rat, CCK appears to inhibit the gastric emptying of liquid meals by multiple mechanisms. Recent work by Raybould and Taché [15] and McCann et al. [7] has demonstrated a role for vagal afferents in this inhibition. Vagal afferent capsaicin lesions result in the elimination of CCK's ability to inhibit the emptying of nonnutrient or glucose test meals. Removal of pyloric CCK receptors by pylorectomy produces a mixed result. While the ability of CCK to inhibit the emptying of a saline test meal was intact following pylorectomy, CCK's ability to inhibit the emptying of a glucose test meal from the rat's stomach was eliminated [12]. Thus, CCK appears to act through both a vago/vagal reflex and directly on pyloric CCK receptors for the inhibition of gastric emptying. If no inhibitory signal to emptying is generated by the gastric contents, an intact vagus is sufficient to mediate the full inhibitory actions of CCK. However, if emptying is already slowed by an inhibitory signal arising from the gastric contents, a further slowing produced by CCK appears to depend both on an intact vagus and an intact pylorus.

The ability of exogenous CCK to inhibit food intake has long been noted [3,4,19], and recent work with CCK antagonists has demonstrated the physiological significance of this action of CCK [16]. Pylorectomy, eliminating pyloric CCK receptors, results in a significant attenuation in the ability of exogenous CCK to inhibit food intake. The nature of this attenuation is such that the dose response curve is truncated [11]. This means that the inhibitory actions of low doses of CCK are intact while higher dosages are unable to produce further inhibitions on food intact (Fig. 3). Thus, an action mediated through pyloric CCK receptors appears to play a role in the effect of CCK on food intake. We have hypothesized that this enhancement is due

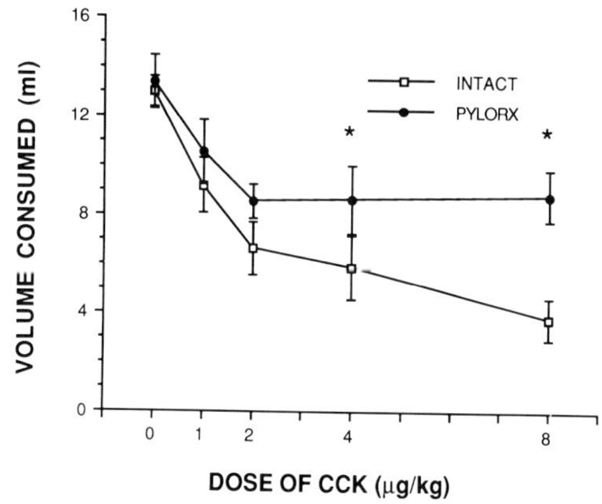

Fig. 3. Suppression of glucose intake before and after pylorectomy by CCK. Values are means ±SE *Significant differences from preoperative intake [from 11]

to, and secondary to, CCK's effects on the gastric emptying. The demonstration that pylorectomy eliminates the ability of exogenous CCK to produce a slowing of the emptying of a glucose test meal from the stomach supports this interpretation.

Summary

The work discussed in this chapter has demonstrated the presence of a subpopulation of CCK receptors localized to the circular muscle layer of the pyloric sphincter. This CCK receptor subpopulation exists in both rodent and primate species, and the pharmacological characteristics of these receptors indicate that they are type A CCK receptors. The interaction of CCK with this receptor population results in the contraction of the pyloric sphincter. CCK's actions at this receptor site appear to play a role in CCK's ability to inhibit the gastric emptying of nutrient test meals and in the inhibition of food intake produced by CCK.

References

1. Bitar KN, Maklouf GM (1982) Receptors on smooth muscle cells: characterization by contraction and specific antagonists. Am J Physiol 242:G400–G407
2. Collins SM Gardner JD (1983) Cholecystokinin-induced contraction of dispersed smooth muscle cells. Am J Physiol 243:G497–G504
3. Gibbs J, Falasco JD, McHugh PR (1976) Cholecystokinin decreased food intake in rhesus monkeys. Am J Physiol 230:15–18
4. Gibbs J, Young R, Smith GP (1973) Cholecystokinin decreases food intake in rats. J Comp Physiol Psychol 84:488–493

5. Jensen RT, Zhou ZC, Murphy RB, Jones SW, Setnikar I, Rovati LA, Gardner JD (1986) Structural features of various proglumide-related cholecystokinin receptor antagonists. Am J Physiol 251:G839–G846
6. Margolis RL, Moran TH, McHugh PR (1989) In vitro response of rat gastrointestinal segments to cholecystokinin and bombesin. Peptides 10:157–161
7. McCann MJ, Verbalis JG, Stricker EM (1988) Capsaicin attenuates multiple responses to cholecystokinin in rats. J Auton Nerv Syst 23:265–272
8. Moran TH, McHugh PR (1982) Cholecystokinin suppresses food intake by inhibiting gastric emptying. Am J Physiol 242:R491–R497
9. Moran TH, McHugh PR (1988) Anatomical and pharmacological differentiation of pyloric, vagal and brainstem cholecystokinin receptors. In: Wang RY, Schoenfeld R (eds) Cholecystokinin antagonists. Liss, New York, pp 117–132
10. Moran TH, Robinson PH, Goldrich MS, McHugh PR (1986) Two brain cholecystokinin receptors: implications for behavioral actions. Brain Res 362: 175–179
11. Moran TH, Shnayder L, Hostetler AM, McHugh PR (1988) Pylorectomy reduces the satiety action of cholecystokinin. Am J Physiol 255:R1059–R1063
12. Moran TH, Crosby RJ, McHugh PR (1989) Effects of pylorectomy on the inhibition of gastric emptying by cholecystokinin (CCK). Soc Neurosci Abstr 14:1280
13. Murphy RB Smith GP, Gibbs J (1987) Pharmacological examination of cholecystokinin (CCK-8) induced contractile activity of the isolated rat pylorus. Peptides 8:127–134
14. Murphy RB, Schneider LH, Smith GP (1988) Peripheral loci for the mediation of cholecystokinin satiety. In: Wang RY, Schoenfeld R (eds) Cholecystokinin antagonists. Liss, New York, pp 73–91
15. Raybould HE, Taché Y (1988) Cholecystokinin inhibits gastric motility and emptying via a capsaicin-sensitive vagal pathway in rats. Am J Physiol 255: G242–G246
16. Reidelberger RD, O'Rourke MF (1989) Potent cholecystokinin antagonist L-364 718 stimulates food intake in rats. Am J Physiol 257:R1512–R1518
17. Robinson PH, McHugh PR, Moran TH, Stephenson JD (1988) Gastric control of food intake. J Psychosom Res 32:593–606
18. Schwartz GJ, McHugh PR, Moran TH (1989) Effects of sulfated and nonsulfated cholecystokinin on pyloric contraction in the developing rat. Soc Neurosci Abstr 14:1279
19. Smith GP, Gibbs J (1981) Brain-gut peptides in the control of food intake. In: Neurosecretion and brain peptides. Ravan, New York pp 389–395
20. Smith GT, Moran TH, Coyle JT, Kuhar MJ, O'Donahue TL, McHugh PR (1984) Anatomic localization of cholecystokinin receptors to the pyloric sphincter. Am J Physiol 246:R127–R130
21. Stromayer AJ, Greenberg D, Moran TH, McHugh PR (1987) CCK receptor binding in the pylorus of genetically obese mice (ob/ob). Soc Neurosci Abstr 13:587

Effects of CCK Antagonists on Intestinal Motility in Dogs*

M. Karaus[1] and C. Niederau[2]

Introduction

The motility of the canine small and large intestine consists of cyclic motor patterns which are controlled by neural and hormonal factors. During the interdigestive state, a specific motor pattern called the migrating motor complex (MMC) occurs rhythmically in the small intestine. The MMC cycle is characterized by four phases: Phase one has little or no activity, phase two has intermittent and irregular contractions, during phase three the bowel contracts at its maximum frequency, and phase four is the following transition period back to quiescence. Phase three of the MMC is migrating aborally along the bowel. A meal sharply interrupts the MMC cycle and causes a prolonged increase in irregular contractile activity similar to phase two activity [2,14,22]. The canine colon also shows a cyclic motor pattern called the colonic motor complex (CMC), consisting of rhythmic bursts of tonic and phasic contractions [16]. After a meal the cyclic motor pattern of the colon is not interrupted but the motor activity is increased in the distal half of the colon. This is called the gastrocolonic response [15].

The neural and hormonal mechanisms which control the cyclic motor patterns of the small and large intestine are not fully understood. Likewise, it is not yet known which factors cause the postprandial changes in the intestinal motor patterns. Cholecystokinin (CCK) is one of the substances which have been suggested as regulatory peptides of small and large intestinal motor activity. CCK is a brain-gut peptide known to act both as a circulating hormone and a neurotransmitter within the the brain and the enteric nervous system (ENS) [13,19]. Exogenous CCK is known to stimulate the motility of both the small and large intestine causing an irregular pattern in the small intestine similar to the fed pattern and inducing an increase in colonic motility resembling the gastrocolonic response. The development of potent and specific CCK antagonists has made it possible to study the role of endogenous CCK in the regulation of the intestinal motor patterns.

---

*Dr. Karaus and Dr. Niederau were supported by grants from the Deutsche Forschungsgemeinschaft (Ka 631/5–1 and Ni 224/2–2).

[1] Freie Universität Berlin, Universitätsklinikum Rudolf Virchow, Standort Charlottenburg, Spandauer Damm 130, 1000 Berlin 19, FRG

[2] Heinrich-Heine-University of Düsseldorf, Department of Internal Medicine, Div. of Gastroenterology. Moorenstr. 5, 4000 Düsseldorf, FRG

G. Adler and C. Beglinger (Eds.)
CCK Antagonists in Gastroenterology

Effects of CCK-Antagonists on Motor Activity of Canine Ileum and Colon In Vitro

Niederau and Karaus [12] investigated the effects of various CCK antagonists on muscle strips from canine ileum and proximal colon in a perfusion apparatus. The muscle strips containing both circular and longitudinal layers were mounted in longitudinal direction. The CCK analogue caerulein and CCK-8 caused a dose-dependent increase of contractile activity with maximal effects seen at $1–3*10^{-8}$ M. The dose-response curves of the longitudinal muscles of colon and ileum were virtually identical for the two different CCK agonists. However, the colon was 2–5 times less sensitive to CCK agonists than the ileum.

The concurrent perfusion of various CCK antagonists dose-dependently inhibited the actions of the CCK agonists on the longitudinal muscle strips of both ileum and colon. L-364718 was the most potent antagonist followed by asperlicin and the peptides CR 1409, CR 1392, CR 1505, and by proglumide. All antagonists except proglumide were able to abolish the stimulation due to maximal effective doses of the CCK agonist. Concentrations of the antagonists ($10^{-5}M$ CR 1409 and $3*10^{-7}$ M L-364718), which markedly inhibited the actions of the CCK agonists, did not alter the spontaneous (basal) motor activity of the muscle strips. The CCK antagonists did not affect either the contractile responses of ileal and colonic muscle strips to substances which are thought to act via different receptors on the intestinal muscle ($10^{-7}M$ acetylcholine, $5*10^{-6}M$ histamine, $3*10^{-8}M$ motilin, $3*10^{-6}M$ substance P). This study further showed that combined application of caerulein and acetylcholine, both at concentrations resulting in near maximal effects of these substances, caused an increase in motor activity which was greater than the responses to either substance alone. The CCK antagonist CR 1409 ($10^{-5}M$) reduced this additory effect to that seen with acetylcholine alone, indicating a noncholinergic action of CCK on intestinal muscle [12]. This corresponds to the in vitro studies from colonic muscle of other species (man and cat) where additional application of atropine did not affect the stimulation of colonic contractions or myoelectrical spike-activity by CCK [4,20]. However, one cannot conclude from these studies that CCK acts directly on colonic smooth muscle. It has been shown in the guinea pig colon that CCK-generated contractions of longitudinal muscle strips are mediated by a neural pathway involving serotonin and substance P [27]. This pathway was atropine-resistant, suggesting substance P as an important final excitatory transmitter of the gastrointestinal tract [27]. In contrast to the colon, the effects of CCK on the small intestine of dogs and guinea pigs seem to be completely neurally mediated, involving a final cholinergic pathway [21,25].

CCK antagonists may be a useful tool for further elucidation of these complex regulating mechanisms of intestinal motor activity involving CCK. A previous study by Niederau and Karaus has shown that the new CCK-antagonists specifically and selectively act at the CCK-receptor in the ileum and the colon [12].

Effects of CCK Antagonists on Motor Activity of the Small Intestine in Dogs In Vivo

CCK given exogenously at doses that mimic the postprandial rise in CCK plasma levels interrupts the interdigestive motor cycle (MMC cycle) and causes an irregular pattern resembling that after feeding [10,17]. CCK further increases the coordination of contractions in the jejunum causing an increase of propagating contractions [19]. There are so far three reports dealing with the effects of CCK antagonists on motor activity of canine small intestine in vivo. Two studies by Thor et al. [23,24] used serosal electrodes to measure myoelectrical spike activity. The third, a study by Niederau and Karaus [11], used extraluminal strain gauges to measure contractile activity. The CCK antagonists tested were CR 1409 and L-364718 [23,24] and CR 1505 (loxiglumide) [11].

Effects on CCK- and Caerulein-Induced Motor Activity

The study by Niederau and Karaus [11] showed that intravenous injection of caerulein caused a burst of phasic contractions resulting in a dose-dependent increase in the area under contractions. This stimulation of motor activity had already occurred at a dose of 10 ng/kg caerulein which increased plasma CCK immunoreactivity to postprandial levels. Simultaneous infusion of CR 1505 at 10 mg kg^{-1} h^{-1}, in addition to caerulein, reduced the area under contractions to control levels. Likewise, Thor et al. [23], showed that the MMC cycle which was disrupted by CCK-8 infusion at 100 pmol kg^{-1} h^{-1} was immediately restored by simultaneous infusion of CR 1409 (2 μmol kg^{-1} h^{-1}). This effect was dose-dependent. Reversal of the mimicked after feeding pattern to the fasting pattern was observed at doses of 1 μmol kg^{-1} h^{-1} or higher.

Effect on Interdigestive Motor Activity

The results from the three studies we have mentioned are conflicting as to the effects of CCK antagonists on fasting motor patterns of the canine small intestine. Niederau and Karaus [11] showed that the contractile activity during phase two of the MMC cycle was diminished by 20% during infusion of CR 1505. In contrast. Thor et al. [24], did not see a change in the percentage of slow waves with spike activity at this phase of the MMC cycle. It is possible that small changes of motor activity are detected more readily by measurement and analysis of contractile activity than by that of spike activity. The characteristics of the MMC cycle under the CCK antagonists

Table 1. Effects of CCK antagonists on postprandial motor patterns of the small intestine in dogs in vivo

	Thor et al. [23]	Niederau and Karaus [11]
Method of motility measurement	Myoelectrical spike activity	Contractile activity
CCK antagonists	CR 1409 (2–8 μmol kg^{-1} h^{-1}) L-364718 (0.5 μmol kg^{-1} h^{-1})	CR 1505 (loxiglumide) (10 mg kg^{-1} h^{-1})
Disruption of the MMC by a meal	No effect	No effect
Motor activity during the fed state	Slow waves with spikes reduced	Area under contractions and contractile frequency reduced

were also seen differently. Thor et al. [23,24] observed a prolongation of the MMC cycle during infusion with the CCK antagonist which was due to a prolongation of phase one. Niederau and Karaus [11], on the other hand, reported no effects of the CCK antagonist on MMC-cycle period and on the percentages of the different phases of the MMC cycle. Thus, the role of endogenous CCK in the regulation of interdigestive cyclic motor patterns is not yet clear. The high variability in MMC-cycle periodicity requires longer recordings of the interdigestive motor activity than were performed in each of the previous studies to finally address this question [7].

Effects on Postprandial Motor Activity

Concerning the effects of CCK antagonists on fed motor patterns of the small intestine, there was agreement between the different studies. As shown in Table 1, infusion of the CCK antagonists did not prevent the interruption of the interdigestive MMC cycle after a meal in these studies. However, both the contractile activity (area under contractions) and the spike activity were significantly reduced in the postprandial state during CCK antagonist infusion [11,23] (Table 1).

These results suggest that CCK plays a physiological role in the regulation of postprandial motor activity of the small intestine in dogs. However, other factors in addition to CCK mediate the meal-induced motor activity. These additional mechanisms are probably more important than CCK. These studies in dogs did not investigate whether CCK is involved in the maintenance of the fed pattern after a meal. The normal duration of the postprandial motor pattern in the dog is about 16h, which makes the investigation of this pattern very cumbersome in the dog model [26]. A study in rats, which have a much shorter MMC-cycle period and a shorter duration of the fed pattern, evaluated the effects of centrally administered CCK antagonists on the postprandial motor pattern. Infusion of a CCK antagonist into the ventromedial hypothalamic region reduced the duration of the postprandial disruption of the MMC by 25% at the duodenum, suggesting an additional physiological role of CCK in regulating intestinal motor activity at the CNS level [8].

Effects of CCK Antagonists on Colonic Motor Activity in Dogs In Vivo

Application of exogenous CCK stimulates colonic motility in vivo. In man, administration of CCK causes an increase in colonic motor activity which mimics the postprandial increase in colonic motor activity, also called the gastrocolonic response [3,5]. These observations indicate that CCK is also involved in the regulation of colonic motility. The role of endogenous CCK in the control of fasting and fed motor activity of the canine colon in vivo was investigated by Karaus and Niederau [6]. They used strain-gauge transducers sutured onto the colon to measure contractile activity. The conscious dogs were studied in the fasting and fed state. CR 1505 (loxiglumide) at a dose of 10 mg kg^{-1} h^{-1} was used for CCK-receptor blockade.

Effects on Caerulein-Induced Motor Activity

The intravenous injection of 10 ng/kg caerulein had no consistent effect on colonic motor activity compared to saline. Caerulein at a dose of 50 ng/kg caused a regular motor complex consisting of phasic and tonic contractions. The area under contractions was significantly increased compared to control. Simultaneous infusion of CR 1505 abolished the stimulating effect of caerulein and reduced the area under contractions to control levels [6].

This means that the colon is less susceptible to CCK than the small intestine which confirms the in vitro results reported before [12]. Similar results were obtained in the anaesthetized dog where physiological doses of CCK-8 could not stimulate colonic motility. Only high doses of CCK-8 injected into an artery directly supplying the colon induced bursts of colonic contractions [1]. One can conclude from these studies that, in dogs, the responses to CCK antagonists in vivo will not indicate a physiological hormonal effect of CCK on the colon. However, a response to the antagonist may indicate a mediation due to neural blockade of CCK receptors in the enteric nervous system where CCK acts as a neurotransmitter.

Effects on Interdigestive Motor Activity

In vivo infusion of CR 1505 (loxiglumide) did not change the cyclic occurrence of colonic motor complexes in the dog [6]. The area under contractions in the fasted state was reduced in the proximal colon as shown in Fig. 1. CR 1505 did not alter the area under contractions in the distal colon [6].

These results suggest a physiological role of CCK in the regulation of colonic motor complexes in the proximal part of the canine large bowel. There may be regional differences in the responses to endogenous CCK, explaining the restriction of the effect to the proximal colon. This would imply a differential distribution of CCK-containing neurons and CCK receptors along the colon. Indeed, in vitro studies from feline colon showed that only the proximal colon responds to CCK [9]. However, this has not been proven for the colon from dog and man.

Effects on Postprandial Motor Activity

In the study by Karaus and Niederau [6] infusion of the CCK antagonist reduced postprandial motor activity in both parts of the colon when compared to the postprandial control experiments without CR 1505 (Fig. 1). During infusion of the CCK-antagonist, the postprandial areas under contractions in the proximal and distal colon were not significantly different from fasting values. Thus, the increase of motor activity in the distal colon after a meal was abolished during CCK-receptor blockade [6].

This indicates that in dogs the gastrocolonic response is at least partially mediated by endogenous CCK. As discussed before, this has to be a neurally mediated mechanism. Within the complex neural network of the ENS, CCK is only one of the neurotransmitters involved in this regulation. More studies are needed, including those of other peptides, if the control mechanisms of postprandial changes in colonic motor activity in dogs are to be fully understood.

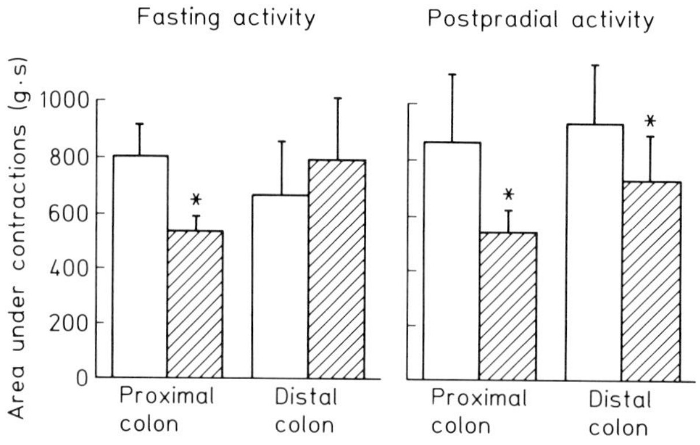

Fig. 1. Effects of the CCK antagonist loxiglumide (CR 1505) on contractile activity of the dog colon measured by implanted strain-gauge transducers and analysed as area under contractions ($n = 7$). Loxiglumide at a dose of 10 mg kg^{-1} h^{-1} reduced significantly fasting motor activity in the proximal colon and postprandial motor activity in both parts of the colon ($*p < 0.05$).
□, control experiments; ▨, experiments with loxiglumide [6]

Summary

The substances that have been proven to act as potent antagonists of CCK on the gallbladder and the pancreas also act as specific and potent antagonists of the CCK effects on the motor activity of small and large intestine in dogs. By using the CCK antagonists the role of endogenous CCK in the regulation of fasting and fed motor patterns of the canine small and large intestine has been evaluated. However, because of conflicting results, the effects of CCK-receptor blockade on fasting activity of small intestine is not yet fully understood. Prolonged monitoring would be necessary to work out the role of endogenous CCK for the cyclic occurrence of intestinal motor patterns. Phase two of the MMC cycle seems to be reduced by CCK-receptor blockade. The postprandial activity of the small intestine is partially controlled by CCK because the antagonists significantly reduced the motor activity after a meal. This may indeed be a hormonal effect because physiological doses of CCK, which increase plasma CCK to postprandial levels, stimulate small intestinal motor activity. However, the disruption of the MMC cycle after a meal is not affected by the CCK antagonists in dogs. This indicates that factors other than CCK play a more important role in the regulation of postprandial motor activity. In the canine colon CCK does not cause any motor effect in vivo at physiological doses. Therefore, CCK-receptor blockade only reveals the role of CCK as a neurotransmitter in the colon. In the fasted state only the proximal colon responds to the CCK-antagonists by reduction of motor activity, suggesting a regional variability in the response to CCK. The postprandial increase in colonic motility, the gastrocolonic response, was inhibited by the CCK-antagonist. This indicates an important physiological role of CCK in the control of this motor pattern in dogs.

References

1. Barone FS, Ormsbee HS, White RF, Labosh TJ (1984) The effects of cholecystokinin and cholecystokinin receptor antagonists on proximal colonic motility of the anaesthetized dog. Dig Dis Sci [Suppl] 29:8S
2. Code CF, Marlett JA (1975) Then interdigestive myoelectric complex of the stomach and small bowel of dogs. J Physiol (Lond) 246:289–309
3. Dinoso VP, Meshkinpur H, Lorber SH, Guitierrez JG, Chey WY (1973) Motor responses of the sigmoid colon and rectum to exogenous cholecystokinin and secretin. Gastroenterology 45:364–367
4. Egberts EH, Johnson AG (1977) The effect of cholecystokinin on human taenia coli. Digestion 15:217–222
5. Harvey RF, Read AE (1973) Effect of cholecystokinin on colonic motility and symptoms in patients with the irritable-bowel syndrome. Lancet 1:1–3
6. Karaus M, Niederau C (1989) Effects of CCK-receptor antagonist on colonic motility in the dog. Gastroenterology 96:A248
7. Kerlin P, Phillips SF (1982) Variability of motility of the ileum and jejunum in healthy humans. Gastroenterology 82:694–700

8. Liberge M, Bueno L (1989) CCK-8 neurons of the ventromedial hypothalamus (VMH) mediated the upper gut motor changes associated with feeding in rats. J Gastrointest Motil 1:54A
9. Merlo A, Cohen S (1988) Neuropeptide responses and mechanics of the proximal and distal feline colon in vitro. Am J Physiol 255:G787–G793
10. Mukopadhyay AK, Thor PF, Copeland EM, Johnson LR, Weisbrodt NW (1977) Effect of cholecystokinin on myoelectrical activity of small bowel in the dog. Am J Physiol 232:E44–E47
11. Niederau C, Karaus M (1989) Effects of CCK-receptor blockade on fed and fasted small intestinal motor activity. Gastroenterology 96:A366
12. Niederau C, Karaus M (1990) Effects of agonists and antagonists of cholecystokinin on contractile and myoelectrical activity of colonic and ileal muscle in the dog and guinea pig in vitro. J Gastrointest Motil 2(3):169–175
13. Niederau C, Heindges T, Rovati L, Strohmeyer G (1989) Effects of loxiglumide on gallbladder emptying in healthy volunteers. Gastroenterology 97:1331–1336
14. Sarna SK (1985) Cyclic motor activity; migrating motor complex. Gastroenterology 89:894–913
15. Sarna SK, Lang IM (1989) Colonic motor response to a meal in dogs. Am J Physiol 257:G830–G835
16. Sarna SK, Condon R, Cowles V (1984) Colonic migrating and nonmigrating motor complexes in dogs. Am J Physiol 246:G355–G360
17. Schang JC, Kelly KA (1981) Inhibition of canine interdigestive proximal gastric motility by cholecystokinin octapeptide. Am J Physiol 240:G217–G220
18. Schemann M, Siegle ML, Sayhoun H, Ehrlein HJ (1986) Computer analysis of intestinal motility: effects of cholecystokinin and neurotensin on jejunal contraction patterns. Z Gastroenterol 24:262–268
19. Schumann MA, Kreulen DL (1986) Action of cholecystokinin octapeptide and CCK-related peptides on neurons in inferior mesenteric ganglion of guinea pigs. J Pharmacol Exp Ther 239:618–625
20. Snape WJ (1983) Interaction of the octapeptide of cholecystokinin and gastrin I with bethanecol in the stimulation of feline colonic smooth muscle. Gastroenterology 84:58–62
21. Steward JJ, Burks TF (1977) Actions of cholecystokinin octapeptide on smooth muscle of isolated dog intestine. Am J Physiol 232:E306–E310
22. Szurszewski JH (1969) A migrating electric complex of the canine small intestine. Am J Physiol 217:1757–1763
23. Thor P, Laskiewicz J, Konturek P, Konturek SJ (1988) Cholecystokinin in the requlation of intestinal motility and pancreatic secretion in dogs. Am J Physiol 255:G498–G504
24. Thor P, Konturek SJ, Laskiewicz J, Maczka M (1990) Role of cholecystokinin in gallbladder and duodenal motility in the interdigestive state of dogs. J Gastrointest Motil 2(1):40–46
25. Vizi SE, Bertacini G, Impicciatore M, Knoll J (1973) Evidence that acetylcholine released by gastrin and related polypeptides contributes to their effect on gastrointestinal motility. Gastroenterology 64:268–277
26. Weisbrodt NM (1987) Motility of the small intestine. In: Johnson LR (ed) Physiology of the gastrointestinal tract. Raven, New York, pp 631–663
27. Wiley J, Owyang C (1987) Participation of serotonin and substance P in the action of cholecystokinin on colonic motility. Am J Physiol 252:G431–G435

The Role of CCK and CCK Antagonists in Human Esophageal and Gastroduodenal Motility

M. KATSCHINSKI[1]

Introduction

The pancreas and the gallbladder are known as the principal target organs of cholecystokinin (CCK) in the gastrointestinal tract. However, CCK receptors are located throughout the entire gut, having been identified on smooth muscle cells of the esophagus, stomach, small intestine, and colon [1]. Therefore it is conceivable that CCK is also involved in physiological modulation of gastrointestinal motility.

However, it has been difficult to establish whether actions of CCK on gastrointestinal motility are truly physiological or only pharmacological. One way to test whether or not a candidate transmitter acts as a hormone is to measure plasma levels of the transmitter simultaneously with its target tissue response. If infusion of exogenous hormone replicating the same plasma levels that occur endogenously brings about the same target tissue response, it is possible to consider this transmitter as a true hormone. However, in the postprandial state many different hormones are concomitantly released together with an activation of neural pathways. Therefore, under physiological conditions, a specific transmitter acts in concert with other stimulatory and inhibitory factors. Of course, this situation cannot be mimicked by exogenous administration of a single transmitter.

An alternative method of investigating the physiological role of candidate hormones is to selectively inhibit the hormone of interest by a specific antagonist. Recently, newly developed, potent and highly specific antagonists of CCK have become available for use in humans. These agents considerably extend the possibility of investigating the significance of CCK as a physiological modulator of gastrointestinal motility. They provide the opportunity of studying the effects of endogenously released CCK acting as hormone and neurotransmitter.

In this chapter, I address human esophageal and gastroduodenal motility. The effect of exogenous CCK on gastrointestinal motility in the respective regions is discussed since these results must be viewed in concert with

[1]Department of Gastroenterology Philipps University, Baldingerstr. 1, 3550 Marburg, FRG.

G. Adler and C. Beglinger (Eds.)
CCK Antagonists in Gastroenterology

studies applying CCK receptor antagonists. This paper mainly focuses on studies with loxiglumide. This pentanoic acid derivative highly specifically binds to CCK receptors and has an affinity constant for this binding site about 7000 times greater than that of proglumide [2,3]. Furthermore, current opinion on the mode of action of CCK is discussed for both regions.

Esophageal Motility

Effect of Exogenous CCK on Esophageal Motility

It is well established that pharmacological doses of CCK given as intravenous bolus or constant infusion decrease lower esophageal sphincter pressure (LESP) [4–7]. It has also been observed that ingestion of a meal with high content of fat can cause a rapid and sustained decrease in LESP [8]. Because fat is a potent stimulant of CCK secretion [9], it has been hypothesized that fat-induced increases in circulating levels of CCK lower LES tone postprandially [4,8]. However, a meal rich in fat also releases other transmitters, potentially lowering LESP (e.g., neurotensin). So from these studies a role for CCK as a physiological regulator of LES tone cannot be directly deduced.

In a recent study, CCK_8 was infused in concentrations bringing about postprandial and supraphysiological levels [10]. Postprandial levels did not significantly inhibit LESP, which was only lowered by supraphysiological concentrations. These results argue against the notion that hormonal CCK is a major physiological regulator of LES tone in the human.

Studies with Loxiglumide

We carried out these studies [11] to investigate the influence of endogenous CCK on esophageal motility by blocking its effects with loxiglumide in both basal and postprandial states.

Methods. Studies were performed on 12 healthy male volunteers. Each subject underwent three different manometric studies on 3 different days. The probe incorporated four recording orifices in the esophageal body and a Dent sleeve sensor to study LESP. In the first series (investigation of basal CCK) saline and loxiglumide (10 mg/kg per hour) were intravenously infused during consecutive 45-min periods on the same day. The loxiglumide recording period was preceded by a loading phase. In the second series (investigation of postprandial CCK) two experiments were carried out on 2 different days: During a background intravenous infusion of saline on 1 day, or loxiglumide at 10 mg/kg per hour on the other day, a Lundh testmeal was intraduodenally perfused at 4 ml/min for 45 min. The testmeal (volume: 300 ml, total caloric content: 367 kcal, i.e., 1.2 kcal/ml) contained 40 g carbohydrate, 15 g protein, and 18 g lipid. Analysis of esophageal motility was computer-assisted by home-made software.

Results: Inhibition of Basal CCK (First Series). As compared to saline, loxiglumide did not significantly change LESP. In terms of esophageal peristalsis it slightly enhanced esophageal motility index (area) by 10.4% ± 4.7% (mean ± SEM; $p < 0.05$), increased duration of contraction by 3.5% ± 1.6% ($p = 0.06$) and slowed velocity of peristaltic progression by 9.9% ± 3.2% ($p = 0.01$). The remaining parameters of esophageal peristalsis were left unaltered.

Effect of Testmeal (Second Series). As compared to basal state, intraduodenal perfusion of the testmeal reduced LES pressure by 30.9% ± 9.8% ($p < 0.01$), but increased motility index by 30.9% ± 9.6% ($p < 0.05$) and duration of contraction by 15.5% ± 2.5% ($p < 0.01$). The remaining parameters of peristalsis were left unaltered.

Inhibition of Postprandial CCK (Second Series). Loxiglumide significantly raised LESP ($p = 0.0005$) approximately restoring the basal interdigestive tone. Values amounted to 24.9 ± 2.9 mmHg (mean ± SE) in the interdigestive state, 16.8 ± 2.5 mmHg postprandially without loxiglumide, and 22.7 ± 2.7 mmHg postprandially with loxiglumide. The drug did not change the parameters of esophageal peristalsis as compared to saline.

Conclusions. In the interdigestive state, the specific antagonist loxiglumide proves CCK to exert a slightly inhibitory effect on esophageal peristalsis but not to change LESP. CCK is no major regulator of interdigestive esophageal motility. This conclusion is substantiated by a study we performed on six patients with reflux esophagitis grades 1/2 according to Savary and Miller. In this group intravenous loxiglumide did not change parameters of interdigestive esophageal motility as compared to saline.

It is suggested that, in the digestive state, CCK plays an important role in the regulation of LES tone, considerably contributing to the postcibal decrease of LES tone. Loxiglumide could arguably be of therapeutic value in patients with postprandially hypotensive LES.

Mode of Action of CCK on the Esophagus

The relaxation of LES is explained by an indirect neural effect via postganglionic inhibitory nonadrenergic, noncholinergic nerves overriding a direct excitatory effect on smooth muscle receptors. Therefore, CCK was proposed as a tool to identify disturbed inhibitory innervation in achalasia [7]. Vasoactive intestinal polypeptide (VIP) and peptide histidine isoleucine may function as the neurotransmitter for this pathway [12,13]. The inhibitory neuronal receptor is quite specific for CCK, whereas the stimulatory smooth muscle receptors do not discriminate between CCK and gastrin. Proglumide shifted the dose-response curves of the inhibitory as well as excitatory effects of CCK analogues to the right [14].

On the one hand, exogenous CCK at postprandial concentrations does not interfere with LESP [10], on the other hand, blockade of postprandially released endogenous CCK significantly elevates LESP [11]. Taken together, these findings render an action of circulating CCK less likely although it cannot be ruled out. Increased vagal input on postganglionic inhibitory neurons in the postprandial state could hypothetically augment their response to circulating CCK acting on receptors located on these inhibitory neurons. This would result in enhanced release of neurotransmitter lowering LES tone. However, the action of neurally released CCK operating via the inhibitory esophageal innervation may conceivably be more important in terms of regulation of LES tone. In animal models there is evidence of such an action as neurotransmitter [15]. In the human LES nerve fibers containing CCK have not been demonstrated yet [16]. Further experiments are clearly necessary to better elucidate the suggested role of endogenous CCK regulating human LES tone by acting as as neurotransmitter.

Gastroduodenal Motility

Effects of Exogenous CCK on Gastric Emptying and Motility

Liquids with nutrient value, particularly fats and protein, empty from the stomach at a slower rate than nonnutrient liquids. As these foods are the primary stimulants of CCK release this finding suggests a role for CCK in the regulation of gastric emptying. It is well established that pharmacological doses of CCK inhibit human gastric emptying [17]. However, whether this is a physiological action of CCK has been a matter of controversy [18,19]. Recent studies have claimed a role for postprandial concentrations of CCK in retarding gastric emptying of liquid and semisolid meals [20,21]. The effect of CCK was suggested to constitute a feedback system whereby CCK would regulate its own release. When food left the stomach and entered the duodenum CCK would be released. The released CCK would in turn inhibit gastric emptying. Consequently, less food would be delivered to the duodenum and the stimulus for subsequent CCK secretion would be decreased [22]. This concept, however, has been challenged by recent studies employing CCK receptor antagonists (see next section).

As to the effects of exogenous doses of CCK on human gastroduodenal contractile activity, data are limited. Relaxation of the gastric corpus by the CCK analogue cerulein has been demonstrated [23]. A suppression of antral contractile activity and an induction of isolated pyloric contractions by CCK have been described [24,25]. These phenomena are motor correlates of retarded gastric emptying. However, at plasma concentrations approximating to postprandial levels effects were minimal, thus rendering the physiological significance questionable [24].

Effect of CCK Receptor Antagonists on Gastric Emptying

Several studies have shown that gastric emptying of nutrient meals is not significantly altered in the presence of a CCK receptor antagonist: Antagonism with loxiglumide did not accelerate gastric emptying of yolk meal [26] or a normal mixed meal [27]. Accordingly, another study applying the nonpeptide CCK receptor antagonist MK-329 showed no effect of this agent on gastric emptying of solids and liquids [28]. These data strongly argue against CCK being a physiological regulator of the gastric emptying of nutrient meals. They suggest postprandial gastroduodenal motility not to be significantly affected by CCK receptor antagonists.

Regarding the effect of CCK receptor antagonists on gastric emptying of nondigestible markers, data are different. Recently, emptying of nondigestible markers was found to be accelerated by loxiglumide [29]. This result would argue in favor of an earlier occurrence of phase III of the migrating motor complex with loxiglumide.

Effect of Loxiglumide on Cephalically Stimulated Human Antroduodenal Motility

The aim of our study was to characterize the regulation of cephalically stimulated antroduodenal motility, and gastric and pancreatic secretion by cholinergic neural input and CCK.

Methods. With sham feeding, three different tests – each on a separate day – were performed on each of six healthy male volunteers. During an intravenous background infusion (random order) of saline, atropine (0.005 mg/kg per hour), or loxiglumide (10 mg/kg per hour) a modified 15 min sham feeding was performed. This cephalic stimulation was done during interdigestive phase I. Gastric and pancreatic secretion and antroduodenal motility were continuously measured for at least 120 min from the beginning of the sham feeding. On a fourth study day gastrointestinal motility and secretion were monitored during a time-adjusted interdigestive period without sham feeding.

Results. Sham feeding brought about a parallel stimulation of gastrointestinal motility and secretion lasting for 30 min as compared to time-adjusted interdigestive recording. During this period, atropine inhibited gastric acid and pancreatic enzyme secretion by approximately 86%. Loxiglumide did not significantly inhibit cephalically stimulated gastric acid and pancreatic enzyme secretion. Atropine completely abolished antral activity and consequently coordinated antroduodenal motor activity. In the duodenum it reduced frequency of contractions by 57% ± 18% (mean ±SE) and inhibited motility index by 80% ± 8%. Loxiglumide reduced contraction frequency and motility index in the antrum by 73% ± 19% and 74% ± 17%, respectively (Figs. 1, 2), did not change these parameters in the duodenum, and lowered absolute number (Fig. 3) and the probability of coordinated antroduodenal contractions by 87% ± 13% and 90% ± 10%, respectively. With atropine there was no reappearance of phase III of the migrating motor complex in the post-sham feeding recording interval. Under loxiglumide, reappearance of phase III was significantly earlier than under saline (mean intervals: 70.7 and 120 min, respectively).

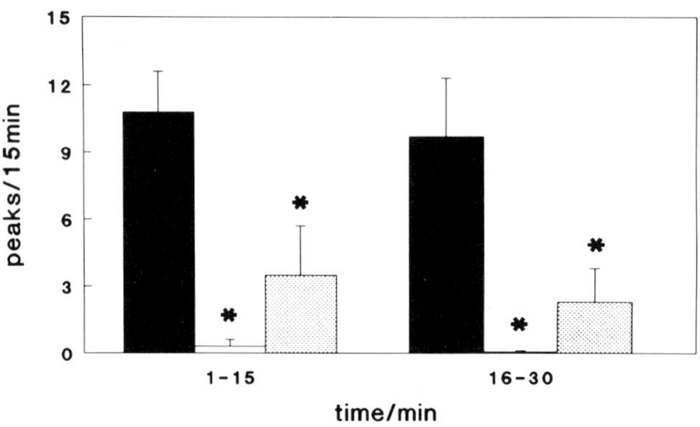

Fig. 1. Atropine (*open bars*) almost abolishes and loxiglumide (CR-1505; *cross-hatched bars*) inhibits cephalically stimulated contraction frequency in the antrum. Mean ±SE. *Asterisks* indicate values significantly different ($p < 0.05$) from saline (*solid bars*)

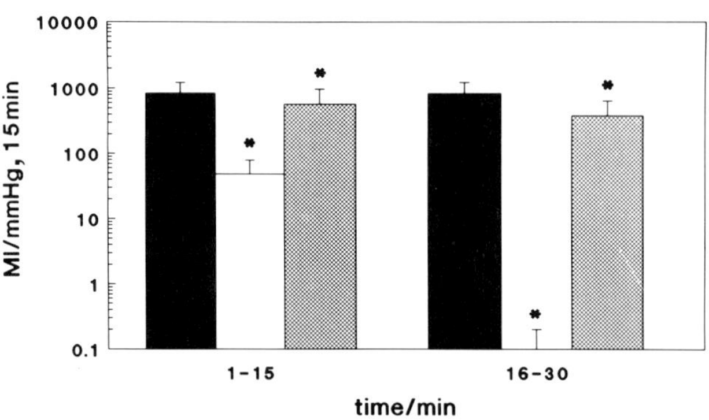

Fig. 2. Atropine (*open bars*) strongly and loxiglumide (CR-1505; *cross-hatched bars*) to a lesser degree reduce cephalically stimulated motility index (*MI*) in the antrum. The motility index is the integral of contractile activity. Mean ±SE. *Asterisks* indicate values significantly different ($p < 0.05$) from saline (*solid bars*)

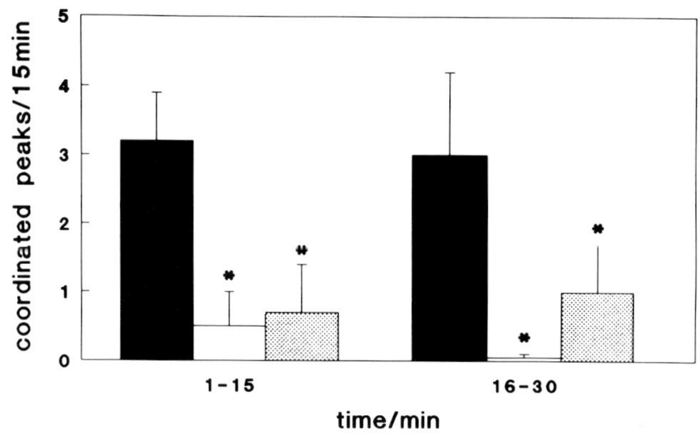

Fig. 3. Atropine (*open bars*) and loxiglumide (CR-1505; *cross-hatched bars*) lower cephalically stimulated antroduodenal coordination. The number of duodenal contractions following an antral one within a 10-s interval is depicted. Mean ±SE. *Asterisks* indicate values significantly different ($p < 0.05$) from saline (*solid bars*)

Conclusions. There is a definite cephalic stimulation of gastrointestinal motility and secretion. It is primarily regulated by the cholinergic system. CCK is suggested to be involved in the physiological regulation of cephalically stimulated antroduodenal motility. The effects obtained with the CCK receptor antagonist suggest that endogenous CCK prolongs the reappearance of phase III following sham feeding and increases antral contractile activity and antroduodenal coordination. As there was no detectable CCK release into the circulation in this study support is given to the notion that neuronally released CCK may act as a local messenger in this setting.

Mode of Action of CCK in the Gastroduodenal Area

It is important to bear in mind that differences in species and experimental models, especially differences of in vitro and in vivo models, have to be considered. Moreover, data on the human are scarce. Derived from experimental models the following mechanisms can be suggested: In the rat, intravenous CCK decreases intragastric pressure by relaxing the body of the stomach leading to an inhibition of gastric emptying [30]. It is suggested that the hormonal action of CCK on the gastric body is exerted in the first place by a direct action on vagal afferents that otherwise mediate gastric mechanoreceptor discharge. Interestingly, there is autoradiographic evidence for the presence of CCK binding sites on vagal fibers [31]. It is suggested, therefore, that CCK stimulates vagovagal reflex mechanisms that relax the body of the stomach. The efferent arm probably involves both increased discharge to preganglionic parasympathetic vagal fibers that terminate on nonadrenergic, noncholinergic (probably VIP-containing) gastric neurons which directly relax the stomach, and decreased discharge of vagal efferent excitatory fibers which terminate on cholinergic postganglionic neurons in the stomach [30].

Concerning antral, pyloric, and duodenal motility, effects of circulating and locally released CCK seem to be different. In man, circulating CCK was shown to inhibit antral and duodenal pressure waves and to stimulate isolated pyloric contractions [25]. In this study the response to CCK was not atropine sensitive.

In experimental models CCK has been intraarterially administered close to the stomach, mimicking the effect of locally released CCK. In such a dog model, in vivo excitatory actions of CCK have been found [32–34]. The response to low concentrations of CCK can be blocked by atropine or tetrodotoxine, suggesting that a receptor for CCK exists at postganglionic neurons and releases acetylcholine when it is occupied [32]. This concept is further supported by another study showing that CCK releases acetylcholine from myenteric neurons, suggesting that this mode of action contributes to the physiological effect of CCK [35]. Higher concentrations of CCK elicit an excitatory response even in the presence of atropine and tetrodotoxine, pointing to the existence of an additional muscle site of action of CCK [32]. This concept is further supported by studies demonstrating CCK to interact directly with pyloric smooth muscle [36] and by use of the glutaramic acid derivative CR-1392. This CCK receptor antagonist still exerted an inhibitory effect on CCK-induced stimulation of antropyloric motility after the cholinergic system had been blocked by atropine [32].

References

1. Walsh JH (1987) Gastrointestinal hormones. In: Johnson LR (ed) Physiology of the gastrointestinal tract. Raven, New York, pp 181–253
2. Makovec F, Christe R, Bani M, Pacini MA, Setnikar I, Rovati LA (1985) New glutaramic acid derivatives with potent competitive and specific cholecystokinin-antagonistic activity. Arzneimittelforschung 35:1048–1051
3. Setnikar I, Bani M, Cereda R, Christé R, Makovec F, Pacini MA, Revel L (1987) Anticholecystokinin activities of loxiglumide. Arzneimittelforschung 37: 1168–1171
4. Resin H, Stern DH, Sturdevant RAL, Isenberg JI (1973) Effect of the C-terminal octapeptide of cholecystokinin on lower esophageal sphincter pressure in man. Gastroenterology 64:946–949
5. Sturdevant RAL, Kun T (1974) Interaction of pentagastrin and the octapeptide of cholecystokinin on the human lower esophageal sphincter. Gut 15:700–702
6. Fisher RS, DiMarino AJ, Cohen S (1975) Mechanism of cholecystokinin inhibition of lower esophageal sphincter pressure. Am J Physiol 228:1469–1473
7. Dodds WJ, Dent J, Hogan WJ, Patel GK, Toouli J, Arndorfer RC (1981) Paradoxical lower esophageal sphincter contraction induced by cholecystokinin-octapeptide in patients with achalasia. Gastroenterology 80:327–333
8. Nebel OT, Castell DO (1972) Lower esophageal sphincter pressure changes after food ingestion. Gastroenterology 63:778–783
9. Liddle RA, Goldfine ID, Rosen MS, Taplitz RA, Williams JA (1985) Cholecystokinin bioactivity in human plasma: molecular forms, responses to feeding, and relationship to gallbladder contraction. J Clin Invest 75:1144–1152

10. Brazer SR, Borislow DS, Liddle RA (1990) Cholecystokinin is not a major hormonal regulator of lower esophageal sphincter pressure. Gastroenterology 99:641–645
11. Katschinski M, Koppelberg T, Wank U, Adler G, Rovati LC, Arnold R (1990) CCK plays a role as a physiological regulator of human esophageal motility (Abstr). J Gastrointest Motil 2:148
12. Biancani P, Walsh JH, Behar J (1984) Vasoactive intestinal polypeptide: a neurotransmitter for lower esophageal sphincter relaxation. J Clin Invest 73: 963–967
13. Biancani P, Beinfeld MC, Hillemeier C, Behar J (1989) Role of peptide histidine isoleucine in relaxation of cat lower esophageal sphincter. Gastroenterology 97:1083–1089
14. Rattan S, Goyal RK (1986) Structure-activity relationship of subtypes of cholecystokinin receptors in the cat lower esophageal sphincter. Gastroenterology 90:94–102
15. Behar J, Biancani P (1977) Effect of cholecystokinin-octapeptide on lower esophageal sphincter. Gastroenterology 73:57–61
16. Aggestrup S, Uddman R, Jensen SL, Hakanson R, Sundler F, Schaffalitzky de Muckadell O, Emson P (1986) Regulatory peptides in lower esophageal sphincter of pig and man. Dig Dis Sci 31:1370–1375
17. Chey WY, Hitanant S, Hendricks J, Lorber SH (1970) Effect of secretin and cholecystokinin on gastric emptying and gastric secretion in man. Gastroenterology 58:820–827
18. Valenzuela JE, Defilippi C (1981) Inhibition of gastric emptying in humans by secretin, the octapeptide of cholecystokinin, and intraduodenal fat. Gastroenterology 81:898–902
19. Konturek SJ, Kwiecien N, Obtulowicz W, Kopp B, Oleksy J, Rovati L (1990) Cholecystokinin in the inhibition of gastric secretion and gastric emptying in humans. Digestion 45:1–8
20. Liddle RA, Morita ET, Conrad CK, Williams JA (1986) Regulation of gastric emptying in humans by cholecystokinin. J Clin Invest 77:992–996
21. Kleibeuker JH, Beekhuis H, Jansen JBMJ, Piers DA, Lamers CBHW (1988) Cholecystokinin is a physiological hormonal mediator of fat-inhibition of gastric emptying in man. Eur J Clin Inv 18:173–177
22. Liddle RA (1989) Integrated actions of cholecystokinin on the gastrointestinal tract: use of the cholecystokinin bioassay. Gastroenterol Clin North Am 18: 135–756
23. Scarpignato C, Zimbaro G, Vitulo F, Bertaccini G (1981) Caerulein delays gastric emptying of solids in man. Arch Int Pharmacodyn Ther 249:98–105
24. Hasler W, Bowling B, Owyang C (1989) Intraduodenal lipids induce pyloric contractions: role of cholecystokinin and the cholinergic and opiate pathways (Abstr). Gastroenterology 96:A200
25. Fraser R, Fone D, Horowitz M, Dent J (1990) Dose related stimulation of pyloric motility in humans by cholecystokinin octapeptide (Abstr). Gastroenterology 98:A351
26. Corazziari E, Ricci R, Biliotti D, Bontempo I, Pallotta N, Torsoli A (1990) Oral administration of CCK antagonist loxiglumide inhibits postprandial gallbladder contraction without affecting gastric emptying. Dig Dis Sci 35:50–54
27. Niederau C, Mecklenbeck W, Heindges T, Lüthen R (1990) CCK hemmt die Magenentleerung einer regulären Mahlzeit unter physiologischen Bedingungen beim Menschen nicht (Abstr). Z Gastroenterol 28:510
28. Liddle RA, Gertz BJ, Kanayama S, Beccaria L, Coker LD, Turnbull TA, Morita ET (1989) Effects of a novel cholecystokinin (CCK) receptor antagonist, MK-329, on gallbladder contraction and gastric emptying in humans: implications for the physiology of CCK. J Clin Invest 84:1220–1225
29. Meyer BM, Werth BA, Beglinger C, Hildebrand P, Jansen JBMJ, Zach D, Rovati LC, Stalder GA (1989) Role of cholecystokinin in regulation of gastrointestinal motor functions. Lancet 2:12–15

30. Green T, Dimaline R, Dockray GJ (1989) Neuroendocrine control mechanisms of gastric emptying in the rat. In: Singer MV, Goebell H (eds) Nerves and the gastrointestinal tract. MTP, Lancaster, pp 433–445
31. Moran T, Smith GP, Hostetler AM, McHugh PR (1987) Transport of cholecystokinin (CCK) binding sites in subdiaphragmatic vagal branches. Brain Res 415:149–152
32. Allescher HD, Daniel EE, Fox JET, Kostolanska F, Rovati LA (1989) Effect of the novel cholecystokinin receptor antagonist CR-1392 on cholecystokinin-induced antroduodenal and pyloric motor activity in vivo. J Pharmacol Exp Ther 251:1134–1141
33. Telford GL, Mir SS, Mason GR, Ormsbee HS III (1979) Neural control of canine pylorus. Am J Surg 137:92–98
34. Kuwahara A, Ozawa K, Yanaihara N (1986) Effects of cholecystokinin-octapeptide on gastric motility of anesthetized dogs. Am J Physiol 251: G678–G681
35. Vizi E, Bertaccini G, Implicciatore M, Knoll J (1973) Evidence that acetylcholine release by gastrin and related polypeptides contributes to their effect on gastrointestinal motility. Gastroenterology 64:268–277
36. Scheurer UL, Varga L, Drack E, Burki HR, Halter F (1983) Mechanisms of action of CCK-octapeptide on rat antrum, pylorus, and duodenum. Am J Physiol 244:G266–G272

Regulation of Gastrointestinal and Colonic Transit by CCK Antagonists

B. Meyer-Wyss, B. Werth, and C. Beglinger[1]

Introduction

CCK is an oligopeptide synthesized within the intestinal mucosa and released into the blood stream in response to the intake of a meal [1]. It is well-established that the main action of the hormone CCK is induction of gallbladder contraction [1] and stimulation of exocrine pancreatic secretion [2]. The recent elaboration of peptide hormone antagonists with CCK as a model has opened the way to conclusively investigate the physiological role of CCK. Thus, studies with loxiglumide, a specific and highly potent receptor antagonist of CCK, have recently shown that CCK is a physiologic mediator of the intestinal phase of meal-stimulated exocrine pancreatic enzyme secretion and gallbladder contraction in humans [3]. CCK binds, however, not only to receptors on smooth muscle cells of the gallbladder or pancreatic acini, but CCK binding receptors have also been found on smooth muscle cells of the stomach, small intestine, and colon [4]. Furthermore, it has been shown that CCK stimulates colonic myoelectric activity [5] and induces contraction of muscle strips from human taeniae coli [6]. Studies on humans have revealed that CCK directly inhibits gastric emptying [7] and radiologists have finally made use of CCK to accelerate the transit of a barium meal through the small intestine [8]. Thus, it is conceivable that CCK has a physiological role not only in stimulating pancreaticobiliary secretion, but it may be involved in the regulation of gastrointestinal motility as well.

Role of CCK Antagonists in the Regulation of Gastric Emptying

The physiological role of the stomach rests on its ability to store ingested nutrients, break them up, and release them in such size and quantity into the duodenum that they can be optimally digested and absorbed [9]. This goal depends on gastric emptying of nutrients, a highly complex phenomenon requiring the coordinated action of the fundus, antrum, pylorus as well as

[1] Division of Gastroenterology, University Hospital, 4031 Basel, Switzerland

G. Adler and C. Beglinger (Eds.)
CCK Antagonists in Gastroenterology

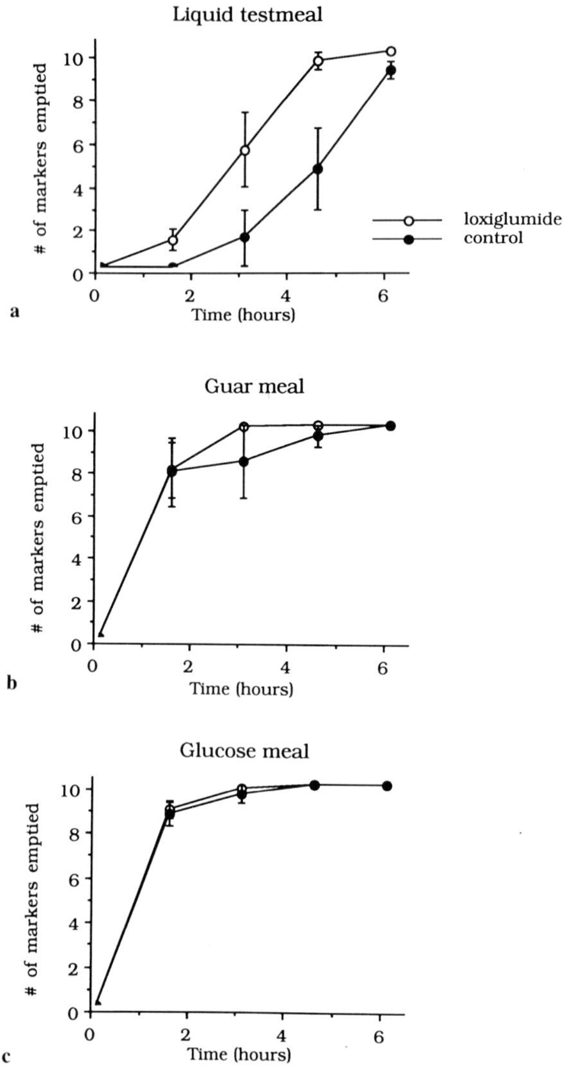

Fig. 1a–c. Cumulative gastric emptying of radio-opaque markers. **a** After administration of a mixed liquid test meal, **b** after the guar meal, and **c** after 5% glucose solution (from [10])

the duodenum [9]. The regulation of these concerted actions in turn depends on the autonomic nervous system, hormones, the intrinsic intestinal nervous system, and finally an intact smooth muscle layer of the gastrointestinal tube. The intestinal peptide hormone CCK administered intravenously to healthy volunteers delays gastric emptying of liquids [7]. This action of the peptide hormone CCK on the stomach forms the rationale for studies designed to investigate its physiological role in regulating gastric emptying.

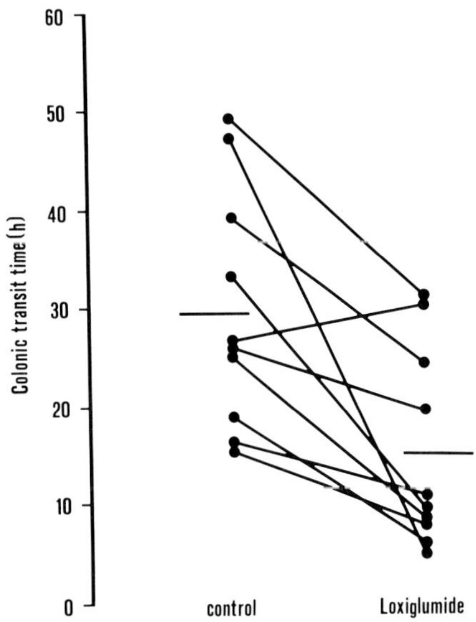

Fig. 2. Colonic transit time of radio-opaque markers in ten healthy volunteers treated for 7 days with oral placebo (control) or loxiglumide (from [10])

As outlined above, the availability of peptide hormone antagonists has made it possible to elegantly design such studies. We have assessed the effect of the potent and highly specific CCK antagonist loxiglumide on gastric emptying of radio-opaque markers [10]. Nineteen healthy volunteers were repeatedly studied in random order after oral intake of loxiglumide (30 mg/kg) or placebo and different types of test meals containing radio-opaque markers. Gastric emptying of the markers was assessed by obtaining plain radiographs of the upper abdomen 1.5, 3, 4.5, and 6 h after ingestion of markers and meals, respectively. Figure 1 shows that markers emptied significantly faster when the volunteers were treated with loxiglumide, the $t_{\frac{1}{2}}$ of marker emptying being approximately 3 h compared to 4.5 h in the control experiments. There was no intrinsic effect of loxiglumide on gastric emptying; the guar meal and glucose meal did not induce CCK release (Fig. 2) and gastric emptying of markers was not affected by loxiglumide treatment (Fig. 1b,c). These experiments therefore suggest that CCK is physiologically involved in the control of gastric emptying. Similar results have been reported by Fried and coworkers [11]. They measured gastric emptying of a liquid test meal labeled with ^{99m}Tc and found that it was significantly accelerated by oral treatment with loxiglumide. By contrast, Liddle and coworkers found that MK-329, a different CCK antagonist, did not affect gastric emptying rates of liquid or solid meal components in healthy volunteers [12]. These authors concluded that CCK possibly has only a limited role in regulating gastric emptying. Further studies are certainly needed to clarify these conflicting results.

Effects of CCK Antagonists on Small Intestinal and Colonic Motility

Hormones have been implicated in inducing changes in gastrointestinal motility. Cholecystokinin infused intravenously in humans produces changes in gastrointestinal motility patterns [13]. In addition to inducing a change in the pattern, CCK also causes a dose-dependent increase in spike potential activity [5,14]. The octapeptide of CCK has furthermore been shown to accelerate transit of contrast material through the human small intestine [8]. CCK, however, probably does not act only as a hormone, as it also exists among many other peptidergic transmitters in enteric nerves [15]. Continuing with this argumentation, CCK directly stimulates colonic myoelectrical and contractile activity when injected intravenously in humans. This effect is probably pharmacological rather than hormonal.

We have investigated the effect of blocking CCK receptors with loxiglumide on small intestinal transit time in healthy volunteers [10]. The subjects who participated in this study received a naso-gastro-duodenal tube. A liquid test meal containing 12 ml of lactulose was then instilled directly into the duodenum over a period of 5 min. Small bowel transit time was measured by breath hydrogen analysis [16]. End expiratory breath samples were collected at baseline before instillation of the meal and then every 15 min for up to 5 h. Small bowel transit time was defined as the time between meal instillation and the initial rise in the breath hydrogen concentration of at least 10 ppm above fasting levels [16]. This rise indicates the arrival of the nonabsorbable meal component lactulose in the cecum and its metabolism by colonic bacteria. The five subjects were studied twice on 2 different days. In random order, they were treated during the experiments with either loxiglumide or saline administered intravenously. The mean small bowel transit time of the liquid test meal assessed by hydrogen breath analysis was similar after loxiglumide and after saline treatment: 117 $\pm$ 21 min vs 115 $\pm$ 48 min, respectively. The failure to demonstrate an effect of loxiglumide on small bowel transit time may, however, be the result of methodological problems [17] and not necessarily reflect a lack of CCK influence on the regulation of small bowel motility. Thus, we have observed a large variability of transit time measurements among our healthy volunteers and it is well-known that large intra-individual differences occur if small bowel transit time is assessed repeatedly by hydrogen breath analysis in the same subjects [17,18]. Furthermore, the hydrogen breath test simply reflects the time gap required for the head of the meal to pass from the duodenum to the cecum. This parameter may not be representative for the time required for the bulk of the meal to travel through the small intestine [16,19], and therefore, studies using radionucleide scanning are needed to evaluate a potential effect of CCK on small bowel transit time.

The effect of the CCK antagonist loxiglumide on segmental and total colonic transit time was investigated in a randomized, double-blind, placebo-

Table 1. Total and regional colonic transit time (h) in ten healthy subjects with and without concomitant oral loxiglumide administration (800 mg t.i.d.). Data are mean ± SEM

Treatment	Right colon	Left colon	Rectosigmoid	Total colon
Placebo	8.8 ± 2.1[a]	11.5 ± 2.9[a]	9.6 ± 4.0	29.4 ± 4.1
Loxiglumide	3.7 ± 1.1	5.6 ± 2.0	5.2 ± 1.2	15.0 ± 3.4[a]

[a] $p < 0.05–0.01$.

controlled cross-over trial in healthy subjects [10]. They were treated for 7 days each with 800 mg loxiglumide or placebo t.i.d. The subjects ingested three sets of 20 radio-opaque markers at 24-h intervals and a single abdominal X-ray was taken of each subject 24 h after ingestion of the last set of markers. The films were evaluated to count the number of markers within the colon, and colonic transit time was calculated according to published methods [20,21]. Figure 2 shows the individual transit times of the ten volunteers during the control period and during loxiglumide treatment. There was a highly significant difference ($p < 0.05$) and mean colonic transit time was much shorter after loxiglumide than after placebo treatment (15.0 ± 3.4 h vs 29.4 ± 4.1 h). The analysis of segmental transit time makes it possible to further characterize the site of action of the CCK antagonist loxiglumide. From Table 1 it is obvious that transit time through the right as well as through the left side of the colon were significantly shortened by loxiglumide treatment. In contrast, the transit through the rectosigmoid colon was not affected by treatment with the CCK antagonist. These findings therefore suggest that CCK is involved in the regulation of the storage capacity of the colon and it does not seem to have an influence on defecation. Moreover, they indicate that CCK antagonists may be used clinically to treat slow transit constipation.

Conclusion

CCK is involved in the physiological regulation of gastric emptying and colonic motility in humans. Blocking CCK receptors with specific CCK antagonists results in dramatic acceleration of both gastric emptying and colonic motility. These findings suggest that CCK blockers may be very potent prokinetic agents. Unfortunately, CCK receptors are found throughout the gastrointestinal tract and long-term blocking of CCK receptors may be associated with significant side effects. Further studies are therefore clearly needed to investigate not only potential benefits of treating patients with CCK antagonists, but also to carefully search for potential adverse effects. Such clinical studies may lead to the development of a new class of potent drugs, the peptide hormone blockers.

References

1. Liddle R, Goldfine I, Rosen M, Taplitz R, Williams J (1985) Cholecystokinin bioactivity in human plasma: molecular forms, responses to feeding, and relationship to gallbladder contraction. J Clin Invest 75:1144–1152
2. Beglinger C, Fried M, Whitehouse I, Jansen JB, Lamers CB, Gyr K (1985) Pancreatic enzyme response to a liquid meal and to hormonal stimulation. Correlation with plasma secretin and cholecystokinin levels. J Clin Invest 75: 1471–1476
3. Hildebrand P, Beglinger C, Gyr K, Jansen JBMJ, Rovati LC, Zuercher M, Lamers CBHW, Setnikar I, Stalder GA (1990) Effects of a cholecystokinin receptor antagonist on intestinal phase of pancreatic and biliary responses in man. J Clin Invest 85:640–646
4. Walsh JH (1987) Gastrointestinal hormones. In Johnson LR (ed) Physiology of the gastrointestinal tract, 2nd edn. Raven, New York, pp 195–206
5. Snape W, Carlson G, Cohen S (1977) Human colonic myoelectric activity in response to prostigmin and the gastrointestinal hormones. Am J Dig Dis 22: 881–887
6. Egberts E, Johnson A (1977) The effect of cholecystokinin on human taenia coli. Digestion 15:217–222
7. Liddle RA, Morita ET, Conrad CK, Williams JA (1986) Regulation of gastric emptying in humans by cholecystokinin. J Clin Invest 77:992–996
8. Levant J, Kun T, Jachna J, Sturdevant R, Isenberg J (1974) The effects of graded doses of C-terminal octapeptide of cholecystokinin on small intestinal transit time in man. Dig Dis 19:207–209
9. Meyer JH (1987) Motility of the stomach and gastroduodenal junction. In: Johnson LR (ed) Physiology of the gastrointestinal tract, 2nd edn. Raven, New York, pp 613–629
10. Meyer BM, Werth BA, Beglinger C, Hildebrand P, Jansen JBMJ, Zach D, Rovati LC, Stalder GA (1989) Role of cholecystokinin in regulation of gastrointestinal motor functions. Lancet I:12–15
11. Fried M, Löchner C, Erlacher U, Beglinger C, Jansen J, Lamers C, Stalder GA (1989) Role of CCK in the regulation of gastric emptying and pancreatic secretion in man. Gastroenterology 96:A159
12. Liddle RA, Gertz BJ, Kanayama S, Beccaria L, Coker LD, Turnbull TA, Morita ET (1989) Effects of a novel cholecystokinin (CCK) receptor antagonist, MK-329, on gallbladder contraction and gastric emptying in humans. Implications for the physiology of CCK. J Clin Invest 84:1220–1225
13. Mukhopadhyay A, Thor P, Copeland E, Johnson L, Weisbrodt N (1977) Effect of cholecystokinin on myoelectric activity of small bowel of the dog. Am J Physiol 232:E44–E47
14. Snape W (1983) Interaction of the octapeptide of cholecystokinin and gastrin I with bethanechol in the stimulation of feline colonic smooth muscle. Gastroenterology 84:58–62
15. Dockray GJ (1987) Physiology of enteric neuropeptides. In Johnson LR (ed) Physiology of the gastrointestinal tract, 2nd edn. Raven, New York, pp 41–66
16. Read NW, Al-Janabi MN, Bates TE, Holgate AM, Cann PA, Kinsman RI, McFarlane A, Brown C (1985) Interpretation of the breath hydrogen profile obtained after ingesting a solid meal containing unabsorbable carbohydrate. Gut 26:834–842
17. Gilmore IT (1990) Orocaecal transit time in health and disease. Gut 31:250–251
18. Staniforth DH, Rose D (1989) Statistical analysis of the lactulose/breath hydrogen test in the measurement of orocaecal transit: its variability and predictive value in assessing drug action. Gut 30:171–175
19. Caride VJ, Prokop EK, Troncale FJ, Buddoura W, Winchenbach K, McCallum RW (1984) Scintigraphic determination of small intestinal transit time: comparison with the hydrogen breath technique. Gastroenterology 86:714–720

20. Chaussade S, Roche H, Khyara A, Couturier D, Guerre J (1986) Mesure de temps de transit colique (TTC): description et validation d'une nouvelle technique. Gastroenterol Clin Biol 10:385–389
21. Metcalf AM, Philipps SF, Zinsmeister AR, MacCarty RL, Beart RW, Wolff BG (1987) Simplified assessment of segmental colonic transit. Gastroenterology 92: 40–47

The Role of CCK in Tumor Growth

T.E. Solomon[1]

Cancers of the gastrointestinal tract, particularly those of colonic, pancreatic, and gastric origin, are major causes of disability and death in the Western world. There has been little progress in our understanding of the causes and progression of these diseases in spite of remarkable advances in the area of tumor biology. One such advance is the realization that "growth factors" may modulate the proliferative rates of malignant neoplasms. Peptides such as epidermal growth factor, the transforming growth factors, and several others may affect tumor growth through direct actions on tumor cell receptors, receptors may be "overexpressed" in tumor cells, and these factors may even be synthesized and released by tumor cells to initiate autocrine growth stimulation. It is also possible that other substances, such as gastrointestinal hormones, may modulate cancer cell growth rates. This idea comes from the well-known trophic effects of gastrointestinal peptide hormones on various target tissues, and the possibility that malignant cells originating from these tissues may retain specific hormonal receptors that still influence proliferation. CCK is a potent growth stimulant of the normal exocrine pancreas [1], and many studies have used this background as an impetus to determine whether CCK also affects pancreatic cancer growth. Several reviews are available on the topic of gastrointestinal hormones and their potential role in pancreatic and other gastrointestinal cancers [2–6].

Pancreatic cancer in humans occurs more commonly in men than women and shows a progressive increase with age; its incidence has increased dramatically in the past 70 years [7]. There are rather vague suggestions that, among several risk factors, diets high in meat and fat increase the incidence of pancreatic cancer [8]. This suggests that the protein and fat components of such diets may elevate plasma CCK levels and predispose subjects to growth promotion of cancer cell clones. Overall, there is no convincing data to support any connection between risk factors and development or course of pancreatic cancer, however. It would be useful to determine whether subjects at risk of developing pancreatic cancer

[1]Kansas City, VA Medical Center, 4801 Linwood Blvd., Kansas City, MO 64068 USA

G. Adler and C. Beglinger (Eds.)
CCK Antagonists in Gastroenterology

have elevated plasma CCK levels over long periods of time and whether patients with pancreatic cancer have altered plasma CCK levels. Whatever the results of such studies, it is still possible that growth rates of pancreatic malignancies may be modulated by normal levels of circulating CCK. It would also be of interest to determine the presence of CCK receptors on primary pancreatic cancers and the presence of CCK gene expression products in such tissue.

Experimental studies on the effects of CCK on pancreatic cancer growth can be broadly divided into those using various animal-derived tumors and those using tumors of human origin. Considerable information can be gained about the general properties of pancreatic cancer growth regulation in experiments with animal-derived neoplasms, but human cancers must ultimately be studied to define potential growth regulatory and therapeutic effects associated with CCK. Thus, most of the work discussed here will involve studies on human pancreatic cancer cell lines grown in vitro or as xenografts in the immunodeprived nude mouse. These two systems each have advantages: in vitro studies allow careful control of the hormonal medium, fairly rapid characterization of growth effects, and the ability to perform many experiments under similar conditions; in vivo studies provide a system in which to determine the effects of dietary manipulation, sex, age, and other host factors.

In the few available studies with xenografts of human pancreatic cancer in nude mice, results suggest that endogenous CCK can modulate tumor growth. Hudd et al. [9] administered an extremely large dose of CCK-8 (50 μg/kg twice per day for 2 weeks) to groups of mice bearing either early passages of four different primary nonpancreatic tumors or two different established pancreatic cancer cell lines. In two of the groups bearing non-pancreatic cancers, tumor growth was suppressed. No effects were seen in the groups bearing pancreatic cancers. The lack of data on lower doses of CCK makes these results difficult to interpret. Smith et al. have examined the effects of CCK, a high fat diet, and the CCK receptor antagonist L-364718 on growth of the established human pancreatic cancer cell line SW-1990 in nude mice [10,11]. Large doses (5, 15 or 25 μg/kg twice per day s.c. in gelatin for 4 weeks) of a synthetic CCK analog increased several measurements of tumor growth after 4 weeks of treatment [10]. In other studies, it was found that tumor xenografts in mice fed a high fat diet grew more rapidly than those in mice fed a normal diet [11]. The CCK receptor antagonist L-364718 reversed the effects of the high fat diet and also slowed the growth of the tumors in mice on a regular diet. Although these findings are suggestive of a growth effect of endogenous CCK, further data on plasma CCK levels would be helpful, as would studies with a greater number of cancer cell lines. In a related study, Alexander et al. [12] found that bombesin, a releaser of CCK in some species, inhibited the growth of a human pancreatic cancer xenograft but stimulated pancreatic growth in the host animals. Again, measurements of plasma CCK in response to bombesin in this model would be helpful in understanding the mechanism of this effect.

There are also a few studies available on growth effects of CCK on human pancreatic cancer cell lines in vitro, but the results are as yet somewhat unclear. It is likely that differences in culture conditions, peptide purity, degradation of peptide during culture, passage number, clonal selection, and other factors can alter the responsiveness of cell lines to peptides such as CCK. For example, it has recently been shown that six human pancreatic cancer cell lines demonstrated growth responses to various molecular forms of CCK, although the magnitude and sensitivity of growth stimulation varied markedly among the different lines [13]. Two of these cell lines (PANC-1 and MIA PaCa-2) were studied at a later time under different conditions and found to be totally unresponsive to growth stimulation by CCK, although clear growth responses to insulin and EGF were found [14]. Pronounced degradation of CCK occurred in the culture medium of both cell lines, as determined by radioimmunoassay; however, even multiple additions of CCK to maintain culture concentrations did not produce any growth response [14]. Another group has reported weak growth responses of an unrelated cell line to high concentrations of CCK [15]. The cell line SW-1990 previously described has also been examined in terms of growth effects of CCK and the receptor mechanisms involved [10]. Tritiated thymidine incorporation into DNA was increased by 24-h exposure to concentrations of a synthetic CCK analog as low as $10^{-10} M$ (lower concentrations were not examined). CCK also increased cell counts when added to culture medium for up to 12 days. The nonspecific CCK receptor antagonist proglumide almost completely reversed the growth stimulation by CCK, and the effective concentrations of proglumide were surprisingly low (10^{-7} and $10^{-6} M$). When proglumide was added to culture medium alone in concentrations from 10^{-8} to $10^{-6} M$, it had no inhibitory effect on cell growth. These results suggest that at least certain human pancreatic cancer cell lines do exhibit a proliferative response to CCK that is mediated by CCK A or B receptors. The lack of an inhibitory effect of proglumide alone on cell growth in the study described above indicates that no autocrine effects of CCK were involved in the regulation of this particular cell line. It has also been reported that secretin stimulated cell growth in the SW-1990 cell line, although very high concentrations were required [10]. Whether this represents a true decrease in sensitivity to secretin or degradation of the peptide (as has been reported for CCK [14]) is unknown. High concentrations of secretin and CCK did not interact to cause potentiated growth, but the effects of lower concentrations were not tested [10].

The one clear result of all of these studies is that the role of CCK in modulating human pancreatic cancer growth is not yet established. More information is required before assessing the importance of CCK as a growth factor. A fruitful approach would be to screen large numbers of primary and established cancer cell lines for the presence of CCK receptors and to characterize the nature of these receptors with other related peptides and specific CCK A and B receptor antagonists. This approach should provide a more logical prediction of growth responses to CCK. The existence of CCK gene expression products in human pancreatic cancer cell lines should also be helpful, as this might indicate that autocrine growth factors are present that may blunt the effects of exogenous CCK. Screening the potential inhibitory growth effects of CCK receptor antagonists in different cell lines would complement these studies. Interactions of CCK and other growth factors might also occur, although this has yet to be determined. As is obvious, this area of research is in a very early stage. The potential importance of CCK receptor antagonists as therapeutic tools in this dismal disease lends some credence to the need for expanding our current knowledge.

References

1. Solomon TE, Petersen H, Elashoff J, Grossman MI (1978) Interaction of caerulein and secretin on pancreatic size and composition in rat. Am J Physiol 235:E714–E719
2. Townsend CM Jr, Singh P, Thompson JC (1986) Gastrointestinal hormones and gastrointestinal and pancreatic carcinomas. Gastroenterology 91:1002–1006
3. Longnecker DS (1987) Interface between adaptive and neoplastic growth in the pancreas. Gut 28 (S1):253–258
4. Longnecker DS, Jamieson JD, Asch HL (1989) Conference report. Regulation of growth and differentiation in pancreatic cancer. Pancreas 4:256–275
5. Townsend CM Jr, Singh P, Thompson JC (1989) Effects of gastrointestinal peptides on gastrointestinal cancer growth. Gastroenterol Clin North Am 18: 777–791
6. Andren-Sandberg A (1989) Peptide hormone influence on exocrine pancreatic cancer. Eur J Surg Oncol 15:236–241
7. Beazley RM, Cohn I Jr (1988) Update on pancreatic cancer. CA 38:310–319
8. Wormsley KG (1985) Aetiology of pancreatic cancer. Ital J Gastroenterol 17: 102–108
9. Hudd C, LaRegina MC, Devine JE, Palmer DC, Herbold DR, Beinfeld MC, Gelder FB, Johnson FE (1989) Response to exogenous cholecystokinin of six human gastrointestinal cancers xenografted in nude mice. Am J Surg 157: 386–394
10. Smith JP, Solomon TE, Bagheri S, Kramer S (1990) Cholecystokinin stimulates growth of human pancreatic adenocarcinoma SW-1990. Dig Dis Sci 35: 1377–1384
11. Smith JP, Kramer S, Bagheri S (1990) Effects of a high-fat diet and L-364 718 on growth of human pancreas cancer. Dig Dis Sci 35:726–732
12. Alexander RW, Upp JR, Poston GJ, Townsend CM Jr, Singh P, Thompson JC (1988) Bombesin inhibits growth of human pancreatic adenocarcinoma in nude mice. Pancreas 3:297–302
13. Smith JP, Kramer ST, Solomon TE (1991) CCK stimulates growth of six human pancreatic cancer cell lines in serum-free medium. Regul Pept (in press)
14. Liehr R-M, Melnykovych G, Solomon TE (1990) Growth effects of regulatory peptides on human pancreatic cancer lines PANC-1 and MIA PaCa-2. Gastroenterology 98:1666–1674
15. Frazier ML, Pathak S, Wang Z-W, Cleary K, Singletary SE, Olive M, MacKay B, Steck PA, Levin B (1990) Establishment of a new human pancreatic adenocarinoma cell line, MDAPanc-3. Pancreas 5:8–16

Part IV: Clinical Potentials of CCK Antagonists

Experimental Pancreatitis

J.H. Grendell[1]

Introduction

The search for a specific, clinically useful treatment to arrest or reverse the autodigestive process believed to be the central pathophysiologic event in acute pancreatitis has so far been frustrating and unsuccessful. One major approach to this problem has been the use of agents such as anticholinergic drugs, glucagon, calcitonin, and somatostatin which have been shown in physiological studies to inhibit pancreatic exocrine secretion. Unfortunately, none of these substances proved to be of value in prospective, randomized clinical trials [1].

With the recent development of new classes of potent cholecystokinin (CCK)-receptor antagonists capable of in vivo administration [2], it has become possible to modulate pancreatic acinar cell function in a new and more specific way, raising the prospect that these compounds might prove of value in the treatment of acute pancreatitis. Cause for hope that this might be the case was the observation that cerulein, a CCK analogue, worsened the severity and mortality of acute pancreatitis produced in rats by intraductal injections of bile salts [3]. In addition, supramaximal stimulation with cerulein in the rat [4] or mouse [5] produces acute pancreatitis. Therefore, it seemed reasonable to investigate whether CCK played a role in the pathophysiology of acute pancreatitis and whether CCK receptor blockade might have a beneficial effect.

CCK Receptor Antagonists in Cerulein-Induced Acute Pancreatitis

Acute pancreatitis produced by supramaximal stimulation with cerulein appears to be due (at least in the rat) to interaction of cerulein with a low-affinity CCK receptor which mediates high-dose inhibition of pancreatic enzyme secretion [6]. Therefore, treatment with CCK receptor antagonists

[1] University of California, San Francisco VA Medical Center, 4150 Clement Street, San Francisco, CA 94121, USA.

G. Adler and C. Beglinger (Eds.)
CCK Antagonists in Gastroenterology

should ameliorate the severity of cerulein-induced acute pancreatitis; and pretreatment with an antagonist of sufficient potency should prevent it. This, in fact, has been demonstrated in experimental studies using both glutaramic acid-derivative [5,7] and asperlicin-derivative CCK receptor antagonists.

CCK Receptor Antagonists in Acute Pancreatitis Produced by a Choline-Deficient, Ethionine-Supplemented Diet

That CCK receptor antagonists can prevent cerulein-induced acute pancreatitis is hardly surprising. However, far more provocative was the observation that proglumide, a glutaramic acid-derivative CCK receptor antagonist, markedly reduced the severity of pancreatitis and improved survivial in the highly lethal, necrotizing acute pancreatitis produced by the choline-deficient, ethionine-supplemented (CDE) diet in mice [8]. Even more remarkably, proglumide was effective whether administered prior to or following initiation of acute pancreatitis (Fig. 1), unlike the potent serine protease inhibitor gabexate which was only effective when administered prior to initiation of pancreatitis. This beneficial effect of proglumide occurred even though plasma CCK concentrations in animals fed the CDE diet were not elevated. That proglumide's beneficial effect was due to CCK receptor blockade was suggested by the ability of CCK-8, at a dose which in itself did not produce pancreatitis, to totally reverse the beneficial effects of proglumide (Fig. 1).

However, whereas lorglumide (CR-1409), a more potent glutaramic acid-derivative CCK receptor antagonist than proglumide, also produced beneficial effects similar to proglumide in CDE diet-induced pancreatitis [9], studies with the asperlicin-derivative CCK receptor antagonist MK-329 (formerly L-364 718), one of the most potent inhibitors of CCK-stimulated enzyme secretion by the pancreas, failed to show a beneficial effect in CDE diet-induced pancreatitis [10,11]. This was true even at doses which markedly reduced the severity of pancreatitis produced by supramaximal stimulation with cerulein.

Indirect support for a therapeutic role for CCK receptor antagonists in CDE-diet-induced acute pancreatitis is provided by studies which showed that the feeding of cholestyramine to mice prior to starting the CDE diet produced both higher plasma CCK levels and higher mortality, whereas feeding with taurocholate strikingly reduced both plasma CCK levels and mortality from CDE diet-induced pancreatitis (Fig. 2) [12]. In addition, the adverse effect of cholestyramine feeding was mitigated by administration of lorglumide (CR-1409), whereas the beneficial effect of taurocholate feeding was reduced by giving CCK-8 (Fig. 2).

It is difficult at present to reconcile the striking beneficial effects of proglumide and lorglumide in this model of pancreatitis with the apparent

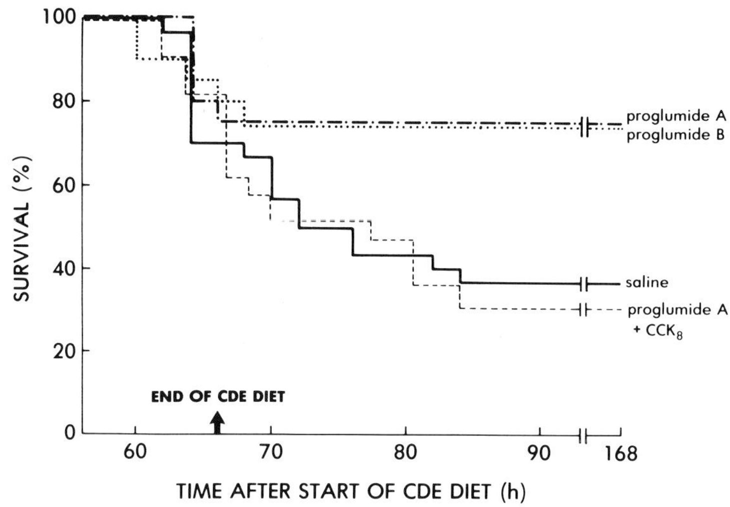

Fig. 1. The effects of proglumide on survival in CDE-diet-induced pancreatitis compared to the saline-treated control (saline). The CCK receptor antagonist proglumide improved survival whether administered before (proglumide A) or after (proglumide B) the onset of pancreatitis. Administration of CCK-8 at a dose which does not produce pancreatitis totally reversed the protective effect of proglumide (proglumide A + CCK-8). [From 8]

lack of effect of MK-329. Although it is possible that the beneficial effects of the glutaramic acid derivatives are unrelated to blockade of CCK receptors, the reversal of the effect with CCK-8 [8] and the studies with cholestyramine and taurocholate feeding [12] suggest otherwise. Alternatively, the deleterious effects of CCK which contribute to the severity of acute pancreatitis may be mediated by an as yet undescribed CCK receptor class for which the glutaramic acid derivatives have a greater affinity than does MK-329. Recent work has suggested the presence on pancreatic acinar cells of CCK receptor classes other than the high- and low-affinity receptors previously described [13].

CCK Receptor Antagonists in Other Models of Acute Pancreatitis

Studies involving the use of CCK receptor antagonists in other models of acute pancreatitis are limited, and the results are mixed. In one report [14] a continuous infusion of MK-329 (L-364718) improved survival and reduced the biochemical and morphological severity in experimental acute pancreatitis produced by perfusion of the pancreatic duct with sodium taurocholate in the rat or by mechanical trauma in the guinea pig. Other investigators have shown a beneficial effect of the CCK receptor antagonist asperlicin in

a b

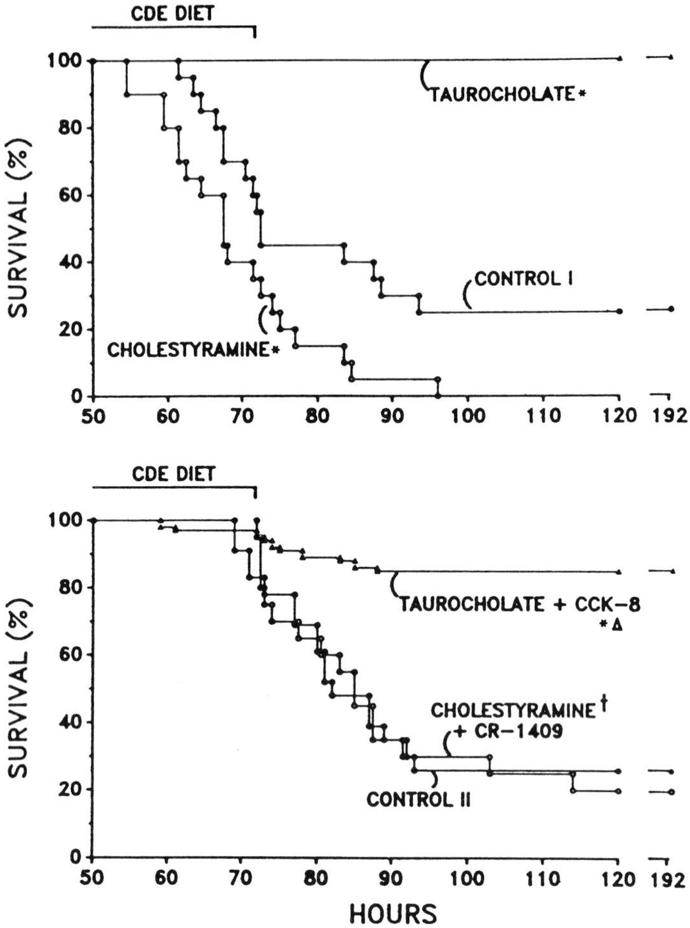

Fig. 2. a The effect on survival in CDE diet-induced pancreatitis of feeding taurocholate or cholestyramine. Taurocholate feeding decreased plasma CCK levels and improved survival compared to the control, whereas cholestyramine feeding increased CCK levels and decreased survival. **b** Administration of CCK-8 (taurocholate + CCK-8) reduced the protective effect of taurocholate feeding, whereas administration of the CCK receptor antagonist lorglumide (cholestyramine + CR-1409) improved survival in cholestyramine-fed animals, suggesting that CCK is contributing to the severity of acute pancreatitis in this model. [From 12]

acute pancreatitis induced by perfusion of the pancreatic duct with sodium taurocholate [15] and of lorglumide (CR-1409) in pancreatitis produced by direct injection of taurocholate into the parenchyma of the pancreas [16]. However, another group of investigators failed to show a beneficial effect for the glutaramic acid-derivative loxiglumide (CR-1505) in pancreatitis produced in the rat by perfusion of the pancreatic duct with taurocholate [17].

Conclusions

Although not all studies show a beneficial effect of CCK receptor antagonists in experimental acute pancreatitis, there are now positive results in four different models (supramaximal stimulation with cerulein, CDE diet, taurocholate perfusion of the pancreatic duct, and trauma) in three different species (rat, mouse, guinea pig). These findings warrant further investigation in experimental models and consideration of clinical trials.

The striking difference in effect in the CDE diet model between glutaramic acid derivatives such as proglumide and MK-329 (L-364 718) suggest that the therapeutic efficacy of proglumide may be mediated by blockade of a CCK receptor unrelated to stimulation of digestive enzyme secretion by the acinar cell but, perhaps, regulating intracellular metabolism in some way. That the beneficial effects of CCK receptor antagonists in acute pancreatitis are unrelated to inhibition of pancreatic secretion would not be surprising given the observation that, in both clinical pancreatitis [18] and in experimental models [19], pancreatic exocrine secretion is already markedly reduced as part of the disease process itself.

References

1. Steinberg WM, Schlesselmann SE (1987) Treatment of acute pancreatitis. Gastroenterology 93:1420–1427
2. Zucker KA, Adrian TE, Modlin IM (1988) Cholecystokinin receptor antagonists. J Surg Res 45:496–504
3. Evander A, Lundquist I, Ihse I (1982) Influence of gastrointestinal hormones on the course of acute experimental pancreatitis. Hepatogastroenterology 29: 161–166
4. Lample M, Kern HF (1977) Acute interstitial pancreatitis in the rat induced by excessive doses of a pancreatic secratogogue. Virchows Arch [A] 373:97–117
5. Niederau C, Ferrell LD, Grendell JH (1985) Caerulein-induced acute necrotizing pancreatitis in mice: protective effects of proglumide, benzotript, and secretin. Gastroenterology 88:1192–1204
6. Saluja AK, Saluja M, Printz H, Zavertnik A, Sengupta A, Steer ML (1989) Experimental pancreatitis is mediated by low-affinity cholecystokinin receptors that inhibit digestive enzyme secretion. Proc Natl Acad Sci USA 86:8968–8971
7. Otsuki M, Tani S, Okabayashi Y, Nakamura T, Fujii M, Fujisawa T, Baba S, Itoh H (1989) Effect of a new cholecystokinin receptor antagonist CR 1392 on caerulein-induced acute pancreatitis in rats. Pancreas 4:237–243
8. Niederau C, Liddle RA, Ferrell LD, Grendell JH (1986) Beneficial effects of cholecystokinin-receptor blockade and inhibition of proteolytic enzyme activity in experimental acute hemorrhagic pancreatitis in mice. Evidence for cholecystokinin as a major factor in the development of acute pancreatitis. J Clin Invest 78:1056–1063
9. McQuaid KR, Niederau C, Ferrell LD, Grendell JH (1988) Effects of chlorglumide alone or with atropine or gastrin on diet-induced acute hemorrhagic pancreatitis in mice (Abstr). Pancreas 3:607
10. Oshio G, Saluja A, Leli U, Sengupta A, Steer ML (1989) Failure of a potent cholecystokinin antagonist to protect against diet-induced pancreatitis in mice. Pancreas 6:739–743

11. Silverman M, Ilardi C, Bank S, Kranz V, Lendvai S (1989) Effects of the cholecystokinin antagonist L-364718 on experimental pancreatitis in mice. Gastroenterology 96:186–192
12. Gomez G, Townsend CM Jr, Green DW, Rajaraman S, Uchida T, Greeley GH Jr, Soloway RD, Thompson JC (1990) Protective action of luminal bile salts in necrotizing acute pancreatitis in mice. J Clin Invest 86:323–331
13. Yu D-H, Huang SC, Wank SA, Mantey S, Gardner JD, Jensen RT (1990) Pancreatic receptors for cholecystokinin: evidence for three receptor classes. Am J Physiol 258:G86–G95
14. Modlin IM, Bilchik AJ, Zucker KA, Adrian TE, Sussman J, Graham SM (1989) Cholecystokinin augmentation of "surgical" pancreatitis. Benefits of receptor blockade. Arch Surg 124:574–578
15. Wisner JR Jr, Renner IG (1988) Asperlicin, a nonpeptidal cholecystokinin antagonist, attenuates sodium taurocholate-induced acute pancreatitis in rats. Pancreas 3:174–179
16. Makovec F, Bani M, Cereda R, Chiste R, Revel L, Rovati LC, Setnikar I, Rovati LA (1986) Protective effect of CR 1409 (cholecystokinin antagonist) on experimental pancreatitis in rats and mice. Peptides 7:1159–1164
17. Tani S, Okabayashi Y, Nakamura T, Fujii M, Itoh H, Otsuki M (1990) Effect of a new cholecystokinin receptor antagonist loxiglumide on acute pancreatitis in two experimental animal models. Pancreas 5:284–290
18. Mitchell CJ, Playforth MJ, Kelleher J, McMahon MJ (1983) Functional recovery of the exocrine pancreas after acute pancreatitis. Scand J Gastroenterol 18:5–8
19. Niederau C, Niederau M, Lüthen R, Strohmeyer G, Ferrell LD, Grendell JH (1990) Pancreatic exocrine secretion in acute experimental models. Gastroenterology 99:1120–1127

Cholecystokinin-Receptor Antagonists in Experimental Pancreatic Tumor Growth*

C.B.H. LAMERS[1], B.R. DOUGLAS, J.B.M. JANSEN, and R.A. WOUTERSEN

Introduction

Cholecystokinin belongs together with gastrin and secretin to the classical gut hormones [1]. Cholecystokinin is produced by the I cells in the upper small intestinal mucosa and is released into the circulation in response to ingestion of nutrients or infusion of the neurotransmitter bombesin/gastrin releasing peptide. The polypeptide hormone is named cholecystokinin because of its property to stimulate gallbladder contraction. In addition to its gallbladder-contracting property, cholecystokinin has been shown to be a potent stimulus of pancreatic growth and pancreatic enzyme and hormone secretion, to affect motility of the gastrointestinal tract, and to play a role in the regulation of satiety. Because of its pancreatic growth promoting action, cholecystokinin has been studied in pancreatic carcinogenesis [2–4]. The recent development of highly effective and specific cholecystokinin-receptor antagonists has enabled to delineate the various actions of cholecystokinin in great detail [5,6]. Two types of cholecystokinin-receptor antagonists can be used for in vivo studies, glutaramic derivates (proglumide, lorglumide, loxiglumide) and non-peptide compounds (asperlicin, L-364 718). Most in vivo studies have been performed using the glutaramic derivates lorglumide (CR-1409) and loxiglumide (CR-1505) and the non-peptide antagonist L-364 718 (MK-329). Studies on the role of cholecystokinin on gastrointestinal tumor growth have been concentrated on the role of cholecystokinin in pancreatic cancer.

Cholecystokinin and Pancreatic Cancer

The effect of cholecystokinin on pancreatic cancer can be studied by various approaches:

* Supported by grant IKW 86-16 from the Netherlands Cancer Society.

[1] Department of Gastroenterology-Hepatology, University Hospital, Leiden and TNO-CIVO Toxicology and Nutrition Institute, Zeist, P.O. Box 9600, 2300 RC Leiden, The Netherlands

G. Adler and C. Beglinger (Eds.)
CCK Antagonists in Gastroenterology

1. Effect of exogenous cholecystokinin on tumor growth
   - Pancreatic cancer in vitro
   - Xenografted pancreatic cancer
   - Chemically induced pancreatic carcinogenesis
2. Effect of endogenous cholecystokinin (surgery, drugs, or nutrients) on tumor growth
   - Xenografted pancreatic cancer
   - Chemically induced pancreatic carcinogenesis
3. Characterization of cholecystokinin receptors on pancreatic tumors
4. Effect of specific cholecystokinin-receptor antagonists on tumor growth
   - Pancreatic cancer in vitro
   - Xenografted pancreatic cancer
   - Chemically induced pancreatic carcinogenesis
   - Advanced pancreatic cancer

Several studies have shown that cholecystokinin not only stimulates the growth of the normal pancreas but also promotes pancreatic carcinogenesis and tumour growth of the pancreas [7,8]. In fact, long-term administration of cholecystokinin to rats induces pancreatic hypertrophy, hyperplasia, and premalignant changes [9]. Furthermore, cholecystokinin has been reported to enhance azaserine-induced pancreatic carcinogenesis in rats [10] and nitrosamine-induced carcinogenesis of the pancreas in hamsters [11]. Two different carcinogenicity models have been used in animals. Azaserine is administered to rats and produces acinar cell-like pancreatic tumors, whereas *N*-nitrosobis (2-oxopropyl) amine provokes ductular cell-like tumors in hamsters. Although histology of human pancreatic adenocarcinomas resembles hamster ductular cell tumors better than rat acinar cell tumors, it cannot be excluded that some human adenocarcinomas also derive from acinar cells. Therefore, both the azaserine rat model and the nitrosamine hamster model should be investigated in studies on the carcinogenesis of pancreatic tumors. In addition, several studies indirectly point to an important role of cholecystokinin in the development of pancreatic cancer. In man, factors suggested to increase the risk of pancreatic cancer, such as high fat and protein intake and previous gastrectomy, are known to be accompanied by a raised plasma cholecystokinin secretion [4]. In animals, especially in rats but also in hamsters, there are numerous studies pointing to a role of cholecystokinin in pancreatic carcinogenesis; tumors can be induced by various manipulations that increase plasma cholecystokinin, such as dietary manipulations (nutrients with trypsin-inhibiting properties such as raw soya flour and camostate), bile salt-binding drugs such as cholestyramine, and surgical interventions inducing deficiency of intestinal proteases or bile salts (pancreaticobiliary diversion), and, possibly, cholecystectomy [12–16]. Furthermore, these plasma cholecystokinin secretion-stimulating manipulations promote pancreatic carcinogenesis induced by chemical carcinogens. It has been shown that azaserine-induced pancreatic carcinogenesis in rats can be enhanced by raw soya flour and a high-fat diet [16–18] and that nitrosamine-induced pancreatic carcinogenesis in hamsters can be stimulated by dietary fat [19]. Furthermore, receptors for cholecystokinin have been demonstrated on human pancreatic adenocarcinomas [20]. Upp et al. [21] have shown that the presence or absence of cholecystokinin receptors on such cancers may predict the responsiveness of the tumor to hormonal treatment. It has further been shown that cholecystokinin stimulates the growth of xenografted human pancreatic cancer [20,22,23].

The recent availability of specific cholecystokinin-receptor antagonists have enabled study of the role of cholecystokinin in pancreatic cancer in more detail. Furthermore, in analogy with the growth-inhibiting effect of steroid-receptor antagonists in breast cancer, the effects of these cholecystokinin-receptor antagonists in pancreatic cancer are presently studied. Recent studies have demonstrated that the specific cholecystokinin receptor antagonists asperlicin and L-364718 inhibit the growth of xenografted human pancreatic carcinomas [22,24,25]. It was shown that a diet high in unsaturated, but not saturated fat, stimulates pancreatic carcinogenesis in the azaserine rat model and growth of a xenotransplanted human adenocarcinoma in the nude mice [17,25]. Interestingly, the cholecystokinin receptor antagonist L-364718 inhibited the growth of a xenotransplanted human pancreatic cancer not only during a high-fat diet but also during standard chow [25]. Furthermore, Douglas et al. [10] have shown that enhancement of asazerine-induced pancreatic carcinogenesis by the trypsin inhibitor camostate in rats can be reduced by treatment with the specific cholecystokinin-receptor antagonist lorglumide (Fig. 1). As shown in Fig. 1, lorglumide inhibited the size, but not the number, of the preneoplastic acidophilic lesions and the drug also reduced the total pancreatic area occupied by these lesions. These workers have also shown that the growth-promoting effect of bombesin was not significantly inhibited by lorglumide, suggesting that the stimulating effect of this neuropeptide on pancreatic carcinogenesis in this model is not fully mediated through the stimulation of cholecystokinin secretion by bombesin [26]. Interestingly, the same group has recently shown that cholecystokinin, but not bombesin or camostate, stimulates the development of advanced ductular lesions in the hamster pancreas [27]. The cholecystokinin-receptor antagonist lorglumide inhibited the effect of cholecystokinin, but had a stimulating effect when given in combination with bombesin or the trypsin inhibitor camostate [27].

It is apparent from the above and several other studies that cholecystokinin may be involved in the development and growth of pancreatic cancer and that the availability of specific cholecystokinin-receptor antagonists may open a new area of research on pancreatic cancer and may ultimately offer new hope to the desperate patients afflicted by this dismal disease.

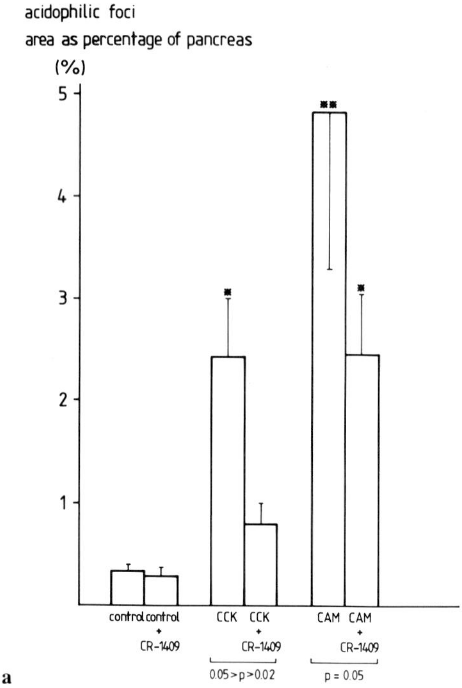

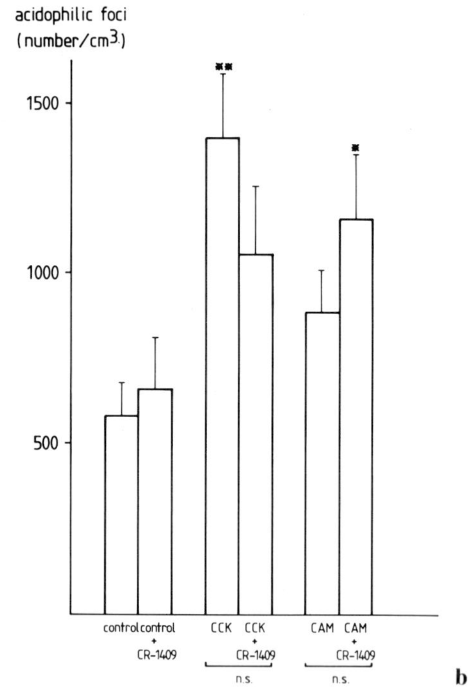

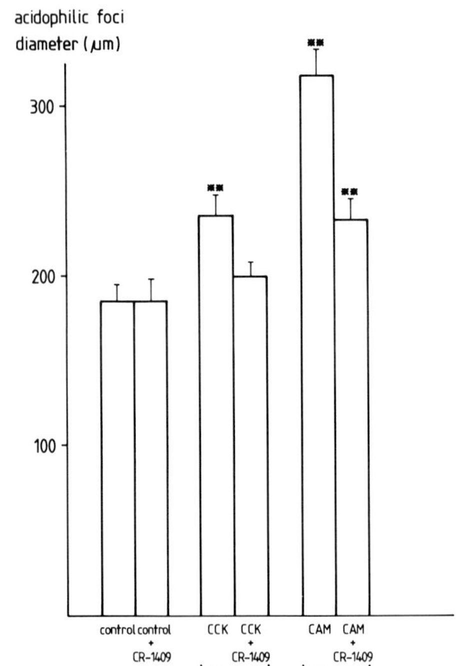

Fig. 1a–c. Stimulation of azaserine-induced preneoplastic acidophilic lesions by exogenously administered cholecystokinin, and by endogenously released cholecystokinin during stimulation by oral administration of the trypsin inhibitor camostate (CAM), and the partial inhibition of cholecystokinin- and camostate-stimulated pancreatic carcinogenesis by the specific cholecystokinin-receptor antagonist lorglumide (CR-1409) in rats. **a** The percentage area of the pancreas occupied by acidophic lesions, **b** the number, and **c** the diameter of these preneoplastic lesions. *Asterisks* denote significant differences from the control studies ($^*P < 0.05$; $^{**}P < 0.01$)

Conclusions

The gut hormone cholecystokinin exerts various actions on the gastrointestinal tract including the regulation of growth. The hormone has been reported to induce hypertrophy and hyperplasia of the pancreas and to enhance chemically induced pancreatic carcinogenesis in animals. Stimulation of endogenous cholecystokinin secretion through the induction of deficiency of intraintestinal proteases and bile salts by trypsin-binding nutrients bile salt-binding drugs, or surgical intervention is also capable of stimulating growth and tumour development in the rat. In man, factors suggested to increase the risk of pancreatic cancer, such as a high-fat and high-protein diet or gastrectomy, are known to stimulate plasma cholecystokinin secretion. Receptors for cholecystokinin have been demonstrated on human pancreatic adenocarcinomas, and cholecystokinin has been demonstrated to enhance the growth of xenografted human pancreatic cancer. The recently developed cholecystokinin-receptor antagonists inhibit not only growth of the normal pancreas, but also pancreatic carcinogenesis in animals and growth of xenotransplanted human adenocarcinomas in nude mice. These new drugs may be valuable new tools for inhibiting pancreatic cancer growth in humans.

Acknowledgements. Secretarial assistance was given by Nelia Koek-van Beelen.

References

1. Walsh JH (1986) Gastrointestinal hormones. In: Johnson LR (ed) Physiology of the gastrointestinal tract. Raven, New York, pp 181–254
2. Lamers CBHW, Jansen JBMJ (1988) Role of gastrin and cholecystokinin in tumours of the gastrointestinal tract. Eur J Cancer Oncol 24:267–273
3. Lamers CBHW, Jansen JBMJ (1988) Hormonal manipulation of gastrointestinal cancer by gut peptides. J Gastroenterol Hepatol 3:379–386
4. Lamers CBHW, Douglas BR, Jansen JBMJ (1988) Cholecystokinin and pancreatic cancer. Scand J Gastroenterol [Suppl 154] 23:103–106
5. Makovec F, Christè R, Pacini MA, Setnikar I, Rovati LA (1985) New glutaramic-acid derivatives with potent competitive and specific cholecystokinin-antagonistic activity. Drug Res 35:1048–1051
6. Freidinger RM (1989) Cholecystokinin and gastrin antagonists. Med Res Rev 9:271–290
7. Solomon TE, Petersen H, Elashoff J, Grossman MI (1978) Interaction of caerulein and secretin on pancreatic size and composition in rat. Am J Physiol 235:E714–E719
8. Pfeiffer CJ, Chernenko GA, Kohli Y, Barrowman A (1981)Trophic effects of cholecystokinin octapeptide on the pancreas of the Syrian hamster. Can J Physiol Pharmacol 60:358–362
9. Fölsch UR, Winckler K, Wormsley KG (1978) Influence of repeated administration of cholecystokinin and secretin on the pancreas of the rat. Scand J Gastroenterol 13:663–671
10. Douglas BR, Woutersen RA, Jansen JBMJ, de Jong AJL, Rovati LC, Lamers CBHW (1989) Modulation by CR-1409 (Lorglumide), a cholecystokinin receptor

antagonist, of trypsin inhibitor-enhanced growth of azaserine-induced putative preneoplastic lesions in rat pancreas. Cancer Res 49:2438–2441
11. Howatson AG, Carter DC (1985) Pancreatic carcinogenesis-enhancement by cholecystokinin in the hamster-nitrosamine model. Br J Cancer 51:107–114
12. McGuinness EE, Morgan RGH, Wormsley KG (1985) Trophic effects on the pancreas of trypsin and bile salt deficiency in the small-intestinal lumen. Scand J Gastroenterol [suppl 112] 20:64–67
13. Stace NH, Palmer TJ, Vaja S, Dowling RH (1987) Long-term pancreaticobiliary diversion stimulates hyperplastic and adenomatous nodules in the rat pancreas. Gut [Suppl 1] 28:265–268
14. Miazza BM, Turberg Y, Guillaume P, Hahne W, Chayvialle JA, Loizeau E (1985) Mechanism of pancreatic growth induced by pancreatico-biliary-diversion in the rat. Scand J Gastroenterol [Suppl 112] 20:75–83
15. Rosenberg L, Duguid WP, Fried GM (1988) Association of cholecystectomy with pancreatic growth and increased plasma levels of cholecystokinin in the Syrian golden hamster. J Surg Res 44:235–241
16. Wormsley KG (1977) Potentiation of the action of azaserine on the rat pancreas by raw soyabean flour. Cancer Lett 3:87–90
17. Roebuck BD, Kaplita PV, Edwards PV, Praissman M (1987) Effect of dietary fats and soybean protein on azaserine-induced pancreatic carcinogenesis and plasma cholecystokinin in the rat. Cancer Res 47:1333–1338
18. Lhoste EF, Roebuck BD, Longnecker DS (1988) Stimulation of the growth of azaserine-induced nodules in the rat pancreas by dietary comostate (FOY-305). Carcinogenesis 9:901–906
19. Birt DF, Salmasi S, Pour PM (1981) Enhancement of experimental pancreatic cancer in Syrian golden hamsters by dietary fat. JNCI 67:1327–1333
20. Smith JP, Mohesky C, Barrett B, Solomon TE (1986) CCK stimulates growth of human pancreatic cancer. Dig Dis Sci 31:1150
21. Upp JR, Singh P, Townsend CM, Thompson JC (1987) Predicting response to endocrine therapy in human pancreatic cancer with cholecystokinin receptors. Gastroenterology 92:1677
22. Alexander RW, Upp JR, Singh P, Hugh T, Poston GJ, Townsend CM, Thompson JC (1987) Asperlicin inhibits the growth of a xenografted human pancreatic carcinoma. Gastroenterology 92:1293
23. Hudd C, LaRegina MC, Devine JE, Palmer DC, Herbold DR, Beinfeld MC, Gelder FB, Johnson FE (1989) Response to exogenous cholecystokinin of six human gastrointestinal cancers xenografted in nude mice. Am J Surg 157: 386–394
24. Maani R, Townsend CM, Gomez G, Thompson JC, Singh P (1988) A potent CCK receptor antagonist (L-364718) inhibits the growth of human pancreatic cancer in nude mice. Gastroenterology 94:A274
25. Smith JP, Kramer S, Bagheri S (1990) Effects of high-fat diet and L364718 on growth of human pancreas cancer. Dig Dis Sci 35:726–732
26. Douglas BR, Woutersen RA, Jansen JBMJ, de Jong AJL, Rovati LC, Lamers CBHW (1989) Influence of cholecystokinin antagonist on the effects of cholecystokinin and bombesin on azaserine-induced lesions in rat pancreas. Gastroenterology 96:462–469
27. Meijers H, Roverts WG, Lamers CBHW, Jansen JBMJ, Rovati LC, Woutersen RA (1989) Modulation of development of (pre)neoplastic lesions in the hamster pancreas by cholecystokinin, bombesin and camostate: effects of the cholecystokinin receptor antagonist CR1409. Digestion 43:162

Efficient Treatment of Biliary Colics with Loxiglumide*

C. Beglinger[1]

Introduction

The recent development of antagonists of cholecystokinin (CCK) has not only generated great interest in the scientific and medical community [1], but the CCK antagonist may also have therapeutic potentials and represent a new class of therapeutic drugs. The role of CCK in regulating biliary motility has been extensively described in various chapters of Part 3 of this book and will therefore not be discussed here. The potent antagonistic effect of CCK blockers on gallbladder motility are the basis for its application in biliary colics [2,3]. Biliary colics are thought to result from intense contractions of the gallbladder when a stone obstructs the outlet. CCK antagonists can then induce relaxation of the gallbladder which forms the basis of the hypothesis that these agents might be beneficial in treating biliary colics. In this pilot trial, the effect of loxiglumide (50 mg by slow i.v. injection or 400 mg orally) was tested in nine patients with biliary colics due to cholecystolithiasis.

Effects of Loxiglumide on Biliary Colics

Nine patients with biliary colics due to gallbladder stones were treated. These patients (3 males, 6 females) were among a group referred for extracorporeal shock wave lithotripsy. After lithotripsy, they were struck by typical biliary colics that were treated in the emergency room with hyoscine-*N*-butylbromide (10–20 mg) given as a suppository or i.v. They all failed to respond to this standard treatment within a prefixed time frame (2 h) and were therefore subsequently given loxiglumide (50 mg i.v. or 400 mg orally). An immediate response was observed in all nine patients who were painfree within 20 min after drug administration. Pain was evaluated by the patient by visual-analogue-scale using a rating system ranging from "no pain" to "unbearable pain." No side effects were recorded in this pilot trial.

* Supported by a grant from the Swiss National Science Foundation (grant 3.890-0.88).

[1] Division of Gastroenterology, University Hospital, 4031 Basel, Switzerland.

G. Adler and C. Beglinger (Eds.)
CCK Antagonists in Gastroenterology

Discussion

The present, limited experience with loxiglumide indicates that CCK antagonists may be an efficient treatment alternative to standard procedures for biliary colics. A randomized, double-blind study is necessary to evaluate the treatment efficacy of these compounds in this disease.

References

1. Snyder SH (1986) Virtuoso design of drugs. Nature 323:292–293
2. Meyer BM, Werth B, Beglinger C, Hildebrand P, Jansen JBMJ, Zach D, Rovati LC, Stalder GA (1989) Role of cholecystokinin in regulation of gastrointestinal motor functions. Lancet 1:12–15
3. Hildebrand P, Beglinger C, Gyr K, Jansen JBMJ, Rovati LC, Zuercher M, Lamers CBHW, Setnikar I, Stalder GA (1990) Effects of a cholecystokinin receptor antagonist on intestinal phase of pancreatic and biliary responses in man. J Clin Invest 85:640–646

The Role of CCK in Chronic Constipation

B. Meyer-Wyss[1], R. Meier[2], K. Gyr[2], and C. Beglinger[1]

Importance of Constipation

The importance of constipation is reflected by the high rate of physician visits for this problem [1]. Constipation is the most common digestive complaint amongst the general population [2].

There is clear evidence that the prevalence of constipation increases with age [1–4], but the mechanisms responsible for this increase, particularly among the elderly, are poorly understood. A diet low in fibre, reduced physical activity, the side effects of medication, and endogenous factors such as increased opioid activity and reduced strength of intestinal smooth muscle contractions are thought to play a role [5]. Only a few studies, however, have attempted to objectively quantify bowel habits in constipated elderly patients [6,7], and furthermore, the results of such studies are conflicting [3,6]. Data from animal experiments suggest, however, that mean colonic transit time increases as animals grow older [8]. There is also evidence of diminished in vitro sensitivity of intestinal smooth muscle cells to cholinergic and electric stimuli and of less frequent bowel innervation with age [8]. Accordingly, electrophysiological experiments with human circular muscle strips from sigmoid colon specimens, removed during surgery from patients with nonobstructing colonic cancer, reveal a strong inverse association between aging and amplitudes of inhibitory junction potentials [9]. From such studies it has been concluded that possibly a form of functional obstruction is present in the colon of aging patients [9].

Hormones as Regulators of Colonic Motility

Little is known about the physiologic regulation of colonic motility and the factors that induce colonic mass movement and consequently induce defecation [10]. Myogenic factors and neural control are certainly important, but

[1] Division of Gastroenterology, University Hospital, 4031 Basel, Switzerland.
[2] Department of Internal Medicine, Kantonsspital, 4410 Liestal, Switzerland.

G. Adler and C. Beglinger (Eds.)
CCK Antagonists in Gastroenterology

hormones may be involved as well. Substance P, gastrin, motilin, and neurotensin have all been shown to exert some effects on colonic motility, but studies with CCK analogues are particularly abundant [11]. They have revealed a wide spectrum of actions on intestinal smooth muscle in vitro and intestinal transit in vivo. For example, CCK directly stimulates colonic myoelectrical and contractile activity in humans when injected intravenously [12]. Moreover, CCK stimulates colonic smooth muscle spike activity and induces contractions of isolated muscle strips from human taeniae coli [13]. These effects seem to be mediated both directly and via neural intermediators. It is thought that CCK does not just act as a hormone but also functions as an exitatory cotransmitter with acetylcholine in the generation of the peristaltic reflex [14].

Treatment of Patients with Chronic Constipation with a CCK Antagonist

The recent elaboration of peptide hormone antagonists using CCK as a model has opened the way for the investigation of putative physiological roles of CCK [15]. We have recently been able to show that blocking CCK receptors with the potent and highly specific antagonist loxiglumide dramatically shortens colonic transit time in healthy human volunteers [16]. We therefore performed a study in chronically constipated nursing home patients [17]. In a randomized, placebo-controlled, double-blind, cross-over study 18 patients were treated for a 3-week period with either 800 mg loxiglumide t.i.d. or placebo. Bowel habits were noted and the colonic transit time determined after each treatment period. Loxiglumide treatment induced a significant increase in stool frequency and a decrease in the need for enemas. The median colonic transit time decreased from 112.8 h (range 57.6 to 144 h) to 80.4 h (range 19.2 to 144.0 h) ($p < 0.0014$). Only 3 of the 18 patients did not have a decrease in transit time while treated with loxiglumide, but all three had more bowel movements and required fewer enemas during loxiglumide treatment.

The principal site of action of the CCK blocker seems to reside in the ascending colon. We observed that segmental colonic transit time was most markedly accelerated by loxiglumide in the ascending colon. These observations fit nicely into the concept that the ascending colon acts as a storage area for colonic contents [18,19] and that in idiopathic chronic constipation the abnormality is usually located in the ascending colon [20]. Therefore drugs working on that part of the colon may particularly be expected to accelerate transit. We speculate from our data that CCK exerts predominantly inhibitory effects on the propulsive motility in the ascending colon in humans and that this inhibitory action can be reversed by CCK antagonists.

The data presented here suggest that blocking CCK receptors with loxiglumide significantly relieves chronic constipation. Peptide hormone antagonists therefore may constitute a new class of potent therapeutic agents.

References

1. Sonnenberg A, Koch TR (1989) Physician visits in the United States for constipation: 1958 to 1986. Dig Dis Sci 34:606–611
2. Hannay DR (1978) Symptom prevalence in the community. J R Coll Gen Pract 28:492–499
3. Connell AM, Hilton C, Irvine G, Lennard-Jones JE, Misiewicz JJ (1965) Variation of bowel habit in two population samples. Br Med J 2:1095–1099
4. Whitehead WE, Drinkwater D, Cheskin LJ, Heller BR, Schuster MM (1989) Constipation in the elderly living at home. Definition, prevalence, and relationship to lifestyle and health status. J Am Geriatr Soc 37:423–429
5. Shamburek RD, Farrar JT (1990) Disorders of the digestive system in the elderly. N Engl J Med 322:438–443
6. Eastwood HDH (1972) Bowel transit studies in the elderly radio-opaque markers in the investigation of constipation. Geront Clin 14:154–159
7. Bassotti G, Gaburri M, Imbimbo BP, Rossi L, Farroni F, Pelli MA, Morelli A: Colonic mass movements in idiopathic chronic constipation. Gut 29:1173–1179
8. Cheskin LJ, Schuster MM (1989) Motility and ageing. Clin Perspectives Gastroenterol 8:4–6
9. Koch TR, Go VLW, Szurszewski JH (1986) Changes in some electrophysiological properties of circular muscle from normal sigmoid colon of the aging. Gastroenterology 90:1497
10. Christensen J (1987) Motility of the colon. In: Johnson LR (ed) Physiology of the gastrointestinal tract, 2nd edn. Raven, New York, pp 665–693
11. Walsh JH (1987) Gastrointestinal hormones. In: Johnson LR (ed) Physiology of the gastrointestinal tract, 2nd edn. Raven, New York, pp 181–253
12. Snape W, Carlson G, Cohen S (1977) Human colonic myoelectric activity in response to prostigmin and the gastrointestinal hormones. Am J Dig Dis 22: 881–887
13. Snape W (1983) Interaction of the octapeptide of cholecystokinin and gastrin I with bethanechol in the stimulation of feline colonic smooth muscle. Gastroenterology 84:58–62
14. Egberts E, Johnson A (1977) The effect of cholecystokinin on human taenia coli. Digestion 15:217–222
15. Snyder SH (1986) Virtuoso design of drugs. Nature 323:292–293
16. Meyer BM, Werth BA, Beglinger C, Hildebrand P, Jansen JBMJ, Zach D, Rovati LC, Stalder GA (1989) Role of cholecystokinin in regulation of gastrointestinal motor functions. Lancet II:12–15
17. Meier R, Thumshirn M, Meyer B, Rovati LC, Gyr K, Beglinger C (1990) Treatment of chronic constipation in geriatric patients with loxiglumide (LOX), a cholecystokinin antagonist. Gastroenterology 98:A374
18. Kamath PS, Phillips SF, O'Connor MK, Brown ML, Zinsmeister AR (1990) Colonic capacitance and transit in man: modulation by luminal contents and drugs. Gut 31:443–449
19. Steed KP, Watts PJ, Blackshaw PE, Barrow L, Wilson CG, Davies MC, Melia C, Spiller RC (1990) Reservoir function of the ascending colon demonstrated scintigraphically: effect of lactulose. Gastroenterology 98:A394
20. Stivland TA, Vassallo M, Camilleri M, Proano M, Rath DM, Brown ML, Thomforde GM, Pemberton JH, Phillips SF (1990) Regional transit in the gut of patients with idiopathic constipation. Gastroenterology 98:A668

The Rational Use of CCK Antagonists in Irritable Bowel Syndrome

N.W. Read[1]

What is Irritable Bowel Syndrome?

The irritable bowel syndrome (IBS) is the name given to a condition that is characterised by the combination of abdominal pain or discomfort and a disorder of bowel habit, for which no pathological cause can be found. The pain is often manifest in the lower abdomen and may be induced or exacerbated by eating a meal, particularly if that meal has a high content of fat. The disorder in bowel habit may vary from diarrhoea to constipation; many patients actually complain of alternating diarrhoea and constipation. Manning et al. [1] have identified a number of symptoms that are characteristic of the irritable bowel; they include abdominal distension, a feeling of incomplete evacuation, abdominal pain relieved by defaecation, looser and more frequent stools with the onset of pain and rectal mucus. These symptoms are also found in inflammatory conditions of the rectum, such as ulcerative colitis [2] and solitary rectal ulcer syndrome [3], and probably indicate rectal "irritation". Patients with the IBS also frequently suffer from symptoms such as nausea, bloating and early satiety that are referable to the upper gastrointestinal tract, and even drowsiness, irritability, headaches, wheeziness and frequency of micturition that may indicate functional disturbances in other parts of the body.

The pathophysiology of the IBS is not well understood. Disturbances in colonic and small intestinal motility have been described [4,5], although most motor disorders described in IBS are not abnormal patterns, but exaggerated responses to stimuli such as luminal distension [6], ingestion of a fatty meal [7] and emotional disturbances [8]. Measurements of bowel transit correspond with the predominant bowel habit; both small bowel and colonic transit tend to be short in patients with diarrhoea and prolonged in patients with constipation, but very few values fall outside the normal range [9].

The variety of symptoms, the poor response to treatment and the absence of physiological or biochemical markers indicate that the IBS is

[1] Sub-Department of Gastrointestinal Physiology and Nutrition, Royal Hallamshire Hospital, Sheffield S10 2TN, UK

G. Adler and C. Beglinger (Eds.)
CCK Antagonists in Gastroenterology

not a single condition but may include several different pathophysiological entities. The challenge is how to recognise and identify different subsets.

One of the commonest findings in patients with the IBS is that the rectum is abnormally sensitive to balloon distension [6,10]. In a recent study [11], we found that 58% of patients with the IBS had abnormal rectal sensitivity in that the threshold volume required to induce a desire to defaecate was outside the normal range. These same patients also had low distension thresholds for other rectal sensations (wind, pain), a low rectal compliance (tight rectum) and showed increased rectal contractile and anal relaxation responses to rectal distension. Values in patients with nonsensitive rectums were very similar to normal controls. It is not known whether patients with a sensitive rectum are the same patients who show an enhanced rectal motor response to ingestion of a fatty meal.

Although more patients with a sensitive rectum present with diarrhoea, about a third of constipated patients also have a sensitive rectum. The latter can be separated from the rest of the constipated patients in that they have a frequent desire to defaecate. The sensitive rectum of these patients generates a desire to defaecate on entry of small faecal pellets, but these patients (like normal subjects) have great difficulty in evacuating the small faecal pellets that they produce [12]. Finally, it is interesting that anxiety scores are much higher in the "sensitive" group than in patients with nonsensitive rectums. We feel these features justify the segregation of patients with a sensitive rectum into a distinct subset for the purpose of epidemiological and therapeutic studies.

Physiology of Cholecystokinin

Cholecystokinin is released into the blood stream from the neuroendocrine cells of the duodenal epithelium following exposure to intraluminal fats, acid and some amino acids. It binds to receptors on the smooth muscle of the gall bladder and the pancreatic acinus to cause gall bladder contraction and pancreatic enzyme secretion. It also directly inhibits gastric emptying, accelerates small bowel transit [13] and, when injected intravenously in humans, stimulates colonic myoelectrical and contractile activity [7]. This effect of CCK on the colon can be inhibited by the opiate antagonist, naloxone [14].

CCK does not just act as a hormone, it exists alongside other transmitters in enteric nerves. It is thought to function, for example, as an excitatory cotransmitter with acetylcholine in the peristaltic reflex [15]. CCK is present in afferent nerves from the colon to the inferior mesenteric ganglion [16] and in afferent vagal nerves from the gastroduodenum [17], where it may play an important role in satiety [18]. CCK may also act as a paracrine agent on afferent nerve terminals in the stomach and duodenum, where it mediates or modulates sensory signals from a meal [17,19]. The possible action of CCK on afferent neurones is supported by the recent observation that the CCK antagonist, L-364 718, delays small bowel transit under basal conditions, but reverses the delay in small bowel transit caused by infusion of fat in the ileum [20]. The best explanation for these data is that the antagonist is acting at a common afferent terminal to blocking the normal acceleration in transit caused by the bulk of the meal as well as the delay in transit induced by fat.

The Gastrocolonic Response

The gastrocolonic response is probably a nervous reflex; it can be inhibited by atropin and naloxone and it is absent in paraplegic patients [21]. The first indication that cholecystokinin may be implicated in the pathophysiology of the IBS came with the pioneering study of Harvey and Read in 1973 [22]. These workers showed that infusion of CCK caused an abnormal increase in colonic motility and pain in patients with the IBS. It is possible that the CCK may have contained impurities that were responsible for the increase in colonic motility. Nevertheless, the essential features of the study were confirmed by Snape and his colleagues [5,7] some years later. Strong support for the involvement of CCK in the gastrocolonic response is provided by the observation that the CCK receptor antagonist loxiglumide abolishes the gastrocolonic response in normal volunteers without diminishing basal colonic motility [23].

In patients with the IBS, colonic motor response to a meal is often delayed [24] and corresponds more closely with the rise in CCK. There are several ways in which CCK could be involved in the exaggerated gastrocolonic response of IBS. Firstly, normal blood levels could increase the response of the sensitised smooth muscle, secondly, more CCK could be released into the blood in IBS and thirdly, CCK could interact with sensitised afferent nervous pathways.

We have recently shown that a drink of coffee can elicit a gastrocolonic response that is associated with a rise in plasma CCK [25].

Gastro-Ileal Response

Eating a meal can increase the activity of the ileum. This response could be mediated by CCK. Kellow and Phillips [26] have shown an exaggerated ileal response to a meal in patients with IBS. These same investigators [27] have also demonstrated that the response of the ileum to CCK is also exaggerated in patients with the IBS. Using intravenous doses of CCK that caused 50% contraction of the gall bladder (assessed by ultrasound), they showed that ileal motility was greater in IBS patients with diarrhoea than in controls. Higher doses elicited prolonged propagated contractions in the patients, but not in the controls, and these contractions were often associated with pain. The authors concluded that CCK octapeptide may unmask dysmotility of the small bowel in IBS.

Action of CCK Antagonists on Intestinal Motility

Administration of the cholecystokinin analogue, caerulein, to conscious dogs increased the motor activity of the small intestine and the large intestine [28]. These effects were blocked by the specific CCK antagonist, loxiglumide, but loxiglumide did not have any effect on the increase in motility induced by neostigmine.

In humans, loxiglumide accelerated colonic transit time, both in normal subjects [29] and in geriatric patients with constipation [30], but is did not affect the transit time of the head of a liquid test meal (Ensure) through the small intestine [29]. The effect on the colon is unlikely to be due to impaired digestion of fat; normal excretion of urinary para-aminobenzoic acid indicated that pancreatic exocrine function was normal. Finally, loxiglumide inhibited the colonic response to a fatty meal in man, but increased basal motility [23]. This strongly implicates CCK in the generation of the gastrocolonic response.

Conclusions

Since CCK may be implicated in the enhanced ileal and colonic motor responses to a meal in IBS and these exaggerated motor responses are associated with symptoms, it seems likely that blocking CCK receptors could reduce postprandial abdominal pain in IBS. Moreover, there is evidence that CCK may play an important role in transducing sensory signals from the gut; if that is the case, then CCK-receptor antagonists may be very useful in reducing sensitivity and reactivity in the subset of IBS patients characterised by a sensitive bowel. Unfortunately, CCK receptors are found throughout the gut and also in the central nervous system and the currently available antagonists may not be sufficiently selective to be useful in clinical practice. Is there a use for a drug that directly reduces colonic motility, but increases the delivery of unabsorbed fat to the colon, resulting in pain and diarrhoea? Further development should be aimed at finding a dose or a compound that can act selectively on gastrointestinal motility.

References

1. Manning AP, Thompson WG, Heaton KW, et al. (1978) Towards positive diagnosis of the irritable bowel syndrome. Br med J 2:653–654
2. Rao SSC, Holdsworth CD, Read NW (1988) Symptoms of stool patterns in ulcerative colitis. Gut 29:342–345
3. Sun WM, Read NW, Bannister JJ, Shorthouse AT, Connelly TC (1989) A common pathophysiology for full thickness rectal prolapse, anterio mucosal prolapse and solitary rectal ulcer. Br J Surg 76:290–295
4. Taylor I, Darby C, Hammond P (1978) Comparison of rectosigmoid myoelectrical activity in the irritable colon syndrome during relapses and remissions. Gut 19:923–929

5. Snape W, Carlsson G, Cohen S (1977) Human colonic myoelectrical activity in response to pro-stigmin and the gastrointestinal hormones. Am J Dig Dis 22: 881–887
6. Whitehead WE, Engle BT, Schuster MM (1980) Irritable bowel syndrome. Physiological and psychological differences between diarrhoea-predominant and constipation-predominant patients. Dig Dis Sci 25:404–413
7. Snape WJ, Materazzo SA, Cohen S (1978) Effect of eating and gastrointestinal hormones on human colonic myoelectrical and motor activity. Gastroenterology 75:373–378
8. Almy T, Hinkle L, Burl B, Kern F (1949) Alterations in colonic function in man in distress. Experimental production of sigmoid spasm in patients with spastic complications. Gastroenterology 12:437–439
9. Cann PA, Read NW, Brown C et al. (1983) The irritable bowel syndrome (IBS): relationship of disorders in the transit of a single solid meal. The symptom patterns. Gut 24:205–211
10. Ritchie J (1973) Pain from distension of the pelvic colon by inflating a balloon in the irritable colon syndrome. Gut 6:105–112
11. Prior A, Sun WM, Read NW (1990) Rectal sensitivity: a rational means of categorising patients with the Irritable Bowel Syndrome. Gastroenterology 90: 1008–1015
12. Bannister JJ, Davison P, Tims JM, Gibbons C, Read NW (1987) Effect of stool size and consistency on defaecation. Gut 28:1246–1250
13. Levant J, Tunn T, Jacknar T, Sturdevant R, Isenberg J (1974) The effect of graded doses of C terminal octapeptide of cholecystokinin on small intestinal transit time in man. Am J Dig Dis 19:207–209
14. Rennie A, Snape WJ, Sun EA, et al. (1983) Role of cholecystokinin in the gastrocolonic response to a meal. Gastroenterology 85:17–21
15. Bartho L, Holzer P, Donnerer J, Lembeck F (1982) Effects of substance P, cholecystokinin octapeptide, bombesin and neurotensin on the peristaltic reflex of the guinea pig ileum in the absence and in the presence of atropine. Naunyn Schmiedebergs Arch Pharmacol 321:321–328
16. Szurzewski JH (1989) Colonic mechanosensory afferent fibres toprevertibral ganglian cells. In: Singer MV Goebell H (eds) Nerves and Gastrointestinal Transit. Kluwer, Norwell, pp 243–251
17. Raybauld HE, Gayton RJ, Dockray GJ (1985) CNS effects of circulating CCK8: involvement of brain stem neurones responding to gastric distension. Brain Res 342: 187–190
18. Smith GP, Jerome C, Cushin BJ, et al. (1981) Abdominal vagotomy blocks the satiety effect of CCK in the rat. Science 213:2111–2124
19. Mei N (1985) Intestinal chemosensitivity. Physiol Rev 65:211–237
20. Brown NJ, Rumsey RDE, Read NW (1990) Effect of cholecystokinin on small bowel transit under control conditions and after ileum infusion of lipid. (Submitted)
21. Glick ME, Meshkinpour H, Holderman S, et al. (1984) Colonic dysfunction in patients with thoracic spinal cord injury. Gastroenterology 86:287–294
22. Harvey RF, Read AE (1973) Effect of cholecystokinin on colonic motility and symptoms in patients with the irritable bowel syndrome. Lancet 1:1–3
23. Jehle EC, Blum AL (1990) The role of cholecystokinin in the regulation of basal colonic motility in the gastrocolonic response. Gastroenterology 98:A361
24. Sullivan MA, Cohen S, Snape WJ (1978) Colonic myoelectrical activity in the irritable bowel syndrome. Engl J Med 298:878–883
25. Brown S, Cann PA, Read NW (1990) The effect of coffee on distal colonic function. Gut 31:450–453
26. Kellow JE, Phillips SF (1987) Altered small bowel motility in the irritable bowel syndrome is correlated with symptoms. Gastroenterology 92:1885–1893
27. Kellow JE, Millar LJ, Phillips SF (1988) Dysmotility of the small intestine is provoked by stimuli in the irritable bowel syndrome. Gut 29:1236–1243

28. Karaus M, Niederau C (1989) Effects of CCK antagonists on motor activity of the small and large intestine. J Gastrointest Motil 1:61
29. Meyer BM, Werth BA, Beglinger C, Hildebrand P, Jansen J, Zach D, Rovati LC, Stalder G (1989) Role of cholecystokinin and regulation of gastrointestinal motor functions. Lancet 1:12–15
30. Meier R, Thumshirn M, Meyer B, Rovati LC, Gear K, Beglinger C (1990) Treatment of chronic constipation in geriatric patients with loxiglumide, a cholecystokinin antagonist. Gastroenterology 98:A374

Cholecystokinin, Cholecystokinin-Receptor Antagonists and the Sphincter of Oddi

J.B.M. JANSEN and C.B.H. LAMERS[1]

As a result of modern techniques like endoscopy, manometry, electromyography and hormonal assays, knowledge of the physiology and pathophysiology of sphincter of Oddi motility is now rapidly increasing. Opening of the sphincter of Oddi, once thought to be a simple passive event is a synchronized, dynamic action, involving both neural and humoral mechanisms.

CCK is believed to play an important role in the regulation of sphincter activity, like it does for gallbladder motility. Therefore, recently developed specific CCK receptor antagonists may contribute to further delineate the role of this hormone to sphincter motility in health and disease. The present review examines recent developments in the understanding of sphincter of Oddi function with special references to the contribution of CCK.

Anatomy of the Sphincter of Oddi

In man, the bile duct and the pancreatic duct usually empty together into the greater duodenal ampulla, located about 7 cm from the pylorus on the concavity of the duodenum. The bile duct often intertwines with the pancreatic duct and in more than one-half of instances the two ducts unite and form a short hepatopancreatic ampulla which opens into the papilla of Vater. In other instances the two ducts meet, but open separately into the duodenum at the mouth of the papilla. Each duct usually acquires sphincteric muscle coats. That about the lower end of the bile duct is known as the choledochal sphincter, which can be divided into a superior portion, encircling the distal choledochal duct just before it enters the duodenum, and an inferior portion, surrounding the submucosal intraduodenal part of the common bile duct. When the choledochal and pancreatic duct form an ampulla, a sphincter of the ampulla may be present surrounding the ampullary duct at the greater duodenal papilla. Variation in extent and thickness of the choledochal and ampullary sphincter is common.

---

[1] Department of Gastroenterology and Hepatology, University Hospital, Building 1, C4-P017, P.O. Box 9600, 2300 RC Leiden, The Netherlands

G. Adler and C. Beglinger (Eds.)
CCK Antagonists in Gastroenterology

The choledochal sphincter, apparently, is not continuous with the musculature of the duodenum, and it has a separate nerve supply. The sphincter is the chief mechanism controlling the flow of bile into the duodenum and preventing reflux of duodenal contents into the biliary tree. These functions are facilitated by a complicated system of mucosal folds in the papilla.

The involvement of a sphincter mechanism in the regulation of bile flow into the duodenum was originally described by Oddi in 1887 [1].

Sphincter Motility

In man, the physiologic sphincter segment is about 4–6 mm in length. In this segment, basal steady state pressure is about 4 mmHg higher than in the common bile duct or pancreatic duct. Spontaneous pronounced contractions are superimposed on this basal steady state pressure with a frequency of 4.1 ± 0.9 per minute, measuring 101 ± 50 mmHg in amplitude and 4.3 ± 1.5 s in duration [2]. Corresponding phasic contractions are absent in the common bile duct, the pancreatic duct and the duodenum.

It has been demonstrated that 60% of these phasic wave activities occur in antegrade direction, 14% are retrograde and 26% occur simultaneously [3]. Although species differences in phasic wave directions make the physiologic purpose of this phenomenon unclear, it is believed that the main mechanism of spontaneous bile duct emptying in opossums, rabbits, guinea pigs, and prairie dogs is antegrade contraction of the sphincter complex [4–7]. These antegrade contractions function like a pump with a systolic phase, during which the contents of the sphincter segment are expelled into the duodenum, and a diastolic phase, facilitating bile flow from the duct into the sphincter segment. Increased antegrade phasic wave activity is initially accompanied by increased flow across the sphincter, but when contractions become more intense and exceed a certain level of about 8–10 per minute [8] the diastolic interval becomes to short for adequate refilling of the sphincter segment and flow ceases. In other species, like cats [9], dogs [10], and man [2], a negative correlation between sphincter activity and bile flow has been reported, in line with the idea that intense motor activity impedes bile flow, whereas less intense activity facilitates bile flow.

Although, the biliary sphincter complex seems to be the major regulator of bile flow into the duodenum, muscular activity of the gastrointestinal tract also contributes to regulation of bile flow, particularly in the fasting state. In several species, bile flow impedes when the amplitude of duodenal contractions is of the same magnitude as those observed during phase III of the migratory motor complex [11]. Further evidence for a link between gastrointestinal and biliary sphincter motility was obtained from studies demonstrating the existence of a reflex mechanism between stomach and sphincter of Oddi [12].

Regulation of Sphincter Motility

The motility of the sphincter of Oddi is regulated by complex interactions between neural and humoral mechanisms.

Neural Mechanisms

It has been demonstrated that the sphincter of Oddi has a separate nerve supply containing cholinergic, adrenergic, and peptidergic neurons.

In guinea pigs, norepinephrine in low concentrations induced a relaxation of the sphincter of Oddi, which could be blocked by either the α-adrenergic-receptor antagonist phentolamine or the β-adrenergic-receptor antagonist propanolol, while norepinephrine in high concentrations induced a contraction of the sphincter which was blocked by phentolamine [13]. This suggests the existence of excitatory α-adrenergic receptors and inhibitory β-adrenergic receptors in the sphincter of Oddi. Although species differences in adrenergic response should be appreciated, it is believed that during sympathetic nerve stimulation mainly α-adrenergic receptors are activated, causing the sphincter to contract.

The biliary sphincter also receives parasympathetic innervations from the vagus nerve. The parasympathetic neurotransmitter acetylcholine and its equivalent bethanochol have been demonstrated to increase the frequency of sphincter contraction in several species [4,14,15]. However, electrostimulation of vagal nerve branches produces less clear sphincter responses [16–18]. Again, species differences may be responsible for these contrasting findings, although, stimulation of non-cholinergic, non-adrenergic neurons in the vagus nerve may contribute to these results [9,19].

Hormonal Influences

Regulatory peptides have been demonstrated to act upon sphincter of Oddi motility. However, interpretation of studies on the effect of regulatory peptides on sphincter motility has been complicated by numerous confounding factors like species differences, electrical versus manometrical studies, and in vitro versus in vivo experiments. As a result of these confusing factors, the function of most regulatory peptides in the regulation of sphincter of Oddi motility is still rather speculative.

Peptides from the secretin-glucagon family have been demonstrated to decrease both electrical and motor activity of the sphincter of Oddi in several species, including man [2,5,20,21]. Consequently, bile flow into the duodenum is increased by these peptides. It remains to be established to what part these effects are mediated by potentiation of the action of CCK on the sphincter.

Bombesin (BBS) and its mammalian counterpart gastrin-releasing peptide (GRP) have also been demonstrated to modify sphincter activity. In rabbits, BBS increased electrical spike activity [5]. In this species, like in guinea pigs, opossums, and prairie dogs, increases in electrical and motor activity in the sphincter complex propel bile actively into the duodenum. After intravenous injection of BBS or GRP into dogs, phasic sphincter contractions disappeared and basal sphincter pressure fell, resulting in increased bile flow into the duodenum [10]. The effects of BBS or GRP on sphincter activity are likely to be explained by the release of CCK [10].

Motilin has also been reported to affect sphincter of Oddi motility. In the prairie dog both motilin and CCK stimulate sphincter of Oddi motility [22]. Motilin may therefore be involved in the regulation of sphincter motility, especially during the interdigestive period.

Somatostatin (SST) has also been demonstrated to modify sphincter motility. In rabbits, SST decreased myoelectrical sphincter activity [23], resulting in decreased bile flow into the duodenum. To what part SST acts by indirect effects via inhibition of the release of other regulatory peptides, such as CCK, remains to be established.

Other regulatory peptides like peptide YY (PYY), neuropeptide Y (NPY), and substance P have also been demonstrated to influence sphincter of Oddi motility. PYY inhibits the effect of CCK on sphincter motility in prairie dogs [24], while NPY has been demonstrated to increase sphincter activity and consequently bile flow in this species [25]. In vitro, substance P has been demonstrated to stimulate sphincter of Oddi contractions in dogs [26]. The physiologic significance of these observations awaits further investigation.

CCK and the Sphincter of Oddi

Among all regulatory peptides, the effect of CCK-like peptides (CCK33, CCK8, caerulein, gastrin) on sphincter of Oddi activity is by far the most extensively tested. Again, the response of the sphincter to CCK varies according to species. In guinea pigs [6,20] rabbits [5], oppossums [21], and prairie dogs [7] CCK increases electrical and phasic wave activity without affecting baseline pressure, resulting in an increased bile flow into the duodenum. In guinea pigs CCK contracts the sphincter by a direct effect on the smooth muscle cells and by an indirect effect mediated by the release of acetylcholine from postganglionic parasympathetic neurons [6].

In other species, like cats [9], dogs [10,16,19], and man [2], bile flow into the duodenum in response to CCK is facilitated by a decrease in baseline pressure and a reduction of phasic wave activity in the sphincter. However, in in vitro experiments CCK has no effect on canine sphincter motility [26,27]. This suggests that intact innervation of the sphincter of Oddi is of importance for the observed effects in vivo. This is supported by studies in cats, demonstrating that sphincter of Oddi relaxation by CCK is abolished by complete denervation induced by tetrodotoxin, but not by selective cholinergic or adrenergic blockade [9]. After complete denervation with tetrodotoxin, CCK causes the sphincter to contract instead of to relax. This indicates that there are at least two receptors for CCK in the sphincter of this species, one that is inhibitory and present at the non-cholinergic, non-adrenergic neurons, and another excitatory at the circular muscle. In vivo the effects of CCK on the non-adrenergic, non-cholinergic receptor predominate over the effects of CCK on the smooth muscle receptor. Similar findings have been reported in dogs. In this species it has been claimed that the mediator of this CCK-stimulated non-adrenergic, non-cholinergic pathway is vasoactive intestinal polypeptide (VIP) [19]. To what part CCK, released after a meal, is responsible for postprandial sphincter of Oddi motility has not yet been demonstrated convincingly. Although some studies have provided evidence for a physiologic role of endogenous CCK in sphincter motility [28,29], other studies have demonstrated less convincing evidence. In several species, fat and protein are potent stimuli for the release of CCK [30]. However, previous studies have failed to demonstrate relaxation of the sphincter of Oddi in response to fat in man, whereas protein was effective [31]. Recent work in prairie dogs has shown that sodium oleate decreases sphincter of Oddi activity, whereas protein stimulated sphincter activity [7,32].

Pathophysiology

Abnormalities in sphincter of Oddi function have been related to several pathological conditions like cholecystectomy, biliary dyskinesia, papillary stenosis, chronic recurrent pancreatitis, and disturbances in nerve supply like vagotomy and Chagas disease.

Cholecystectomy may alter sphincter of Oddi function since it has been demonstrated that sphincter activity in prairie dogs is at least in part mediated by the degree of gallbladder distension via a cholecystosphincteric reflex [7]. Furthermore, it has been demonstrated in this species that the sphincter response to intravenous CCK is blunted after cholecystectomy, while resting sphincter motility is unaltered [7]. Since CCK release is negatively influenced by the concentration of bile salts in the lumen of the small intestine in several species [33], the blunted response to CCK may have been compensated for by an increased release of CCK after cholecystectomy. However, the sphincter response to endogenously released CCK by intraduodenal oleate was also blunted [7]. This suggests that alterations in neural pathways after cholecystectomy rather than alterations in CCK release are related to possible disorders in sphincter function after removing the gallbladder in this species.

Increases in luminal pressure in [34] and dilatation of the bile duct [35] have also been reported after cholecystectomy. However, studies in man did not convincingly confirm these effects [36,37].

Although a clear-cut effect of cholecystectomy on sphincter of Oddi functions has not been demonstrated with certainty in man, at least two pathological conditions of the sphincter of Oddi have been related to cholecystectomy, that is, papillary stenosis and biliary dyskinesia. Papillary stenosis has been defined as a fibrotic narrowing of all or part of the sphincter, while biliary dyskinesia is a disorder of the tonic or phasic motor activity of the sphincter [38]. Papillary stenosis may result from operative procedures, infection, or impacted stones, while biliary dyskinesia is a primary disorder responsible for pain after cholecystectomy.

To distinguish papillary stenosis from biliary dyskinesia, a classification based on clinical, laboratory, radiological, and manometrical findings has been proposed [38]. In papillary stenosis, pathological manometric findings are not influenced by CCK [39], while in biliary dyskinesia at least two subgroups of patients can be identified [40]. One group of patients has a normal response of sphincter motility to CCK, while a second group of patients showed a paradoxical response to CCK resulting in an increase in basal sphincter pressure and/or an increase in the amplitude of phasic wave contractions.

Abnormalities in sphincter of Oddi motility may also play a role in idiopathic recurrent pancreatitis, since elevated basal sphincter pressure, increased numbers of retrograde phasic wave contractions, absence or increased frequency of phasic wave contractions, and paradoxical responses to CCK have been reported in these patients [41].

Abnormalities in nerve supply have also been related to a disturbed sphincter of Oddi function. Increased resistance in the sphincter due to alterations in phasic wave activity has been reported in the prairie dog after vagotomy [42]. In man, autonomic denervation due to Chagas disease resulted in marked increases in basal sphincter of Oddi pressure and in minor increases in the amplitude of phasic wave activities [43]. The response to CCK is not disturbed in these patients. This suggests that neural impairment is limited to preganglionic fibers in these patients.

CCK-Receptor Antagonists and the Sphincter of Oddi

Although CCK has been demonstrated to have important effects on sphincter of Oddi motility in several species including man, the physiologic importance of this peptide in the regulation of sphincter of Oddi function has not yet been fully established. Therefore, studies with recently developed specific CCK-receptor antagonists like CR-1505 and L-364 718 may explain the contribution of CCK to sphincter motility under basal and stimulated conditions.

CCK-receptor antagonists may not only be of value in elucidating the physiologic and pathophysiologic role of CCK in sphincter of Oddi function, but may also contribute to treatment of biliary disorders associated with abnormal responses of the sphincter to CKK, such as biliary dyskinesia and chronic recurrent pancreatitis. Studies with these receptor antagonists are now in progress.

References

1. Oddi R (1887) D'une disposition à sphincter spéciale de l'ouverture du canal cholèdoque. Arch Ital Biol 8:317–332
2. Geenan JE, Hogan WJ, Dodds WJ, Stewart ET, Arndorfer RC (1980) Intraluminal pressure recording from the human sphincter of Oddi. Gastroenterology 78:317–324
3. Toouli J, Hogan WJ, Geenan JE, Dodds WJ, Arndorfer RC (1982) Action of cholecystokinin-octapeptide on sphincter of Oddi basal pressure and phasic wave activity in humans. Surgery 92:497–503
4. Toouli J, Dodds WJ, Honda R, et al. (1983) Motor function of the opossum sphincter of Oddi. J Clin Invest 71:208–220
5. Sarles JC, Delacourt P, Castello H, et al. (1981) Action of gastrointestinal hormones on the myoelectric activity of the sphincter of Oddi in living rabbit. Regul Pept 2:13–24
6. Harada T, Katsugari T, Furukawa T (1986) Release of acetylcholine mediated by cholecystokinin receptor from the guinea pig sphincter of Oddi. J Pharmacol Exp Ther 239:554–558
7. Grace PA, Pitt HA (1987) Cholecystectomy alters the hormonal response of the sphincter of Oddi. Surgery 102:186–194
8. Toouli J (1984) Sphincter of Oddi motility. Br J Surg 71:251–256
9. Behar J, Biancani P (1980) Effect of cholecystokinin and the octapeptide of cholecystokinin on the feline sphincter of Oddi and gallbladder. Mechanisms of action. J Clin Invest 66:1231–1239
10. Sievert CE, Potter TJ, Levine AS, Morley JE, Silvis SE, Vennes JA (1988) Effect of bombesin and gastrin-releasing peptide on canine sphincter of Oddi. Am J Physiol 94:755–761
11. Mochinaga N, Sarna SK, Condon RE, Dodds WJ, Matsumoto T (1988) Gastroduodenal regulation of common bile duct flow in the dog. Gastroenterology 94:755–761
12. Webb TH, Lillmoe KD, Pitt HA (1988) Gastro-sphincter of Oddi reflex. Am J Surg 155:193–198
13. Nakata K, Kurahashi K (1981) Effect of C-terminal octapeptide of cholecystokinin and prostaglandins on adrenergic functions of the guinea pig gallbladder and sphincter of Oddi. Jpn J Pharmacol 31:77–83
14. Crema A, Berte F (1963) Actions of sympathomimetic drugs on the isolated junction of the bile duct and the duodenum. Br J Pharmacol Chemother 20: 221–229
15. Persson CGA (1971) Adrenoreceptor functions in the cat choledocho-duodenal junction in vitro. Br J Pharmacol 42:447–461
16. Funch-Jensen P, Stadkilde-Jurgensen H, Kraglund K, Lugreen NA (1981) Biliary manometry in dogs. Influence of selective electrostimulation of the right and left vagus nerves. Digestion 22:89–93
17. Hopton D, White TT (1972) Effect of hepatic and celiac vagal stimulation on common bile duct pressure. Am J Dig Dis 16:1095–1101
18. Tansey MJ, Lunes DL, Martin JS, Kendal FM (1974) An evaluation of neural influences on the sphincter of Oddi in the dog. Dig Dis 19:423–437

19. Wiley JW, O'Dorisio TM, Owyang C (1988) Vasoactive intestinal polypeptide mediates cholecystokinin – relaxation of the sphincter of Oddi. J Clin Invest 81:1920–1924
20. Kamata M (1980) Electrical and mechanical properties of smooth muscle cells of the guinea pig biliary tree. Jpn J Physiol 30:179–204
21. Honda R, Toouli J, Dodds WJ, Geenan JE, Hogan WJ, Itoh Z (1983) Effect of enteric hormones on sphincter of Oddi and gastrointestinal myoelectric activity in fasted conscious opossums. Gastroenterology 84:1–9
22. Muller EL, Grace PA, Conter RL, Roslyn JJ, Pitt HA (1987) Influence of motilin and cholecystokinin on sphincter of Oddi and duodenal mobility. Am J Physiol 253:G679–G683
23. Adani GF, Leandri R, Sarles JC (1986) Effect of somatostatin on the rabbit Oddi's sphincter in vivo. Interrelation of somatostatin and cholecystokinin. Gastroenterol Clin Biol 10:108–811
24. Grace PA, Couse HF, Taylor IL, Pitt HA (1988) Peptide YY inhibits cholecystokinin-stimulated sphincter of Oddi activity in the prairie dog. Surgery 104:546–552
25. Lillemoe KD, Webb TH, Pitt HA (1988) Neuropeptide Y: a candidate neurotransmitter for biliary motility. J Surg Res 45:254–260
26. Guo YS, Singh P, Gomez G, Rajaraman S, Thompson JC (1989) Contractile response of canine gallbladder and sphincter of Oddi to substance P and related peptides in vitro. Dig Dis Sci 34:812–817
27. Lluis F, Fujimura M, Lonovics J, Guo YS, Gomez G, Greeley GH, Townsend CM, Thompson JC (1988) Peptide YY and gallbladder contraction. Studies in vivo and in vitro. Gastroenterology 94:1441–1446
28. Ono K, Suzuki H, Hada R, Sasaki M, Endoh M (1985) Gastrointestinal hormones and motility of the human sphincter of Oddi. Nippon Heikatsukin Gakkai Zasshi (Suppl 12) 21:69–75
29. Allescher HD (1989) Papilla of Vater: structure and function. Endoscopy (Suppl 1) 21:324–329
30. Hopman WPM, Jansen JBMJ, Lamers CBHW (1985) Comparative study of the effects of fat, protein and starch on plasma cholecystokinin in man. Scand J Gastroenterol 20:843–847
31. Bergh GS (1942) The sphincter mechanism of the common bile duct in human subjects. Its reactions to certain types of stimulation. Surgery 11:299–330
32. Webb TA, Lillemoe KD, Pitt HA (1987) Intraduodenal protein stimulates resting but inhibits CCK stimulated sphincter of Oddi motility. Gastroenterology 92:1687
33. Gomez G, Lluis F, Guo YS, Greeley GH, Townsend CM, Thompson JC (1986) Bile inhibits release of cholecystokinin and neurotenisn. Surgery 100:363–368
34. Judd ES, Mann FC (1917) The effect of removal of the gallbladder. Surg Gynaecol Obstet 24:437–442
35. Mahour GH, Wakim KG, Soule EH, Ferris DO (1988) Effect of cholecystectomy on the biliary ducts in dogs. Arch Surg 97:570–574
36. Longo MJ, Hodgson JR, Ferris DO (1967) Size of the common bile duct following cholecystectomy. Ann Surg 165:250–253
37. Mahour GH, Wakim KG, Ferris DO, Soule EH (1967) The common bile duct after cholecystectomy. Ann Surg 166:964–967
38. Hogan WJ, Geenan JE (1988) Biliary dyskinesia. Endoscopy 20:179–183
39. Yasui A, Nimura Y, Kamiya J, Hayakawa T, Shibata T, Shionoya S (1989) Sphincter of Oddi response to caerulein after endoscopic sphincterotomy for papillary stenosis. Surg Endosc 3:216–219
40. Rolny P, Arleback A, Funch-Jensen P, Kruse A, Ravnsbaeck J, Jarnerot G (1986) Paradoxal response of the sphincter of Oddi to intravenous injection of cholecystokinin or cerulitide. Manometric findings and results of treatment in biliary dskinesia. Gut 27:1507–1511

41. Toouli J, Roberts-Thomson IC, Dent J, Lee J (1985) Sphincter of Oddi motility disorders in patients with idiopathic recurrent pancreatitis. Br J Surg 72:859–863
42. Pitt HA, Doty JE, DenBesten L, Kuchenbecher SL (1982) Altered sphincter of Oddi phasic activity following truncal vagotomy. J Surg Res 32:598–667
43. Guelrud M, Bettarello A, Cecconello I, Pinotti W, Mantelmacher H, Velasquez T (1983) Sphincter of Oddi pressure in Chagasic patients with megaesophagus. Gastroenterology 85:584–588

Subject Index

Printing: Druckerei Kutschbach, Berlin
Binding: Buchbinderei Lüderitz & Bauer, Berlin